THE PROSTATE HEALTH PROGRAM

A Guide to Preventing
and Controlling
Prostate Cancer

Daniel W. Nixon, M.D.
PRESIDENT, INSTITUTE FOR CANCER PREVENTION

and Max Gomez, Ph.D.
HEALTH EDITOR, WNBC

Free Press
New York London Toronto Sydney

ƒP

FREE PRESS
A Division of Simon & Schuster, Inc.
1230 Avenue of the Americas
New York, NY 10020

Copyright © 2004 The Institute for Cancer Prevention, Max Gomez,
and The Reference Works, Inc.
All rights reserved,
including the right of reproduction
in whole or in part in any form.

Photo of Max Gomez courtesy of WNBC.

Recipes in Chapter 7 are from *The Cancer Recovery Eating Plan* by Daniel Nixon,
copyright © 1994 by Daniel Nixon, M.D., and Alison Brown Cerier Book Development, Inc.
Used by permission of Times Books, a division of Random House, Inc.

FREE PRESS and colophon are trademarks
of Simon & Schuster, Inc.

For information regarding special discounts for bulk purchases, please contact Simon & Schuster Special Sales at 1-800-456-6798 or business@simonandschuster.com

Designed by Karolina Harris

Manufactured in the United States of America

10   9   8   7   6   5   4   3   2   1

Library of Congress Cataloging-in-Publication Data
Nixon, Daniel W.
    The prostate health program : a guide to preventing and controlling prostate cancer /
Daniel W. Nixon and Max Gomez.
       p.   cm.
    Includes bibliographical references and index.
    1. Prostate—Diseases—Prevention—Popular works.   2. Prostate—Diseases—Diet therapy—
Popular works.   3. Prostate—Cancer—Prevention—Popular works.   4. Prostate —Cancer—
Diet therapy—Popular works.   I. Gomez, Max.   II. Title.
RC899.N595   2004
616.6'5—dc22   2004040377

ISBN 0-7432-5348-5

This publication contains the opinions and ideas of its authors. It is intended to provide helpful and informative material on the subjects addressed in the publication. It is sold with the understanding that the authors and publisher are not engaged in rendering medical, health, or any other kind of personal or professional services in the book. The reader should consult his or her medical, health, or other competent professional before adopting any of the suggestions in this book or drawing inferences from it.

   The authors and publisher specifically disclaim all responsibility for any liability, loss, or risk, personal or otherwise, that is incurred as a consequence, directly or indirectly, of the use and application of any of the contents of this book.

To the late Dr. Bill Fair,
a world-famous urologist who was a pioneer
in improving the quality of life of cancer patients.

ACKNOWLEDGMENTS

The authors wish to thank: Richard Rivlin, Robert Thompson, Jarrett Kroll, Rachel Kessler, Gayle Nixon, Mark Erickson, William Turner, and Nabil Bissada.

Produced by The Reference Works, Inc.
224 West 30th Street
New York, NY 10001

Robert McCann, senior health editor
Robert Byrne, managing editor
Roslyn Siegel, executive editor
Paul Meehan, advisory editor
Stephen Smith, developmental editor
Peter Cusack, illustrations

The publisher and producer wish to thank Robert McCann for his tireless efforts in overseeing the complex production and completion of this work.

CONTENTS

V. ALTERNATIVES

INTRODUCTION

Max Gomez, Ph.D., Health Editor, WNBC

How's your prostate? What do you think it will be like in five years? In ten? In fact, as long as I'm asking—how's your health in general? How is your cholesterol? Your blood pressure? Your PSA?

Sound a little nosy? Even rude? Sort of like asking what your bank balance is or whether you'll be able to afford to retire at age sixty-five or put your kids through college. I would never dream of asking about your private finances, but I'll bet you have at least a pretty good idea of how much you have in the bank. You may even read money magazines, newsletters, follow the stock market, or get financial advice from friends or professional advisors. But I'd be willing to bet just as much that you *don't* know your blood pressure, cholesterol, or, since this book is about prostate health, your PSA number.

Most men are serious about providing for the financial needs of themselves and their family. But when it comes to their personal health, their level of concern or interest is nowhere near the same. How many men subscribe to health newsletters or confer with nutritionists, never mind see their doctors regularly? Think about the financial straits your family would be left in should you develop a serious illness or, God forbid, die from a disease *that could have been treated and even prevented!* When you consider what you mean to your family, maybe you should be paying more attention to your health; at the very least, it should be as much as you pay to your finances.

In the United States—a country with some of the best doctors, hospitals, and medicine in the world—the majority of men never visit a doctor regularly. For many men, years can go by without their having their blood pressure taken, cholesterol checked, or urine analyzed. Men in America don't go to the doctor until they are sick, figuring that "if it ain't broke, don't fix it." The trouble is, this attitude is like closing the barn door after the horse is gone. By that I mean that, often, by the time you get sick enough to force you to go to the doctor, there may be precious little a doctor can do to help. The problem may have been treatable or even *preventable* had you gone sooner; but in a later stage, treatments may be painful, devastating, or may not be able to "fix" the problem.

Remember the old Geritol commercial slogan that proclaimed, "When you've got your health, you've got just about everything"? Sounds trite, but it's really true. When you're sick, nothing else matters; when you're healthy, everything else is possible. The fact is that the single most important thing a man can do to provide for the security of his family—both financial and emotional—is to take care of his health. Caring for your family means caring for your health, pure and simple.

But visiting a doctor is only one part of taking control of your health. An equally important part is learning everything you can about preserving your health with preventive care—learning about the foods and nutrients that enhance your health as well as the substances that can harm it. The dirty little secret no one wants to talk about when it comes to health is that most of the diseases Western man dies of are largely self-inflicted. I know this sounds like blaming the victim, but we have to own up to the fact that the heart attack or cancer we suffer from at age sixty probably had its roots in the cheeseburgers we were eating (and other bad habits we were practicing) throughout our twenties, thirties, and beyond.

But let's get back to prostate cancer, which has been a topic of special interest to me for some time. It has long struck me that men just don't take prostate cancer as seriously as women take breast cancer. Men are certainly are not as vocal about it, yet prostate cancer is very similar in terms of the numbers affected, while treatments are nowhere near as advanced as they are for breast cancer. Far more research dollars flow into breast cancer research than into prostate cancer research primarily because women have mobilized and lobbied for it. This in no way means that we have conquered breast cancer or even that we have adequate means of treating, detecting, or preventing it—just that the current state of knowledge on prostate cancer lags well behind what we know about breast cancer.

My opinion stems partly from my recent prostate cancer news segments, which have focused on such topics as:

- Mobile health units that spread the word to men on this silent but often deadly disease
- A recent study confirming that men who undergo vasectomies are no more likely to develop prostate cancer than men who do not
- The controversy over the effectiveness of PSA testing for finding prostate cancer
- How researchers at several institutions are currently testing vaccines that may save countless lives from prostate cancer

Of all the newsworthy topics relating to prostate cancer and health, arguably none is more important than the role of proper nutrition in preventing or controlling prostate cancer, yet it is the least well understood by the general public. Few men, for example, have ever heard that Asian men, who eat more soy, have a lower prostate cancer rate than other ethnic groups, another recent news segment I reported. That's a big reason why in this book you will find additional leading-edge information from America's top researchers on how to prevent various kinds of prostate problems—from an enlarged prostate to prostate cancer. I would venture to guess that one of the most surprising yet important things you will discover in these pages is this: the same plan of prevention that helps stave off cancer in the first place should be continued and is still effective even *after* prostate cancer is diagnosed.

In the pages of this book you will get that crucial information from the Institute for Cancer Prevention's top researchers, including potentially life-saving information on treatment options after diagnosis. The Institute for Cancer Prevention (the new name of the American Health Foundation) is America's premier cancer prevention research organization. In fact, it is the only national research organization devoted specifically to the prevention of cancer and has been studying the nutritional factors in cancer prevention with multidisciplinary research since 1974.

In case the significance of the word "prevention" in the Institute's name hasn't quite registered, think about the following: It is estimated that fully 70 percent of cancers are preventable through lifestyle changes, primarily diet and the avoidance of tobacco. Seventy percent! That means that if we could just change a few bad habits and adopt a few preventive measures by modifying our diets, we could well see cancer become an unusual occurrence instead of the scourge it has become today.

More important, we're talking *prevention*, not treatment. As good and promising as some new cancer therapies are, any candid oncologist (cancer specialist) will admit that it is *far* better never to get cancer than to treat it. Even successful cancer treatment will likely be a damaging ordeal. How much better to *prevent* cancer in the first place than to go through disfiguring surgery, brutal chemotherapy, and energy-sapping radiation! That's the potential we present here.

In the course of this book, we present the Transition Diet. It is a program based on the pioneering effort made over many years by my coauthor, Dr. Daniel Nixon, President of the Institute for Cancer Prevention. Dr. Nixon explains that the changes that we need to make in our diet should be undertaken gradually and systematically—that we should dismantle our old, unhealthy eating habits one nasty habit at a time and introduce healthy substitutions in the same systematic way.

This may well be the most sensible diet plan you'll ever see, and it offers not only the best hope of preventing prostate cancer but also of treating the disease in its early stages.

Let me take a more personal perspective, if I may, that I hope will drive home my reasons for believing in cancer prevention as a better way. I was born in Cuba and grew up with the Caribbean equivalent of "bicoastal"; that is, for all intents and purposes, my immediate family lived both in Miami and Havana until Fidel Castro came to power. Then virtually all of my extended family—aunts, uncles, cousins, grandparents—were trapped in Cuba, prohibited from emigrating for years. It was shortly thereafter that my grandfather, after whom my father and I were named, developed prostate cancer. Prevented from coming to America for treatment, he died never again having seen his son or grandchildren.

Recently my father and I returned to Cuba for the first time in nearly forty years. I did a bittersweet story on how my father was able to, after all these years, visit his father's grave and finally bid him rest in peace. But as the senior health correspondent for the flagship NBC television station, I was also particularly interested in the Cuban health system. While the standard of living in Cuba is poor by Western standards, Cuba has achieved remarkable success in health care despite the fact that its medical system lags behind ours in many respects. Cubans living on the island have nearly the same life expectancy as people living in the United States, their infant mortality rates are actually better than in many cities in this country, and they die of the same degenerative diseases of the Western world: cancer, heart disease, and stroke.

Yet when I visited a hospital or clinic in Cuba, I was struck by the lack of medical supplies—many clinics hardly had two aspirins to rub together. So how had Cuban medicine managed to achieve many of the same health milestones we have in this country?

There are many answers to this question. In Cuba's version of socialized medicine, doctors work for the government public health system. Every school, factory, farm, workplace, apartment complex, and neighborhood is assigned a physician; Cuba has more than twice as many doctors per capita as we do in the States. Not only do these doctors work in the neighborhoods they serve, they actually live in their practice area. A common arrangement is for a doctor to live above his office, often with his nurse living in the same apartment complex or the same small stand-alone clinic.

Because these doctors are neighbors of the people they treat, they see whether Señor Rodríguez is smoking again, whether Señora González has been coming in for prenatal care, and that Señorita López may be getting too heavy. The doctor can then help his or her patients before they get really sick. In other words, they may not have high-tech medicine, but they practice good old-fashioned hands-on preventive medicine! Granted that much of this is born out of necessity, but there are lessons here for all of us.

One area that Cuban doctors have developed—again, partly out of necessity but partly out of a long tradition of herbal medicine and healing—is *medicina verde*, literally "green medicine." (I still remember my grandmother brewing up a cup of *manzanilla* tea—chamomile in America—to ease my upset stomach.) Because they have a tremendous shortage of modern drugs and medications, Cuban doctors use herbal medicine for a wide range of ailments. In fact, the government publishes a pamphlet detailing the uses of herbal preparations, and every pharmacy has an entire section devoted to *medicina verde*.

Perhaps as a consequence of our scientific achievement in America, we have forgotten the ancient lessons learned by less technologically advanced cultures when it comes to the value of good nutrition and the appropriate use of herbal medicine. In recent years, we have discovered more and more about the science behind Chinese herbal medicine and Indian Ayurvedic medicine, both of which utilize food and herbs for good health. But we still tend to treat people after they get sick rather than work at keeping them healthy.

Not only is it often too late to really help people after disease has taken hold, but our propensity to look to science to fix a problem has become counterproductive when it comes to our health. America still has the space-age attitude that to every problem there's a technological answer. We expect to be able to eat a lousy diet, never exercise, smoke, drink to excess, and fry in the sun, and that modern medicine will give us a pill or an operation to make us all better when we suffer a heart attack or stroke—or develop skin, lung, breast, colon, or prostate cancer. Well, I'm here to tell you that modern medicine often *won't* be able to help you. You have to acknowledge some responsibility for your own health; not only are a lot of the diseases we suffer from partly due to our lifestyles, but *we can do something about them!!*

Eating foods today that will protect you tomorrow is really as simple and logical as planning the finances today that will help you live better when you retire—or changing the oil in your automobile now so that it won't need a complete engine overhaul later. When it comes to both your car and your health, the mechanic in the commercial had it right—you can pay me now or you can pay me later—and later it's going to be a lot more painful.

Recently I learned something that made preventive medicine even more compelling. I started studying prostate cancer rates around the world. Autopsies show that even young men—as young as their early thirties—have signs of prostate cancer. If even thirty-year-olds have the seeds of prostate cancer but live out their whole lives and die in their eighties and nineties of something else, what is going on?

It could be genetic, of course. But Dr. Nixon and the researchers at the Institute for Cancer Prevention and others found otherwise.

The difference is diet and nutrition. When Asian men move from Japan or China to Hawaii and begin consuming our Western diet, their rate of prostate cancer rises to meet that of men in the United States. And not only is the incidence of prostate cancer lower among Asian men (in Asia), their death rate from the disease is also far lower. The lesson here is that we in America can do a lot to protect ourselves against the number two cancer-killer of men.

Both as a health reporter and as a man, I know that the information in this book is crucial to all men of all ages and to their families. It is far more important than almost any of the other things you spend time and energy worrying about. You must play a part in protecting your most precious possessions, your own body and health. After all, there will always be another stock and another car. But you only have one body and your family has only one you. The time to care for your health is now.

I.

PREVENTING PROSTATE PROBLEMS AND DISEASES

1. An Overview

Liberating Yourself

Ask people what causes cancer, and chances are you'll hear about air pollution, toxins, and the environment. They'll also mention electromagnetic fields, nuclear power plants, and genetic predisposition.

But the hard fact is that the vast majority of cancer doesn't just happen to us, we do it to ourselves. The Institute for Cancer Prevention estimates that 70 percent of all cancers are lifestyle-related. This means that you have the power not only to lower your risk of cancer but to control and minimize the course of the disease simply by making a few lifestyle changes.

In fact, one of the most exciting recent discoveries made by the scientists at the Institute for Cancer Prevention is that for prostate problems and even prostate cancer, **prevention, control, and treatment contain similar elements.** They all depend on lifestyle issues associated with the environment, nutrition, habits bad and good, age, weight, and physical exercise.

To clear up any misunderstanding about its position and function, the prostate gland is located around the neck of the bladder and the urethra. Its primary function is to secrete most of the fluid in the semen. There are basically two common maladies associated with the prostate: Lower urinary tract symptoms (we can call them LUTS for short; these make up the bulk of prostate problems), and cancer. The most common cause of LUTS is benign (that is, noncancerous) prostatic enlargement (BPH for short). But since cancer—of any kind—is so frightening, benign conditions such as prostatitis and BPH are often mistaken for harbingers or precursors of prostate cancer.

Scientists still know far less than they need to about how prostate cancer begins, grows, and spreads. They still lack the ability to distinguish between potentially lethal and nonlethal prostate cancer cells. Treatment for localized prostate cancer varies with the individual case. When the cancer is advanced, the disease is all but incurable.

Despite this, the past decade has seen momentous advances in the understanding and treatment of prostate cancer on a multitude of levels. Not only has detection at an earlier stage been improved and medication proven more effective, but simple adjustments in behavior have been shown to be one of the most powerful weapons of both prevention and management of the disease.

SENSITIVITIES AND SEXUAL POLITICS OF THE DIGITAL RECTAL EXAM

Many men are understandably sensitive when it comes to having a digital rectal exam (DRE). (No, it doesn't have anything to do with computers.) For some there may well be homophobia involved. For some it's simply the discomfort of having even a board certified urologist stick his finger in their rectum.

A few years back I did a news segment about a new procedure for treating BPH that included a few shots of men in a position most women would recognize from a visit to the gynecologist.

The story aired a couple of times, and pretty much without exception, the anchormen introducing the piece cringed visibly when they talked about it. It occurred to us then that their reaction might be at the heart of (or perhaps a little lower) men's reluctance to keep tabs on their prostate health.

All of which led to another story about why men won't go get their prostate checked. And since that checkup involves a digital rectal exam, we called the story "Fear of the Finger." We talked to women about their similar experiences at the gynecologist (didn't find much sympathy there), and ended with a sound bite from General Norman Schwarzkopf, a prostate cancer survivor and vocal advocate of prostate cancer screening. He said, "Look your doctor straight in the eye and tell him, 'Bring me to my knees if you have to, Doc, but check my prostate.' "

While it clearly shouldn't be quite that difficult, the message, I think, was clear. Regardless of the psychosexual issues, here's the point: GET OVER IT!

But the purely physiological aspects of prostate cancer are only one aspect of a man's difficulty in dealing with the disease. Psychological and sociological issues involving any sort of prostate disease and testing cut to the heart of a man's psyche.

The myth of the alpha male is that a man is too virile to seek, or to feel he needs to seek, help. It keeps many men from seeing their doctors, barring outright physical collapse—and not just for prostate problems but for a universe of potential ailments and conditions. The old "what I don't know won't hurt me" and "maybe it'll just go away" attitudes come into play.

The stark fact is that tens of thousands of men die each year from what amounts to fear and embarrassment—fear of visiting their physician to check their prostate health and embarrassment about the digital rectal exam (DRE).

Prostate disease is the single most prevalent problem in men's health. Eight in ten men will eventually develop an enlarged prostate, and one in ten will be diagnosed with prostate cancer. Those are significant numbers, truly "it could happen to me" numbers. Fortunately, we are finally seeing an increased public and media focus on prostate problems (thanks to such courageous trailblazers as former senator and presidential candidate Bob Dole, one of the first significant media names to go public). Prostate disease is finally coming out of the closet. Fear and embarrassment will no longer be considered insurmountable barriers to effective diagnosis, prevention, and treatment.

BREAST CANCER AND PROSTATE CANCER: A PARALLEL UNIVERSE

There are a number of parallels between breast cancer and prostate cancer that teach us a lot about both—and, not so incidentally, a lot about the bond between men and women. In many ways, prostate cancer is to men what breast cancer is to women. Both cancers have approximately the same annual mortality rate. The risk of contracting both increases with age. When these cancers occur in younger men and women, they tend to be of a more aggressive nature. Another key parallel is that early detection is vital in arresting both forms of cancer.

The root causes of prostate and breast cancer also reveal similarities. Both are linked to hormonal factors (breast cancer to estrogen, prostate cancer to androgens). Both can exist furtively in the body for many years.

Trigger factors can include diet, environment, aging, and declining immunity levels. And both breast cancer and prostate cancer can be prevented and controlled by simple lifestyle changes.

Finally, prostate and breast cancer have one other thing in common: a traditional reluctance of individuals and the society at large to acknowledge them and to discuss them frankly. Cancer sufferers become victims twice over: once as a result of the physical consequences of their disease and again by becoming second-class citizens, strangers even to their own body. Fortunately, this situation is undergoing a rapid evolution for the good. There has already been a huge positive change in how society looks at breast cancer, most of it happening over the last generation. Now, like breast cancer, prostate cancer is being reconsidered in a more honest, liberating light.

THE NUTRITION CONNECTION

As foods are increasingly put to the test in the lab and in clinical trials, more doctors are beginning to view nutrition and diet as a vital,

WHERE DO BREAST CANCER AND PROSTATE CANCER DIVERGE?

As someone who interviews "the man on the street" on a regular basis, I know that despite progress, there's still a long way to go in how men regard prostate cancer. While women have become very outspoken about breast cancer in the past decade or so, men remain far more reluctant to discuss their prostates, whether enlarged or cancerous. Men, by and large, remain embarrassed.

And this leads me to another important difference between breast cancer and prostate cancer. While treatment choices for breast cancer are relatively well defined and research has moved ahead at a brisk pace, prostate cancer has lagged far behind. In many ways, prostate cancer is where breast cancer was ten years ago: we know much less about appropriate ways to treat prostate cancer than we do breast cancer.

That's why Rudy Giuliani, former mayor of New York City and certainly one of the most decisive public figures in recent history, and thousands of men like him, agonize over whether to have surgery, external beam radiation, hormone treatments, or radioactive seed implantation, or even simply to watch and wait.

all-important part of a prostate health program. The late Dr. Ernst Wynder, the founder of the American Health Foundation (now known as the Institute for Cancer Prevention), one of the first and still most respected national organizations devoted to researching the effect of nutrition on general health, invented the term "nutritional therapy" and was a pioneer in its strategic use. Researchers at the institute have been working for years towards finding a specific diet, matched to a man's risk for prostate disease. A major step in that direction is our groundbreaking Prostate Health Pyramid and the Transition Diet, two of the cornerstones of this book.

It is estimated that up to 70 percent of all cancers are preventable, and some 35 percent may be related to diet. Other data indicates that certain nutritional factors can substantially influence *existing* cancer as well. The evidence is clear: following the Prostate Health Pyramid will help prevent, control, and even minimize the effects of prostate cancer.

THE PROSTATE HEALTH PYRAMID

The Prostate Health Pyramid emphasizes lowering fat and increasing fiber, fruits, and vegetables. Since dietary fat is the leading source of excess calorie consumption in the average American's diet, we should concentrate not on how many overall calories we are ingesting but on reducing the amount of fat in our diet to 20 to 30 percent, in some cases even 15 percent of ingested calories.

Inspired by the United States Department of Agriculture's (USDA's) famous Food Guide Pyramid, the Prostate Health Pyramid has been specially developed to target and alleviate prostate problems and diseases. It improves on the USDA's pyramid in that it is body-part specific and nutrient-, rather than food-group specific. It

OBESITY AND CANCER

Obese and overweight individuals simply have more cells in which cancer can form. Continued caloric excess stimulates these cells to divide faster, creating a domino effect called metabolic overdrive. The faster cells divide and the more cells that exist, the more likely there will be spontaneous or carcinogen-induced cell transformation. Fat cells also produce substances that promote cancer cell growth. In late-stage cancer, calories that once would have supported a healthy body are appropriated by ravenous cancer cells.

differentiates among various vegetables and fruits and links together an assortment of foods that provide the same nutrients.

THE TRANSITION DIET

Drawing on the guidelines from the Prostate Health Pyramid, the Transition Diet shows how to make sustained, long-term changes in eating patterns that may not only cut down your risk of ever getting prostate cancer but can help manage, control, and minimize the effects of the disease if you already have it. The Transition Diet helps you gradually and comfortably make the long-term changes—introducing less fat and more fiber, vegetables, fruits and grains—that will make all the difference not just to your prostate health but to your overall health as well.

The Transition Diet will teach you to:

• Learn new cooking techniques
• Sharpen your shopping techniques: learn how to read labels on food products
• Learn how to switch to nonfat snacks
• Totally rethink your meat consumption
• Find the most painless way to integrate more fruits and vegetables into your diet
• Learn how to eat appropriately in restaurants—including fast-food restaurants
• Discover herbs and spices, the secret ingredients of healthy, tasty cooking

THE EXERCISE/FITNESS/LIFESTYLE CONNECTION

While it is premature to say that diet and exercise can prevent prostate cancer from developing or progressing, a study at UCLA's Jonsson Comprehensive Cancer Center strongly suggests that a low-fat diet and exercise regimen appear to favorably affect the levels of hormones or growth factors that influence prostate cancer. We feel this combination is the best approach to prostate cancer prevention and prostate health maintenance, and for helping control existing prostate problems and diseases.

There is a virtually universal consensus in the medical community

PROSTATE PROTECTORS

- **Lycopene:** This carotenoid is a potent antioxidant widely touted for its cancer-protective effects. "You can give someone who has prostate cancer large doses of lycopene through tomato products and find that the actual structure of the prostate tumor can change to a less damaging and less dangerous structure," says Dr. Leonard Cohen of the Institute for Cancer Prevention.
- **EGCG (epigallocatechin gallate):** This powerful cancer-preventive, cancer-fighting antioxidant is found in green tea. EGCG is a phytonutrient (plant-based nutrient) that, according to Dr. Mitchell Gaynor of the Strang Cancer Prevention Institute, "is one of the major protectors against the development of cancer over the long term. It is twenty times more potent than vitamin E and five hundred times more potent than vitamin C."
- **Selenium:** This antioxidant guards against cancer cell formation.
- **Vitamins E and C:** Antioxidants that neutralize cell-damaging free radicals.
- **Glycine, alanine, and glutamic acid:** These amino acids are effective for treating prostatitis and its attendant urinary conditions.
- **Zinc and magnesium:** Minerals necessary for prostate health and potency.
- **Lecithin:** A phospholipid containing the nutrient choline that has been successfully used to treat enlarged prostates and related urinary problems.

that exercise has many generalized anticancer effects. These include improving immune function and antioxidant defenses, regulating blood sugar, and lowering body fat percentage. There also seems to be a clear relationship between exercise and prostate cancer. Although the cause of prostate cancer is not known, the potential risk factors are. These include improper diet, obesity, and a sedentary lifestyle.

The most prevalent theory as to why exercise "works" against prostate cancer is that a pronounced degree of physical activity lowers circulating testosterone levels. Studies have shown that men who exercise have a rise in testosterone levels during the workout and lower testosterone levels immediately following the workout, followed by a significant postexercise drop of as much as 25 to 50 percent.

Moreover, men who are obese are more likely to die of prostate cancer than those who are not, according to a study in *Cancer Epidemiology Biomarkers and Prevention*. Researchers who have examined the relationship between body mass index (BMI), height, and incidence of death from prostate cancer in two large study groups found that the prostate cancer death rate was 27 percent higher in men who were obese. At the very least, exercise is beneficial in weight control, which ultimately helps keep cancer risk down.

EXERCISE AND STRESS

When we're feeling stressed or anxious, stress related and adrenaline hormone levels shoot up. Aerobic exercise has been shown to lower stress hormone levels.

We recommend that you exercise for at least thirty minutes on most days of the week. Walking is a good form of exercise.

Exercise is also important after prostate removal surgery.

THE IMPORTANCE OF REGULAR CHECKUPS

Middle-aged and older men need to get regular prostate health updates. In 2002, nearly 190,000 men were told they had prostate cancer. Many more have an enlarged prostate.

It is very helpful to make a list of questions you want to ask your physician or urologist when you go for a checkup. Take notes during the session if you can.

Although screening for prostate cancer is a common part of a routine checkup, a study by the U.S. Preventive Services Task Force published in *Annals of Internal Medicine* concluded that there is insufficient scientific evidence to endorse routine screening for all men and inconclusive evidence that early detection improves health outcomes. While tests are effective for detecting disease, there is insufficient evidence that they improve long-term health outcomes. And therein lies one of the major unanswered questions—and controversies—in prostate health.

But this we do know: **Since the use of early detection tests for**

EXERCISE AND PSA LEVEL

Refrain from exercising—particularly an aerobic activity such as cycling—for a minimum of three days before getting a prostate checkup. Exercise might artificially increase your PSA level, the prostate cancer marker discussed in the section above.

prostate cancer became relatively common (in about 1990), the prostate cancer death rate has dropped. It has not been proven that this is the direct result of screening—at least not yet—but long-term clinical studies will soon give us a good estimate of how effective screening is in this regard.

THE PSA TEST AND THE DRE

Two critical tests for detecting men at higher risk for prostate cancer and other prostate problems are the digital rectal exam (DRE) and the prostate-specific antigen test (PSA). *Never have your PSA level tested* after *having a DRE. Your PSA level will be elevated by the DRE procedure.* Having a DRE after a PSA test is not a problem. A high PSA level in the blood can indicate the presence of prostate cancer. But a high PSA does not *necessarily* mean that cancer is present. Neither the DRE nor the PSA test can tell if you have cancer; they can only suggest the need for further tests. Many men with BPH also have elevated PSA levels. Any condition involving inflammation of the prostate (prostatitis) can cause PSA levels to rise. Thus, while the PSA level will usually rise in the face of growing cancer, an elevated PSA does not necessarily mean that cancer is the cause.

The benefits of PSA testing include the all-important early detection of cancer, but the downside includes a fairly high percentage of false-positive and false-negative results. The fallout of false-positives includes unnecessary anxiety (which cannot be overestimated!), unneeded biopsies, and the potential complications of overtreating early cancers.

Exactly what can we find out by measuring PSA levels? PSA is a protein found in blood serum that is specific to the prostate. Malfunction of, say, the liver won't make your PSA level rise, which is why we say that this protein level is prostate-specific.

The normal prostate cell retains most of its PSA, letting very little leak into the bloodstream. Current studies indicate that a PSA level of 4.0 or less is normal in men not at high risk. Recent studies suggest that a 20 percent rise in PSA in one year should raise a red flag that a patient should be tested more closely. When we talk about "normal," however, we are already getting into a gray area. There is such a thing as a "high normal" PSA—"high" because the number seems relatively elevated and "normal" because adequate testing has been done to rule out the presence of suspicious nodules. Testing would very likely include a digital rectal exam and a transrectal ultrasound, with or without specific or random biopsies. The only way to definitively determine the presence of cancer is by examining tissue taken from a biopsy of the prostate gland.

The "free PSA" test has begun to replace the more conventional PSA test. Free PSA represents the current cutting edge of prostate cancer screening tests. Free PSA measures the amount of PSA that is not bound to albumin or other proteins. The *lower* your free PSA,

PROSTATE DISEASE: THE BIG THREE

The three most common conditions affecting the prostate are benign prostatic hyperplasia, prostatitis, and prostate cancer.

- **Benign prostatic hyperplasia (BPH),** a noncancerous enlargement of the prostate, is the most common prostate condition. In fact, more than 50 percent of men age sixty and 80 percent of men age eighty are estimated to have BPH. The enlargement often squeezes the urethra where it runs through the prostate, blocking the normal flow of urine from the urinary bladder. Symptoms of BPH include difficulty initiating urination, having a weak urinary stream, and waking up several times a night to urinate. BPH is more common among older men: as a man ages, his prostate naturally tends to enlarge. BPH can be treated by a variety of methods, including prescription medications and surgery.
- **Prostatitis** is an acute or chronic, bacterial or nonbacterial inflammation of the prostate. It is not contagious, but modern medicine does not clearly understand the mechanism by which the prostate becomes infected. One popular theory is that the bacteria that causes prostatitis may get into the prostate from the urethra because of the backward flow of infected urine. Both acute and chronic prostatitis can be treated with antibiotics. Noninfectious prostatitis is not treatable with antibiotics, although muscle relaxants, hot sitz baths, periodic prostatic massage, and other treatments may offer some measure of relief.
- **Prostate cancer** is mutated cells that evolve into a malignant tumor, most often beginning in the outer part of the prostate. As the tumor grows, it may spread to the inner part of the prostate and beyond that into other regions of the body (the spread of cancer is called metastasis). Treatment options for prostate cancer include "watchful waiting," hormonal therapy, chemotherapy, radiation, brachytherapy (radioactive seed implantation), cryotherapy, and surgery.

the *higher* the likelihood you have prostate cancer. If your free PSA level is less than 10 percent, there is more than a 50 percent chance that cancer will be detected by a prostate biopsy. Free PSA should be tested when the regular PSA level is between 4.0 and 10.0.

PROSTATE MYTHS AND REALITY

Misinformation and misconceptions about the prostate gland abound. Men should educate themselves about the nature of their prostate; learn about prostate problems and disease; and, most of all, realize the necessity for checkups and for preventive prostate health measures.

PROSTATE FUNCTION
The prostate's primary function is regulating urine flow through the urethra.

Wrong. Although the prostate surrounds the urethra and may restrict the flow of urine if it becomes enlarged, its main function has to do with reproduction: the prostate produces most of the fluid that carries and nourishes sperm through the urethra. At one time, the prostate was thought to protect against urinary tract infections (the word "prostate" is from the Greek word for "protector").

GENERAL PROSTATE SYMPTOMS
Trouble with urination automatically equals prostate problems.
No, there are a variety of causes for most urinary symptoms.

Frequent urination is due to "weak" kidneys.
This is one of the great myths of folk medicine.

BENIGN PROSTATIC HYPERPLASIA (BPH): ENLARGED PROSTATE
If your physician discovers that your prostate is enlarged, you will most likely want to request a biopsy to check for cancer.

No, an enlarged prostate doesn't signify cancer. It's a typical occurrence as men grow older, although it can cause significant complications if it continues to enlarge.

Are most prostate problems cancer-related?

Not by a long shot. Noncancerous prostate enlargement is by far the most common prostate condition. Even though it is not easily diagnosed or classified, approximately 2 million cases of prostatitis (inflammation of the prostate) are diagnosed each year.

You should consider medication or surgery for an enlarged prostate as soon as it's detected.

Certainly not. Drugs and surgery can have side effects and risks. It's usually best to leave an enlarged prostate alone unless symptoms become bothersome.

Massage can help an enlarged prostate.

It can ease its symptoms, especially when combined with proper supplementation and hot baths.

PROSTATITIS

Prostatitis leads to prostate cancer.

There is no relationship whatsoever between prostatic infection or inflammation and prostate cancer.

Prostatitis is caused by too little or too much sex.

Excessive sexual activity does not generally contribute to prostatitis, but congestion or buildup of semen in the prostate can cause some of the symptoms of prostatitis. So a healthy sex life helps maintain a healthy prostate.

PROSTATE CANCER

All cancers pose an equal risk.

No. Cancers of different organs and within specific organs carry very different prognoses and grow at widely differing rates. While some cancers progress rapidly without treatment, others progress at a very slow, one might almost say leisurely, pace. This includes certain skin cancers (basal cell carcinoma), thyroid cancer, and prostate cancer. It may take years before these cancers become threatening, if ever. Scientists do not yet know how to tell which men with a small focus of prostate cancer cells are most likely to go on to develop a clinically significant disease.

Prostate cancer is an older man's disease.

It is true that the risk and incidence of prostate cancer increases with age, but 25 percent of prostate cancers are found in men under age sixty-five, representing 40,000 to 50,000 men every year. At any rate, old age is relative. At the turn of the twentieth century, the average male life expectancy was fifty-seven years; by the end of the twentieth century, it was seventy-two years. An extra 26 percent was added to the lifespan of the average man in the course of a single century. As the male population's general health improves and men avoid or postpone dying from a number of other diseases, the risk of prostate cancer as a disease time bomb looms larger. Awareness of its potential risks thus becomes even more vital.

Frequent urination is a common symptom of prostate cancer in its earliest stages.

No. In its early stages, prostate cancer rarely exhibits any symptoms, which is why annual prostate cancer screenings are so important when a man reaches middle age. Once symptoms do appear, it is often already too late to treat the cancer effectively. Symptoms such as frequent or difficult urination are more typically caused by prostate enlargement.

Every man, if he lived long enough, would eventually get prostate cancer.

Quite possibly. According to some statistics, 40 percent of all eighty-year-old men have it, as established through postmortems. Many men don't even know they have prostate cancer, as it tends to develop slowly. Chances are they simply die of something else first. Since we know that incidence does increase with age, it's possible that if a man lived a very long time, he would get prostate cancer sooner or later—*but not necessarily die from it.*

A vasectomy increases the risk of prostate cancer.

A study funded in part by the U.S. National Institute of Child Health & Human Development (NICHD) in New Zealand found that men who undergo vasectomies are no more likely to develop prostate cancer than men who do not.

Eating a proper diet will prevent prostate cancer.

Many clinical studies have shown that diet positively affects the incidence and virulence of prostate cancer. A prostate-healthy diet will help prevent, manage, and control the progress of the disease. **In the war against prostate cancer, there is no greater weapon than nutrition.**

An early transurethral resection of the prostate helps a man avoid prostate cancer later in life.

No. Transurethral resection removes primarily the transitional zone of the prostate, rarely a cancer site. The peripheral zone, where cancers usually develop, is not removed.

Prostate cancer is a genetically based disease.

Only about 5 to 10 percent of patients with prostate cancer have a strong family history of age-specific-onset prostate cancer.

Dribbling after urination is a sign of prostate cancer.

Dribbling is a common occurrence in older men and does not signify that cancer is present.

Prostate removal or radiation treatment will cure prostate cancer. The patient has little to worry about from that point on.

Retreatment is needed in 35 percent of cases.

Testosterone replacement therapy causes prostate cancer.

The relationship between testosterone and prostate cancer isn't as clear as we would like it to be. It is true, however, that patients with existing prostate cancer should not receive testosterone replacement therapy, as it could make matters worse. Scientists are beginning to consider the possibility that estrogen plays a role in the hormonal regulation of the prostate. If that proves true, there could be a connection between prostate cancer and high dietary and environmental estrogen levels.

A fall or injury can cause prostate cancer.

There is absolutely no cause-and-effect relationship between the two.

A sexually transmitted infection (STI) can cause prostate cancer.

STIs don't cause prostate cancer.

THE PSA TEST

The PSA test has improved the survival rate for prostate cancer.

The jury is still very much out on this. In the United States, prostate cancer deaths have dropped 10 percent since the early 1990s. Both experts and patient groups attribute this to the prostate-specific antigen test, which is a simple blood test. But not everyone is convinced, pointing out the test's relatively low accuracy level, which produces what many consider to be an unacceptable number of false-positives and false-negatives. And one of the big problems is determining just how aggressive a particular PSA-detected prostate cancer tumor really is.

An elevated number in a PSA test causes a great degree of stress in men who may, in fact, turn out not to have prostate cancer.

It's true that the PSA test is not a prostate cancer–specific test. That is, the PSA level may go up for a number of reasons, such as prostate enlargement, or even intercourse. Other possible causes of a rise in PSA have to be definitively excluded before cancer can be diagnosed. But the PSA level remains the best prostate cancer marker science has yet to develop. In fact, the PSA level is able to detect cancer seven to nine years before it becomes clinically significant.

People who eat a lot of dairy products have a higher risk of prostate cancer.

Some observational studies link a high intake of dairy foods with an increased risk for prostate cancer, according to a review by the American Institute for Cancer Research. However, observational studies do not show a cause-and-effect relationship. Some recent studies link certain components in milk and dairy products to a *lower* risk of developing certain types of cancer, including colon cancer.

Prostate cancers detected by PSA alone (with a normal DRE) are as biologically significant as those detected by an abnormal DRE (with or without PSA elevation).

True. Assessments at the Mayo Clinic and Baylor University show that the prognostic determinants are almost identical.

SEX, IMPOTENCE, AND INFERTILITY
Sex is not good for the prostate.

A loving sex life with a regular partner is one of the best medicines for the prostate. A recent study (covered in Chapter 9) also indicates that masturbation is healthful for the prostate. Celibate men have the highest incidence of prostate cancer. However, sexual promiscuity with multiple partners is also seen as a risk factor.

Impotence is what men fear most about prostate cancer treatment.

That's a very real fear, but many men faced with treatment for prostate cancer are also concerned about the possibility of long-term urinary incontinence.

Surgery for an enlarged prostate will make you impotent.

A TURP or an open prostatectomy will reduce or eliminate the discharge of semen with orgasm, but it rarely diminishes the erection of someone who did not have that problem prior to surgery.

Postsurgical prostate cancer problems, particularly incontinence and impotence, occur only in a limited number of cases.

Unfortunately, these problems are common. Incontinence and impotence occur because of nerve and muscle damage during surgical or radiation treatment. However, those statistics can vary dramatically with the skill of your surgeon.

PSYCHOLOGICAL ASPECTS OF PROSTATE PROBLEMS AND DISEASE
Men don't know how to support other men the way women support other women.

Most men do tend to look primarily to a woman—usually their spouse—during time of illness. But male-centered prostate cancer support groups have sprung up across America, and their number is growing every day, giving the lie to the myth that men don't know how to close ranks and support each other. Anyone who has ever watched a touch football game can vouch for that.

2. The Healthy Prostate

Prostate Power

Prepare to meet your prostate. You need to get a sense of what your prostate gland looks like; where it is located; how it functions in relation to the rest of your body; and how to recognize when you may be experiencing prostate problems.

The Prostate Gland

The prostate is a gland or, more accurately, a cluster of glands, that secretes fluids the body needs to function properly. Glands come in two varieties: those that secrete substances into the bloodstream (*endocrine* glands, such as the thyroid gland) and glands whose secretions are delivered into a duct system for direct delivery into an organ (*exocrine* glands, such as the salivary glands). The prostate is an exocrine gland located in the urogenital system that secretes fluid and vital nutrients of semen, the milky ejaculate that nourishes sperm, which are produced by the testicles. Sperm travels up from the testicles through long tubes called the vas deferens.

During orgasm, the prostate fluid mixes with fluid from the seminal vesicles, located on each side of the prostate. Muscles squeeze this fluid into the urethra, where it carries sperm through the penis during orgasm. To make sure semen doesn't move in the wrong direction and back up into the bladder, a ring of muscle at the neck of the bladder (the internal sphincter) remains tightened during ejaculation.

The prostate is located just below the bladder and in front of the rectum. The prostate surrounds the urethra, the tube that carries urine from the bladder out through the tip of the penis as it emerges from the bladder. This accounts for many of the urinary symptoms that arise from an enlarged or inflamed prostate.

A thin capsule of fibrous tissue, and then a layer of fat, surrounds the prostate gland. To work properly, the prostate needs male hormones (androgens). Hormones are responsible for most sex characteristics. The primary male hormone is testosterone, manufactured mainly by the testicles. Some male hormones are also produced in small amounts by the adrenal glands.

In newborns, the prostate gland is about the size of a pea. This tiny pea continues to grow until about age twenty, when it reaches normal adult size, the size of a walnut or chestnut. It remains that size until, on average, age forty-five, at which time it often begins to grow again, as testosterone levels begin to decline.

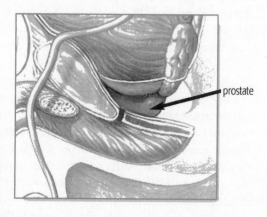

prostate

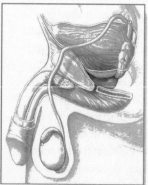

The prostate gland surrounds the urethra just below the bladder. When enlarged it may squeeze the urethra closed, making urination difficult.

THE MALE UROGENITAL SYSTEM

THE LYMPH NODES

The front wall of the rectum lies only a few millimeters behind the prostate gland. Lying on each side in the space between the prostate and the rectum are nerves and blood vessels.

Prostate veins drain toward the heart via connections along the spine. Lymph, a watery fluid found in all tissues, flows away from the prostate via small channels (lymphatics) to lymph nodes along the wall of the pelvis on both sides. Lymph nodes filter out bacteria, viruses, and other impurities as well as cancer cells before the lymph flows further upstream toward veins that eventually empty into the heart.

THE URINARY SYSTEM

The urethra extends through the "core" of the prostate and is part of the system that handles waste removal and maintenance of the body's fluid and electrolyte balance, consisting also of the kidneys, ureters, and bladder. The kidneys cleanse the blood and produce urine. Urine travels from the kidneys to the bladder—which stores the urine—through long, thin muscular tubes (ureters). The bladder is behind and slightly above the pubic bones when full and is separated from the rectum by paired seminal vesicles. For the bladder to work effectively in passing urine, its muscle, controlled by nerve impulses, must contract, while muscles of the urinary sphincter must relax. The bladder also works as a storage organ, allowing urine to collect without discomfort. It's very hard to give an exact measurement of the volume of the bladder. Each person's ability to hold a given amount of urine differs. When the bladder is full, urine exits through the urethra. This urinary channel is a tube about as wide as a pencil.

The prostate isn't a primary component of the urinary system, but because of its location, it impacts urinary health. For example, conditions such as prostate enlargement can seriously impact urine flow, squeezing the urethra and affecting the ability to urinate.

The urethra also plays a role in the reproductive system, composed of the testes and its duct systems, and the prostate gland and its seminal vesicles.

When we are young, the prostate plays its role in the body largely unremarked upon and unnoticed. Unnoticed, that is, until we begin developing prostate problems.

DO I HAVE A PROBLEM?

Having a prostate problem is one thing; knowing you have a prostate problem is another. **If you suspect you have a prostate problem, see a physician.** Don't rely on self-diagnosis or self-treatment. It is estimated that 80 percent of men keep their prostate symptoms and problems under wraps. That's a shame, since early detection and treatment make all the difference.

Prostate problems usually don't occur until after age thirty, at the earliest. The prostate may become inflamed due to the presence of bacterial infection; in men over fifty, an enlarged prostate may press on the urethra, interfering with urination; prostate cancer occurs most often in older men (by age eighty, some cell mutation has occurred in most men).

Those who say that prostate problems are connected with aging are, in the main, right. That doesn't mean a young man shouldn't be concerned about prostate health. **It is when you are young that you most need to address the preventive measures that will provide insurance against future prostate problems.**

Men with lower urinary tract symptoms (LUTS for short) will often think they are having prostate trouble. Not all urinary symptoms relate to the prostate; in fact, that is far from the case.

SYMPTOMS: IT'S NOT ALL ABOUT THE PROSTATE

Some symptoms are prostate-related and some are not. Obstruction of normal urine flow and pressure in the lower back may be due to an enlarged prostate. Other symptoms include a feeling that your bladder is not emptying completely; persistent urine dribbling, even after you feel you have already finished urinating; and the need to urinate frequently. However, frequent urination may be unrelated to prostate problems. After all, elderly women who have no prostate may also need to visit the bathroom a number of times each night.

Changes in the bladder muscle and its innervation can be caused by aging, illnesses such as Parkinson's disease, diabetes, stroke and other neurological conditions, and the effects of certain medications. An "overactive" bladder can cause urgency symptoms, as well as the frequent need to urinate. Other conditions, such as urinary tract infection or kidney stones, can produce similar symptoms. Just as the bladder can be overactive, so can it be underactive, leading to incomplete emptying and a weak urine stream.

Infection and inflammation of the lower urinary tract can cause symptoms including a burning sensation when urinating and the need to urinate frequently. Men in their forties and fifties sometimes interpret these symptoms as indicants of prostate disease. These other conditions need to be clearly distinguished from prostate problems, as treatment options differ widely, depending on the cause.

SYMPTOMS IN YOUNGER MEN

Many lower urinary tract problems experienced by men under forty tend to resolve on their own. The cause may not always be found or even known. Whatever your age, see your doctor, especially if you have recurring urinary tract problems.

CHANGE IN PROSTATE SIZE

It can be seen from the location of the prostate—just beneath the bladder and surrounding the urethra—that a change in prostate size is bound to affect the urinary function in some way. An increase in tissue caused by benign enlargement usually occurs on the inner part of the gland, where it is most likely to squeeze the urethra and cause obstruction. Tissue increase caused by a cancerous growth usually occurs in the outer part of the gland, where it is less likely to cause urinary symptoms.

PAIN

Pain originates in the prostate when a prostate infection causes swelling and inflammation. It is usually described as a dull pain, a constant aching, and has its center in the perineum, the region between the anal opening and the scrotum. Pain originating in the prostate gland can radiate to the lower back, the groin, and even the penis and legs. Lower abdominal pain may occur when the prostate is infected or when prostate infection leads to a bladder infection.

RISK FACTORS OF PROSTATE CANCER

A risk factor is anything that may increase a person's chance of developing a disease. From 1973 to 1991, prostate cancer mortality in the United States increased at a rate of 1 percent per year among white males and 1.8 percent among black males. But considerable progress has been made over the last decade due to earlier screening and better testing procedures.

Although risk factors increase a person's risk, they do not necessarily *cause* the disease. This is an important distinction. Some men with one or multiple risk factors may never develop prostate cancer; others develop prostate cancer or other prostate problems with no discernible risk factors.

Knowing the risk factors of prostate cancer—and knowing which factors are considered more significant than others—can provide guidelines for a preventive, prostate-healthy lifestyle. Risk factors are of two types, controllable and uncontrollable. Controllable factors include diet, environment, and hormone supplementation; uncontrollable factors include age, family history, and ethnicity.

DIET

Diet is a major risk factor, specifically a diet high in saturated fat and low in fiber. The dangers of a Western diet with its emphasis on red meat are something we will emphasize again and again in this book.

OBESITY

Statistics from the Centers for Disease Control and Prevention estimate that over 60 percent of Americans are overweight or obese. Men who are obese are more likely to die of prostate cancer than men who are not overweight, according to a study reported in *Cancer Epidemiology Biomarkers and Prevention*. Obesity increases the risk of death from prostate cancer by an estimated 25 to 33 percent.

Researchers at the American Cancer Society examined the relationship between body mass index (BMI), height, and death from prostate cancer in two large study groups. Researchers found that prostate cancer mortality rates were 27 percent higher in obese men. As many as 90,000 cancer deaths a year in the United States may be linked to obesity, including 14 percent of *all* cancer deaths among men. The greater a man's weight, the higher his risk of developing cancer.

AGE

Sixty percent of all newly diagnosed prostate cancer cases, and almost 80 percent of all deaths, occur in men seventy years of age or

IS "LINK" THE SAME AS "CAUSE"?

Whenever you read a scientific study—okay, whenever you hear about a scientific study on TV or the radio or read about it in the newspaper—there's one very important thing to keep in mind. And that is whether the study shows a "link" between Factor A and Result B . . . or does it actually show that Factor A *caused* Result B? It sounds like a small difference, but it's at the very heart of figuring out how much stock to put in a particular study.

Here's what I mean. Simply because something is "linked" to something else doesn't mean that it actually "caused" it. For example, people who live in Miami have a lot more skin cancer than people who live in Toronto. So living in Miami is "linked" to an increased risk of skin cancer. What is it about Miami that leads to more skin cancer? Is it the ocean? The number of Spanish-speaking residents? That the residents drink more orange juice because they live closer to orange groves? Or could it be the *latitude* at which they live? In other words, the closer to the equator you live, the more skin cancer the population will suffer because the sun's rays hit the earth more directly and therefore there's more cancer-causing ultraviolet radiation. Miami is "linked" to skin cancer, but it doesn't *cause* it!

Similarly, some years ago the brain cells of Alzheimer's disease sufferers were found to contain increased levels of aluminum. Aluminum was *linked to* Alzheimer's, and so many people jumped to the conclusion that it was the excess aluminum we were being exposed to in antiperspirants and aluminum cookware that was responsible for the increase in Alzheimer's disease.

It turns out that the aluminum was not causing the Alzheimer's at all. Rather, the aluminum in the brain cells was there because whatever *was* causing the disease had damaged the cells enough so that they could no longer keep aluminum out, as they normally would, and the aluminum was able to seep into them, later to be found when researchers analyzed victims' brains.

So there's a big difference between something being *linked with* or *to* a particular disease or cancer and actually *causing* it. In science, we call that the difference between *causation* and *correlation*.

older. After age fifty, the chance of being diagnosed with prostate cancer increases rapidly.

GENETIC PREDISPOSITION

Numerous studies point to family history as a major risk factor, responsible for an estimated 5 to 10 percent of all prostate cancer cases. Prostate cancer's hereditary aspect has been studied extensively only over the last generation or so. An overview of all genetic studies suggests that family history is a very strong risk factor, with a pronounced effect on the incidence of, and perhaps even the virulence of, prostate cancer.

According to a study in *The Journal of Urology*, men who have a family history of prostate cancer develop the disease at a younger age and die from it more often than men without such a history. This study reinforces the notion that men with a family history of prostate cancer should be screened on a regular basis.

Chromosomes (genetic material) are found in the center of every cell of the body. Most cells of the body normally contain 46 chromosomes, or 23 pairs, half inherited from one's mother and half from one's father.

Chromosomes contain the body's blueprint, the genes. Some cells, when altered or mutated, create a higher risk for uncontrolled cell growth, which in turn can lead to tumor development. These genes are referred to as cancer susceptibility genes. Approximately 9 percent of all prostate cancers, and 45 percent of cases in men younger than fifty-five, can be attributed to a cancer susceptibility gene that is inherited as a dominant trait (that is, passed on from parent to child).

The exact genes that cause prostate cancer or increase a man's

THE IMPACT OF FAMILY HISTORY

It is estimated that having a father or brother with prostate cancer doubles a man's risk of developing the disease. The risk is even higher when there are several relatives diagnosed with prostate cancer, particularly if the relatives were young at the time of diagnosis. Geneticists divide families into three groups, depending on the number of men who have exhibited prostate cancer, and their ages at onset of the disease:

- **Sporadic:** A family with prostate cancer present in one man, at the typical age of onset for the disease.
- **Familial:** A family with prostate cancer present in more than one person, but with no definitive pattern of inheritance and usually an older age of onset.
- **Hereditary:** A family with a cluster of three or more affected relatives among parents and their children; a family with prostate cancer in each of three generations on either the mother's or father's side; or a cluster of two relatives affected at a young age (fifty-five or less).

"IT DOESN'T RUN IN THE FAMILY"

Family history is a powerful predictor of your risk of developing prostate cancer. But don't make the mistake of thinking that because you don't have prostate cancer (or any other cancer, for that matter) in your family, that you're out of the woods.

I can't tell you the number of people I have interviewed over the years who tell me they're not in such a rush to get a prostate exam (or a mammogram or colonoscopy, and so on) because "it doesn't run in my family."

Even sadder are the cancer patients I've met who tell me essentially the same thing: "I was shocked; no one in my family ever had this cancer. I don't know how I got it."

The fact is that although family history tells you whether you are at *increased* risk for developing a particular cancer, it cannot tell you that you have *no* risk. If you have a prostate, a colon, or whatever, you have at least some risk of developing cancer, especially as you grow older.

All family history means is that a person who has cancer in the family has to be even more careful and vigilant about diet, lifestyle, and screening tests than a person who doesn't. But the latter guy still has to be careful too!

chances of developing it have not been identified, although many genes that may play a role are being closely studied.

HORMONES

Hormones are essential for normal prostate development and function. Hormone therapy is an important part of prostate cancer treatment. Although the trigger for prostate cancer development is not well understood, factors such as elevated testosterone levels seem to play an important role. We know that hormone levels play a substantial role in the development of prostate cancer in laboratory animals.

Increased estrogen level is fast gaining credibility as another hormonal risk factor.

What we refer to as estrogen is actually a collective of three similar hormones. As men age, their testosterone levels go down and they begin to lose muscle mass at the same time that they are gaining fat. Fat cells convert testosterone to estrogen. Estrogen levels remain at the same level as men age or may actually rise a little, thus altering the testosterone-to-estrogen ratio.

An estrogen imbalance encourages the regrowth of prostate cells that have already suffered a type of damage called oxidative free-radical damage. It seems feasible that this can prompt cancer cells to grow in a man's prostate, just as they do in a woman's breast.

The best way to address the potential estrogen risk factor is to have your estrogen level checked and to take the appropriate steps to lower it if necessary. Indole-3-carbinol, found in cruciferous vegetables and thought to have a cancer-protective effect on women's breast tissue, may also have a protective effect on the prostate.

On the other side of the ledger, researchers at the University of Connecticut Health Center concluded that small amounts of estrogen therapy can actually help reduce osteoporosis caused by testosterone suppression treatment.

TESTOSTERONE: GOOD OR BAD?

As you read through this book, you may say, "I'm confused. First testosterone is good, then it's bad, then it's good again." Well, it *is* confusing.

Testosterone is vital for normal prostate development in boys. It's also important in puberty, for muscle development, for normal sex drive, and so on. Yes, I know there are those who think that testosterone is responsible for everything from road rage to wars to the inability to ask for directions. But let's just talk prostate physiology for now.

We're also told that testosterone is a key hormone in the causation of prostate cancer. Yet prostate cancer rates climb as we get older—precisely the time when our testosterone levels are dropping! Go figure. And just to make it really confusing, testosterone seems to "feed" prostate cancer cells. A mainstay of hormonal therapy for prostate cancer is some variation of testosterone blockage or withdrawal.

Some of this is still being worked out, but here's a plausible way to think of testosterone and prostate physiology: as guys age, there's a drop in blood testosterone levels; dihydrotestosterone (DHT) levels remain relatively steady (testosterone is converted to DHT by an enzyme called 5alpha-reductase); and estrogen levels rise slightly (diminishing the ratio between testosterone and estrogen levels).

So why does the prostate enlarge and become more susceptible to cancer in so many older men? One theory is that an aging prostate may be more susceptible to the effect of hormones, even though the testosterone level is lower. A higher estrogen ratio plus an aging prostate might equal a prostate that is more affected by testosterone.

But when all is said and done, we'll just have to bear with medical science until the relationship between testosterone and the prostate is cleared up once and for all.

Another hormone-based threat to prostate health is DHT, a potent form of testosterone. Until recently, it was believed that DHT was the primary, and perhaps the only, hormonal threat to the prostate. It is now believed by some scientists that DHT is a threat in conjunction with poor diet and increased estrogen levels as men age.

SMOKING

Prostate cancer tends to be more advanced and virulent in smokers. According to a recent study, among younger men with prostate cancer, current or former smokers are more likely to have cancer that spreads beyond the prostate.

Researchers from Johns Hopkins University found that for men under age fifty-five the risk was even higher for current smokers than for former ones.

Researchers collected data on the smoking histories of 350 men who had undergone prostate cancer surgery in the 1990s. All the operations had been performed by a single physician. The study found that men who had ever smoked were 66 percent more likely to have cancer spread (metastasize) outside the prostate by the time of surgery. Men who had smoked within the last ten years had 2.5 times an increased risk. The risk for those who were still smoking was more than 3.5 times as high.

The risk of developing a more virulent cancer was also related to the number of cigarettes smoked. The risk was highest among men with a history of at least forty pack-years, that is, the number of packs per day times the number of years smoked. Men who quit smoking before they're diagnosed with prostate cancer may improve their chances of developing a less virulent form of the disease.

The majority of large studies have not found a link between smoking and prostate cancer. In the studies that have detected a connection, one plausible explanation is that substances in cigarette smoke may act as cancer promoters and/or activators. They may enter the bloodstream and concentrate in the prostate. While these substances may not be the root cause of the cancer, they may affect DNA in a way that makes cancerous cells grow more rapidly.

BONE MASS

Preliminary findings suggest that men with higher bone mass may be at a greater risk of developing prostate cancer. Some studies indicate that male hormone levels and calcium and vitamin D intake may play a role. It is well known that these factors influence bone mass.

In a recent study, a team from Boston University School of Medicine monitored the health of more than 1,000 white males over the course of thirty years. The subjects were all free from prostate cancer at the beginning of the study, and they all were given bone mass analyses.

As the study evolved, 100 of the men were diagnosed with prostate cancer. When researchers divided the men into four groups based on bone mass, they found that those with higher bone mass were more likely to have prostate cancer than those with lower bone mass and concluded that there could be a risk factor involved. Researchers also suggested that levels of the compound insulin-like growth factor-I (IGF-I), which plays a role in bone development, could be a risk indicator.

CALCIUM INTAKE

According to a study in *The American Journal of Clinical Nutrition*, the risk of prostate cancer may increase with calcium intake. Researchers investigated the connection between dairy products, calcium consumption, and prostate cancer in a group of 20,885 physicians. They created a dairy score for each participant by summing up the daily calcium contributions of five common dairy foods. The group of completed questionnaires concerned diet and lifestyle between 1982 and 1995. During eleven years of follow-up, 1,012 incidents of prostate cancer were reported among the group.

Men with a high daily calcium intake had a 34 percent higher risk of developing prostate cancer than men with a low daily intake of dairy products. The risk was 30 percent higher for advanced prostate cancer and 47 percent higher for localized cases.

STRESS!

Men with high levels of stress and those with limited or poor contact with friends and family members tend to have higher blood levels of prostate-specific antigen (PSA), according to a study reported in *Health Psychology*. Investigators at the State University of New York at Stony Brook's medical school studied 318 men recruited through a prostate cancer screening program. They were tested for blood PSA levels, and each man received a digital rectal exam. The men also completed standard psychological scales assessing their feelings of anger, nervousness, and ability to cope, as well as their level of satisfaction with family members and friends.

Stress levels and degree of social support seemed to clearly predict subjects' PSA levels. After researchers controlled for age, a factor known to influence PSA levels, they found that the incidence of elevated PSA was higher for men with high stress levels than for men with low levels.

DHEA

The supplement DHEA may aggravate BPH or increase the risk of developing prostate and other cancers. DHEA is a naturally occurring androgen (male hormone). It is a precursor hormone—one that converts into other hormones, such as androstenedione and androstenediol; it can also convert into estrogen. DHEA levels increase sharply at puberty, peak during adulthood, and decrease gradually as we age.

DHEA supplements are touted to slow aging, burn fat, build muscle, strengthen immunity, increase libido and sex drive, and treat other illnesses, including Alzheimer's and Parkinson's diseases. In addition to the prostate risks, the list of side effects can include hair loss, development of female characteristics in men, skin problems, irritability, and restlessness.

THE ENVIRONMENTAL QUESTION

Studies of occupational groups have shown farmers to be at consistently higher risk for prostate cancer, although it is unclear if this finding is the result of occupational factors, lifestyle factors, or a combination of factors. Other studies have hinted at associations between prostate cancer and the work environment in rubber manufacturing, iron and steel foundries, and other manufacturing environments. Other studies have suggested a weak association between prostate cancer and exposure to cadmium.

THE DANGERS OF HERBAL SUPPLEMENTS

Herbal supplements should be used with caution. The effects of many herbal preparations have not been adequately studied, and herbal supplements are not FDA-approved.

VASECTOMY

Some studies have raised questions about a possible relationship between vasectomy (an operation to cut or tie off the two tubes that carry sperm out of the testicles) and the risk of developing cancer, especially prostate and testicular cancer. One in six men over age thirty-five in the United States has had a vasectomy. The evidence linking vasectomy to increased risk of prostate cancer is flimsy at best.

DOES SIZE MATTER AFTER ALL?

After age fifty, tall men have a moderately higher risk of developing prostate cancer than their shorter peers, according to a recent study presented at the national meeting of the American College of Preventive Medicine.

Men who were six feet tall and over the age of fifty had a 32 percent greater risk of prostate cancer than shorter men of the same age group. Men six feet tall and over and past the age of sixty had a 24 percent greater risk of developing the disease than shorter men in the same age group. Men younger than age fifty showed no increased risk of prostate cancer related to height.

IGF-I

Insulin-like growth factor–I (IGF-I) may contribute to the growth of prostate tumors in men over the age of forty. IGF-I is a growth factor found in blood serum that resembles insulin but is not recognized by the antibodies that react with insulin. According to a research study, men with the highest levels of growth factor had up to 4.3 times an increased risk of prostate cancer as men with lower IGF-I levels. This growth factor increases the risk of mutations in prostate cells and protects mutated cells from programmed cell death.

AN INSTITUTE FOR CANCER PREVENTION RISK FACTOR SAMPLER

INCREASED RISK
- Family history
- Race (if African American)
- High-fat, low-fiber diet
- Hormone levels

No Definitive Clinical Risk Assessment
- Vasectomy
- Occupation
- Smoking

Risk Factor Specifics
- **Age.** In the United States, prostate cancer is found mainly in men over age fifty-five. The average age of patients at the time of diagnosis is seventy.
- **Family history of prostate cancer.** A man's risk for developing prostate cancer is higher if his father or brother has had the disease.
- **Race.** Much more common in African-American men than in white men; less common in Asian and American Indian men.
- **Diet and dietary factors.** A diet high in fat may increase the risk of prostate cancer; a diet rich in fruits and vegetables may decrease the risk. Studies are in progress to discern whether men can reduce their risk of prostate cancer by taking certain dietary supplements.
- **Obesity.** America's obesity plague starts with its children. According to a new report issued by the National Institutes of Health and the U.S. Census Bureau, 15 percent of children aged six to eighteen are overweight (compared to 6 percent in 1980). The figure is 22 percent for African-American children, and 25 percent for Mexican Americans.
- Physical inactivity is another suspected risk factor, since it leads to obesity and other health problems.

Risk Factoids
- About 80 percent of all diagnosed prostate cancers occur in men aged sixty-five or older.
- Fewer than 10 percent of men with prostate cancer die within five years of the diagnosis.
- African-American men have the highest rates of prostate cancer incidence and mortality.

Aspirin and Prostate Cancer

A Mayo Clinic study indicates that aspirin, ibuprofen, and other NSAIDs (nonsteroidal anti-inflammatory drugs) may help prevent prostate cancer. The study found that men sixty and older could re-

THE INSTITUTE FOR CANCER PREVENTION: STUDYING
POPULATION CLUSTERS FOR CLUES TO RISK FACTORS

The Institute for Cancer Prevention, in collaboration with the Beaufort Jasper Hampton Comprehensive Health Services and the Disease Prevention and Control Access Network, both in South Carolina, initiated a program designed to enhance prostate cancer control in the rural, substantially African-American and poor populations of the state. South Carolina's prostate cancer rates are among the highest in the nation.

The goals of the Institute for Cancer Prevention are to reduce prostate cancer incidence and mortality through early detection; increase access to treatment; and disseminate preventive health education. Its Prostate Cancer Telehealth Program provides a high-technology link through a state-of-the-art computer network and video conferencing system between the scientific and medical community at the institute and the medically underserved communities in South Carolina. IFCP plans to use this high-tech linkage to enhance prostate cancer control in the state by establishing more localized screening procedures, providing easier access to medical guidance and evaluation, and delivering comprehensive health education interventions. In turn, the health information gained through the program should provide IFCP scientists with answers to crucial questions about prostate cancer risks and prevention.

duce their risk of prostate cancer by as much as 60 percent by taking one 325 mg aspirin a day. The study also determined that the older the individual, the more benefits he would derive.

It was not known if the findings were applicable to African Americans, since the study focused only on Caucasian men in the Midwest. It was also not determined what would be the ideal aspirin dosage to provide maximal benefit, and what cumulative effect the duration of doses would have.

3. THE PROSTATE CHECKUP

WARNING SIGNS

Regular checkups are important even though there is disagreement over the value of certain tests. **The Institute for Cancer Prevention endorses a man's right to discuss the pros and cons of prostate cancer screening and treatment with his physician, but the Institute urges that all middle-aged and older men be screened on a regular basis. The Institute strongly recommends that once a man reaches fifty (earlier if he's in a higher-risk group), he should have his prostate examined at least once a year.**

Prostate cancer mortality rates have dropped since 1990, when PSA tests for the early detection of prostate cancer became common. It has not yet been proven that this drop is due to early detection, but large-scale, long-term studies are under way in both the United States and Europe to determine if there is a positive connection between early detection and lower mortality rates.

Whatever your age, there are warning signs indicating when you should schedule an immediate prostate checkup. These include any of the following symptoms:

BENIGN PROSTATIC HYPERPLASIA (BPH)
- Frequent urination
- Incomplete emptying of the bladder

- A weak or interrupted urine flow
- Difficulty starting urination

PROSTATITIS
- Frequent urination
- A typical sensation of having a full bladder
- A burning sensation during urination
- A burning sensation during ejaculation
- Blood in the semen

PROSTATE CANCER
- Frequent urination, especially at night
- A weak or interrupted urine flow
- Difficulty urinating
- A painful or burning sensation during urination
- A painful sensation during ejaculation
- Blood in the urine or semen
- A nagging pain in the back, hips, or pelvis

While the symptoms of prostate gland and lower urinary tract problems are relatively clear cut, a variety of prostate and other conditions exhibit similar symptoms, "mimicking" one another.

Early-stage prostate cancer doesn't produce any symptoms, largely because of the cancer's location. Benign enlargement occurs in the part of the prostate that surrounds the urethra, gradually working outward. Malignant growth usually starts in the outer part of the gland. When symptoms finally do appear, they're often an indication of advanced cancer. That's why early detection through screening is so important.

Although many common urinary symptoms are caused by enlargement or inflammation of the prostate, many urinary symptoms are unrelated to the prostate. Disorders that can cause similar symptoms include inflammation of the urethra (the tube carrying urine from the bladder out of the body), as well as infections of the bladder and kidneys, diabetes, and sexually transmitted infections.

BASIC DIAGNOSTIC TESTS

Doctors' recommendations for screening vary. Some encourage yearly screening for men over fifty; others recommend against routine screening; still others counsel men about the risks and benefits of screening, encouraging patients to make a personal decision.

THE DIGITAL RECTAL EXAM (DRE)

The DRE has been recommended for years as a "red flag" test for an enlarged prostate or prostate cancer. It is not a primary diagnostic tool for either condition but rather a useful screening test. The DRE is limited in its ability to detect specific problems or to distinguish a cancerous from a benign condition.

When performing the DRE, the doctor wears a thin rubber glove and inserts a lubricated finger into the patient's rectum. He checks the size and firmness of the prostate, feeling the surface of the gland through the wall of the rectum to detect any hardness, lumps, or irregularities. **Never have a PSA test within forty-eight hours after you've had a DRE. The DRE may elevate your PSA level.**

THE PROSTATE-SPECIFIC ANTIGEN (PSA) TEST

A PSA test detects possible prostate cancer cell activity. A biopsy will confirm that an elevated PSA level is the result of cancer and not due to any of a variety of other causes.

PSA is a protein sugar enzyme produced by epithelial cells in the prostate gland for the digestion of proteins found in semen, which liquefies the ejaculate. PSA is also present in the blood. Since PSA can be used to detect disease, it is referred to as a biological marker or tumor marker. Based on a blood sample, normal PSA levels indicate a low risk for prostate cancer; higher levels may indicate the need for a prostate biopsy to determine if cancerous cell activity is present. Your PSA level is measured in the laboratory (in more technical terms, the blood sample is assayed). The average man's normal PSA level ranges from 0 to 4 nanograms per milliliter (ng/ml). A PSA level of 4 to 10 ng/ml is considered slightly elevated; levels between 10 and 20 ng/ml are considered moderately elevated; and anything above that is considered highly elevated.

PSA levels can rise due to cancerous or benign conditions, including prostate enlargement. Remembering this can save you a lot of unnecessary anxiety. Although the PSA level alone does not give physicians sufficient information to distinguish between benign prostate conditions and cancer, your doctor will take the results of the test very seriously when deciding whether to recommend a biopsy (tissue sampling). If your PSA levels have increased over the course of time, or if a suspicious texture or lump is detected in the DRE, the doctor will recommend a biopsy to tell for sure if cancer is present.

If your PSA level is within normal range, ask your physician when it should be tested again. You may not need to repeat the test as frequently as previously thought, according to data from the Prostate, Lung, Colorectal and Ovarian (PLCO) Cancer Screening Trial, sponsored by the National Cancer Institute (NCI). The Institute for Cancer Prevention recommends that you continue to be PSA-tested on a regular basis—too often is far preferable to too infrequently.

There are now at least six different ways to interpret PSA: total PSA, free PSA, age-adjusted PSA, ethnically adjusted PSA, PSA velocity, and PSA density. Each of these tests has unique characteristics.

PREPARING FOR THE PSA TEST

Ejaculation can cause a brief elevation of PSA level: you should abstain from sexual activity for at least forty-eight hours prior to having your PSA level tested. Do not schedule a PSA if you have recently had a cystoscopy or needle biopsy. A cystoscopy or biopsy can raise your PSA level for as long as several weeks. Also, PSA testing should not be performed until several weeks after successful treatment of a urinary tract infection.

REFINING AND REDEFINING THE PSA TEST

Research is being done to improve the PSA test. Scientists are researching ways to distinguish between benign and cancerous conditions, and between slow- and fast-growing cancers. Variations in the PSA test include:

• **PSA velocity:** Based on changes in PSA levels over time. A sharp rise in PSA level raises the suspicion of cancer as long as the PSA tests were done more than six months apart.

• **Age-adjusted PSA:** Age is an important factor in increasing PSA levels. Some doctors use age-adjusted PSA levels to determine when a biopsy may be needed. When age-adjusted levels are used, different PSA levels are defined as normal for each ten-year age group. Not all physicians are in agreement about the accuracy of age-adjusted PSA levels.

• **Ethnically adjusted PSA:** This adjustment factors in ethnic variations in PSA levels.

• **PSA density:** This calculation considers the relationship of the PSA level to the weight and size of the prostate. An elevated PSA might not arouse as much suspicion when a man with a very enlarged prostate is tested. There is, however, a danger that prostate cancer might be overlooked if too heavy an emphasis is placed on relative PSA density.

• **Free versus attached (bound) PSA:** PSA circulates in the blood in two forms: free or attached to a protein molecule. With benign prostate conditions, there is more free PSA present in the blood. Cancer may be indicated if more PSA is attached to protein molecules. This is called the percent free PSA (%fPSA) test.

• **PSA doubling time:** This is the amount of time it takes for a patient's PSA value to double. This may be useful to help determine the extent and nature of prostate cancer treatment.

• **Other screening tests:** Tests are being developed for other biological markers, but they are not yet widely or commercially available (see a few examples below).

Some variant PSA tests may be more sensitive in identifying patients with prostate cancer, and others may be more specific—meaning that fewer patients without cancer will test false-positive. The more sensitive the test, the higher the percentage of false-positive results. However, none of the variant PSA tests can claim to be completely accurate. All will miss a percentage of cancers (false-negative), and all will incorrectly identify some patients as showing a possible

MORE ON THE PERCENT FREE PSA TEST

As noted, the percent free (%f) PSA test indicates how much PSA is circulating freely in the blood, as opposed to that which is attached to protein molecules. If your PSA results are borderline, a low percent free PSA (less than 10 percent) means that your likelihood of having prostate cancer is about fifty-fifty and you should have a biopsy. A recent study found that if men with borderline PSA results had prostate biopsies only when their percent free PSA was 25 percent or less, about 20 percent of unnecessary prostate biopsies could be avoided, sparing up to 200,000 men a year the inconvenience and anxiety associated with the procedure.

cancer who will prove not to have cancer (false-positive). Accurate diagnosis can involve testing for more than just one PSA value.

THE PSA TEST AND RECURRENT PROSTATE CANCER

The Food and Drug Administration (FDA) has approved the PSA test to monitor patients who have already had prostate cancer to see if the cancer has returned. But an elevated PSA level in a patient who has experienced prostate cancer does not always mean that the cancer has come back. This is why the doctor may repeat the PSA test or perform a biopsy for evidence of recurrence. A patient who is receiving hormone therapy for prostate cancer may have a low PSA reading during or immediately after treatment. In turn, this low level may not be a true measure of PSA levels in the patient's body.

WHEN DOES A MAN NEED TO KNOW?

Is it sometimes actually counterproductive for a man to be aware he even has initial-stage prostate cancer? There's really no simple answer to that question. In addition to the anxiety this knowledge creates, the patient will need to consider surgery or other treatment options, which could lead to impotence or incontinence, or simply opt for "watchful waiting"—keeping an eye on the cancer through frequent testing—which carries its own psychological burden. Clearly the psychological toll is great, but the physical result of not knowing could be fatal.

FOLLOW-UP TESTS
Biopsy

A biopsy is undertaken on an outpatient basis. It does not require the patient to be hospitalized. For at least a week prior to the biopsy, the patient should stop taking any medications that affect blood clotting (for example, aspirin or anti-inflammatory drugs).

A core needle biopsy is the main method of definitive diagnosis of prostate cancer. The doctor uses transrectal ultrasound (TRUS) for guidance, inserting a narrow needle through the wall of the rectum into several regions of the prostate gland. In a transperineal biopsy, a needle is inserted through the skin between the scrotum and the rectum into the prostate. The needle removes a piece of tissue, usually about ½ inch long and 1/16 inch across.

Anywhere from six to thirteen samples are needed to get a representative sample to see how much the prostate may possibly be affected by cancer. As many as eighteen samples may be taken from some patients. When the biopsy sample is sent to the laboratory, a pathologist—a doctor who specializes in the analysis, interpretation, and diagnosis of disease in tissue samples—will examine the sample under a microscope to determine if there are cancer cells present. Analysis usually takes from one to three days. If cancer is present, the pathologist will assign it a grade.

The biopsy procedure sounds painful, but it isn't all that bad. The patient is given an antibiotic prior to the biopsy to reduce the risk of infection. The doctor numbs the area with an anesthetic and an instrument called a biopsy gun quickly inserts and removes the needle. The procedure takes about fifteen minutes and is usually done in the doctor's office. Following the biopsy, some rectal bleeding and perhaps some bleeding from the penis can be expected. Sometimes blood is seen in the semen up to several weeks after the procedure.

Some doctors perform the biopsy through the perineum, the skin between the rectum and the scrotum. The doctor places his finger in the patient's rectum to feel the prostate and then inserts the biopsy needle through a small incision in the skin of the perineum. A local anesthetic is used to numb the area.

Ultrasound Testing: Transrectal Ultrasound (TRUS)

When a suspicious lesion is detected, an ultrasound-guided biopsy may be recommended. Since the prostate gland is located directly in front of the rectum, the ultrasound (US) exam is performed through the rectum.

Ultrasound equipment consists of a transducer and a computerized monitoring system. A transducer is a small, handheld device that resembles a microphone. Sound waves that can't be heard by human ears (ultrasound) are emitted by the transducer. A lubricated protective cover is placed over the transducer, and this probe is placed in the rectum. The sound waves travel only a short distance, creating an image on a video screen (a sonogram) as they echo off the prostate.

Sonogram images are captured in real time (as they happen), showing the actual movement and structure of internal tissues and organs.

Prostate tumors and normal prostate tissue typically reflect sound waves in different ways: TRUS is used to guide the biopsy needle into the tumor region, where it samples cells for microscopic laboratory examination.

Transrectal ultrasound is done in the doctor's office or in an outpatient clinic. If no biopsy is required—that is, if the test is purely exploratory—the procedure is no more uncomfortable than a DRE (the patient might feel some pressure when the probe is placed in his rectum). If a biopsy is performed—and it usually is—additional pain or discomfort due to insertion of the biopsy needle is generally minimal: the rectal wall is relatively insensitive in the prostate region. The biopsy needle removes a number of slivers of tissue, usually about ½ inch long and ¹⁄₁₆ inch across, which are sent to a lab to see if cancer is present.

Whole-Body Bone Scan

If prostate cancer is diagnosed, the patient may have a whole-body bone scan to help determine if the prostate cancer has spread (metastasized) to the bones. This process is not painful, but it can understandably cause some anxiety. The test involves injection of a small amount of radioactive tracer, which goes into the bloodstream and is absorbed into the patient's bones in the areas affected by the cancer. There is usually about a two-hour wait after the injection before the patient is placed under a scanner, which provides images of the affected regions. The spine is the most common site outside the pelvis for prostate cancer to spread to.

CAT Scans and MRIs

A urologist may recommend other investigative procedures, such as a CAT (computerized axial tomography) scan or an MRI (mag-

---

THE BENEFITS OF ULTRASOUND IMAGING

- It's a painless or minimally painful, relatively low cost procedure, widely available and easy to perform.
- Ultrasound uses no ionizing radiation. The procedure evaluates a variety of reproductive system disorders without even the risks associated with X-ray exposure. There are no known harmful side effects of standard diagnostic ultrasound.
- Real-time video imaging makes ultrasound a good tool for guiding minimally invasive objects such as biopsy needles.

netic resonance imaging). A CAT or CT scanner uses X rays linked to a computer, producing a series of detailed pictures from inside the body. An MRI scanner uses magnetic energy and radio waves linked to a computer to create detailed pictures of internal organs and bones, detecting changes in tissue molecules as they are subjected to an intense magnetic field.

The PSTF-1 Test

The former Medical College of Pennsylvania in Philadelphia has developed what it hopes is a better, less invasive test by targeting a marker called prostate-specific transcription factor–I (PSTF-I). PSTF-I is present in the urine of patients with cancer and not present in the urine of patients with benign disorders.

Researchers developed a simple urine test doctors could use to

BIOPSY VERSUS MRI

After elevated PSA numbers and/or a DRE suggest the possibility that there may be cancer present in the prostate, the next step is usually a biopsy.

The limitation of this technique is that the needle samples a pretty small part of the prostate. And even with multiple needle punctures, the biopsies may well miss the cancerous nodule(s). This is especially possible when the cancer is small and/or the gland is large. This "finding the needle in a haystack" approach is illustrated by the fact that biopsy results are reported as "3 out of 6" or "5 out of 8" positive samples.

I recently reported on a new device that may one day make the "hit-and-miss" needle biopsy a thing of the past. It's an MRI scanner, much like the one you may have been in to diagnose a slipped disk or a torn ligament. But it has a variety of modifications that allow it to do a spectroscopic analysis of the prostate gland—a fancy way of saying that it analyzes the chemical composition of the gland (while it's still inside your body, mind you!).

Several studies have shown that the chemical composition of the prostate changes in areas where cancerous cells are present. The diagnostic changes occur in two prostate chemicals called choline and citrate.

I have seen MRIs of the prostate that found cancer missed on biopsies and that also indicated the aggressiveness of the tumor. Still, the technology is young. But as more studies compare the MRI findings to the "gold standard" of needle biopsies, it may eventually turn out that you'll be able to have a reliable prostate biopsy and tumor staging done without any uncomfortable needle punctures.

screen men for this marker. Initial results reportedly proved accurate in more than two hundred urine sample tests. All the positive results were from patients who did have cancer; the vast majority of those who had no cancer tested negatively.

One of the significant findings of the clinical trials was that the amount of PSTF-I in the urine was a strong indicator of the severity of the individual's cancer. If this proves true, the PSTF-I test could also be used to monitor how effectively prostate cancer treatment is working.

The DNA Test

This new test may be able to identify prostate cancer cells in urine samples by detecting changes in DNA in cells shed from the prostate into the urine. Researchers at the Free University of Berlin's department of urology reported that the test was positive in 73 percent of men with prostate cancer; in 27 percent of those with PIN (prostatic intraepithelial neoplasia); and in only 2 percent of men with benign prostate enlargement. The DNA test will reportedly show positive results if only a handful of abnormal cells are present among as many as 100,000 normal cells.

Currently, the test is available only in a handful of research centers and is very expensive.

Further study is needed to confirm the initial clinical trials and to assess the test's efficacy in the early detection of prostate cancer.

PSA Home Testing Kits

Unless it's difficult to get to a health care professional, these blood sample collection kits, which you send to a lab for analysis (often included in the cost of the kit), are more of a gimmick than anything else. Only a primary care physician or urologist can help assure that nothing has compromised the blood sample in your test or that your test results weren't artificially elevated by any number of factors.

New Diagnostic Procedures

Optical dye sensors are special dyes that, when injected, seek out and "stain" only cancer cells. The dye is observable by current scanning equipment and can reportedly pinpoint even minute quantities of cancerous cells. When a surgeon is operating, he or she can see if any cancerous cells are remaining.

Positron emission tomography (PET) is a sensitive scanning procedure that reportedly detects faint traces of cancer cells. A compound called C-11 methionine is injected intravenously. This compound has a half-life of only twenty minutes, and the patient must be very close to the scanning equipment for the scan to be successful.

Doctors at the University of Maryland Medical Center were among the first to use *ProstaScint*. This test was approved by the FDA in 1996. The test uses an antibody designed to find and attach itself to the wall of prostate cancer cells. The antibody is combined with a radioactive tracer, indium 111, to form a drug that is injected into the patient. After four days, the patient's body is scanned; lymph nodes that have been invaded by prostate cancer cells appear as "hot spots" on the test. Through this analysis, doctors can determine whether the cancer has remained localized or if it has spread to lymph nodes or other structures in the body. It can reportedly find tumors in lymph nodes as small as a quarter of an inch in length.

See Chapters 10 and 11 for other diagnostic tests for prostatitis and enlarged prostate.

WHEN SHOULD YOU SEE A UROLOGIST?

See a urologist when you are exhibiting symptoms of possible urinary tract or reproductive system conditions.

Here are some of the common tests a urologist may administer to

PROSTATIC INTRAEPITHELIAL NEOPLASIA (PIN)

Sometimes when a pathologist looks at prostate cells under a microscope, they don't look cancerous, but they're not quite normal either. These results are often reported as "suspicious." This may indicate a condition known as prostatic intraepithelial neoplasia (PIN).

PIN is divided into low-grade and high-grade. Many men begin to develop low-grade PIN at an early age but do not necessarily develop prostate cancer. The relationship of low-grade PIN to full-blown prostate cancer is still unclear.

With an "atypical" finding, or high-grade PIN, cancer may already be present somewhere else in the prostate gland. With high-grade PIN, there is a 30 to 50 percent chance of finding prostate cancer in a subsequent biopsy. For this reason, repeat prostate biopsies are often recommended in such cases.

help determine the nature of your problem, which will often be un-related to the prostate:

- A **urinalysis and urine culture check** to determine if there's an infection or any sign of blood in the urine.
- A **cystoscopy,** which looks into the urethra and bladder through a thin, lighted tube inserted through the penis.
- **Filling cystometry,** which is primarily geared toward patients who can't urinate and in whom nerve injury or other damage to the bladder is suspected.
- A **serum creatinine level check,** a blood test that measures how well the kidneys are working. An elevated creatinine level may indi-cate that prostate enlargement is blocking or limiting the bladder outlet, in turn affecting kidney function. Kidney problems exist in many cases of enlarged prostate.
- A **postvoid residual urine test (PVR),** which measures the amount of urine remaining in the bladder after urination, usually with a simple ultrasound probe pressed against the abdomen.
- **Intravenous pyelogram (IVP),** which creates a series of X rays of the organs of the urinary tract.
- A **uroflowmetry test,** which measures the speed of urine flow out of the bladder electronically.
- **Urethrocystoscopy,** which is performed on men already diag-nosed with an enlarged prostate. A fiber-optic tube (endoscope) is in-serted into the urethra to let the urologist observe the lower urinary tract.
- **Intravenous excretory urography,** an invasive X-ray procedure used only when complications in the upper urinary tract, especially the kidneys, are suspected.
- **Transabdominal ultrasonography,** a test in which a probe is placed over the lower abdomen. This procedure, based on sound-wave echoes, gives an accurate measure of postvoid residual urine, without being as invasive as transrectal ultrasonography, and can look at the kidneys as well.
- **Transrectal ultrasonography,** in which sound waves emanate from a probe inserted into the rectum. These waves bounce off the prostate, and a computer translates the echoes to create a sonogram image.

II.

THE PROSTATE HEALTH PYRAMID AND THE CANCER PREVENTION DIET

4. THE PROSTATE HEALTH PYRAMID AND THE NUTRITION CONNECTION

THE PROSTATE HEALTH PYRAMID AND THE BASIC FOOD GROUPS

The Prostate Health Pyramid is a unique, scientifically based, prostate-specific guide to nutrition developed by research from the Institute for Cancer Prevention. It is the first *disease-specific* nutritional pyramid developed for the general public.

Prostate-specific health and overall health are closely linked. The Prostate Health Pyramid is an excellent general nutrition pyramid, as well as the surest current nutritional guide to prostate health. The same foods recommended in the pyramid can lower your cholesterol level; help manage your weight or help you overcome obesity; and lower your risk of getting other diseases, including other types of cancer.

While no single food, food group, or supplement can protect you from prostate cancer, a variety of cancer-preventive and cancer-fighting foods, combined with a low-fat diet, will help dramatically to ensure prostate health. The Institute for Cancer Prevention estimates that 35 percent of all prostate cancers may be preventable through dietary modification. The pyramid is a scientific formula for prostate health that can be a powerful "magic bullet" in the battle against prostate cancer.

Even if you already have prostate cancer or are showing elevated PSA levels, by making the Prostate Health Pyramid your daily diet guide you'll take a proactive role in slowing down the progress of the disease—or stopping it in its tracks.

The Prostate Health Pyramid is meant to be used in conjunction with the Transition Diet (discussed at length in Chapter 6) and the Healthy Prostate Fitness Regimen (Chapter 8). Diet must always go hand in hand with a regular exercise program in order to be maximally effective. Indeed, exercise is the "invisible foundation" of the Prostate Health Pyramid, as it should be of any nutritional plan.

In some ways, what you don't eat is as important as what you do. The Institute for Cancer Prevention stresses avoiding dietary elements that weaken the immune system, promote cellular mutation, and increase the production of free radicals (we'll discuss free radicals shortly). These include processed and smoked foods, refined foods, food additives, margarine, vegetable shortening, red meats, and fruits and vegetables with pesticide residues.

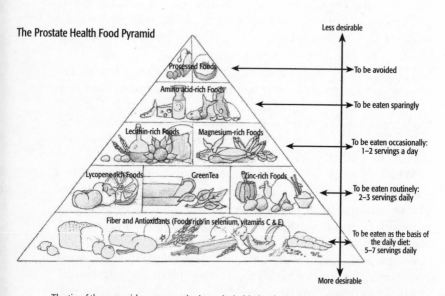

The Prostate Health Food Pyramid

Less desirable

Processed Foods → To be avoided

Amino-acid-rich Foods → To be eaten sparingly

Lecithin-rich Foods | Magnesium-rich Foods → To be eaten occasionally: 1–2 servings a day

Lycopene-rich Foods | GreenTea | Zinc-rich Foods → To be eaten routinely: 2–3 servings daily

Fiber and Antioxidants (Foods rich in selenium, vitamins C & E) → To be eaten as the basis of the daily diet: 5–7 servings daily

More desirable

The tip of the pyramid represents the least desirable foods, the base of the pyramid the most desirable. Processed foods and fats should be avoided. Fiber and antioxidant-rich foods are highly desirable and should form the foundation of your daily diet. Foods rich in amino acids, lecithin, magnesium, lycopene, and zinc are also excellent for prostate health. Also, drink at least two to three cups of green tea a day.

NUTRITIONAL ELEMENTS OF THE PROSTATE HEALTH PYRAMID

FIBER

Dietary fiber is sometimes referred to as roughage or bulk. Fiber is a complex mixture of carbohydrates derived from the structural components of plants, found in the storage and cell walls of vegetables, fruits, and grains.

There are two categories of fiber, water-soluble and water-insoluble; soluble fiber can be digested, insoluble fiber cannot. In addition to aiding overall digestion and possessing a laxative effect that facilitates bowel movement, fiber has other beneficial effects, some of them quite remarkable. Water-insoluble fiber has been associated with a inhibiting effect on carcinogenic cellular activity and polyp formation. It can bind with carcinogens and other harmful compounds and eliminate them from the body. Fiber has demonstrated the ability to inhibit prostate cancer progression. By eating generous quantities of soluble fiber, men may be able to lower their plasma testosterone levels, so that testosterone will not be present at elevated levels that stimulate tumor growth. In addition, water-soluble fiber lowers blood cholesterol levels.

Many fiber-rich foods contain both types of fiber. Sources of insoluble fiber include fruits (strawberries, bananas, pears), fresh and cooked vegetables (green beans, broccoli, peppers), and wheat bran and whole grains (bread, crackers, breakfast cereals). Sources of soluble fiber include some fruits (apples, citrus fruits), some vegetables (winter squash, carrots, potatoes), bran (barley, oat and rice bran), and legumes (pinto beans, kidney beans, black-eyed peas).

Fiber and PSA

In a recent clinical study, healthy men were fed diets high in either soluble or insoluble fiber. The subjects' prostate-specific antigen (PSA) levels decreased by 10 percent after only four months on the high-soluble-fiber diet. Men on the high-insoluble-fiber diet showed declines in plasma testosterone levels. The lower testosterone levels were due to increased testosterone excretion in the feces. Researchers believe that consuming fiber to decrease testosterone levels is an effective way to prevent the progression of primary prostate cancer.

COMPLEX CARBOHYDRATES

The primary role of carbohydrates is to genarate energy. Starches and sugars are broken down into glucose (blood sugar), which provides fuel for the body. Carbohydrates are divided into two classes, simple and complex, depending on their chemical structure. Simple carbohydrates are sugars including fructose (fruit sugar), sucrose (table sugar), and lactose (milk sugar). Foods that contain mainly simple carbohydrates are fruit, fruit juices, milk products, candies, honey, molasses, and syrups. Processed foods such as cookies, high-sugar cereals, pastries, and sodas are also sources of simple carbohydrates in our diet.

Complex carbohydrates are starches and fiber and include grains, grain products, and vegetables. Whole-grain starches such as brown rice and whole-wheat breads are better choices because they are minimally processed; fiber and vitamins and minerals have been retained. Starches such as white bread, pasta, and white rice are refined and have lost much of their fiber content. While whole fruits contain simple carbohydrates, the fiber remains, making them resemble complex carbohydrates.

Starches and sugars stimulate the body to produce substantial amounts of the hormone insulin. Insulin is the catalyst responsible for removing sugar from the blood. Reduction in the cells' ability to respond to the action of insulin to take up glucose is called insulin resistance. Studies have indicated that insulin is a growth factor for the prostate cell. Elevated levels of blood sugar and blood fats provide cancer cells with extra fuel to grow.

The steps men may take to help lower their insulin levels are in many cases the same steps they would take to help prevent against prostate cancer: eating high-fiber foods, limiting saturated fats, and eating fewer refined carbohydrates.

Here are some other tips to see you through the carb controversy:

• **Choose carbs from the Prostate Health Pyramid.** Many carbs in the pyramid are easy on your blood sugar level. Prostate-healthy carbs that are relatively low in glucose include tomatoes, rice bran, tortillas, grapefruit, apples, soybeans, kidney beans, pinto beans, lentils, chickpeas, and whole-wheat spaghetti.

- **Cut sugars and starches.** Refined sugars and starches break down quickly and elevate blood sugar levels.
- **Substitute slow-release carbohydrates.** These are carbohydrates that have the least effect on the blood sugar level (beans, vegetables, fruits, whole grains). Although the glycemic response to food varies from person to person and depends somewhat on the *combination* of foods consumed, you should choose carbs with a low glycemic effect.

The glycemic index (GI)—which measures the rate at which glucose enters the bloodstream—was developed to assist diabetics in stabilizing blood glucose levels. The GI is also used as a tool in the treatment of obesity and hypoglycemia.

ANTIOXIDANT-RICH FOODS

Antioxidants include a number of organic substances, such as vitamin A (converted from beta-carotene), vitamins C and E, the mineral selenium, and a group known as the carotenoids.

Antioxidants are considered effective in helping prevent cancer, heart disease, and stroke. They protect cells by deactivating particles called free radicals.

Free radicals usually take the form of oxygen molecules and are the product of oxidative reactions inside and outside the body. Oxidation and free radicals are normal, necessary biological phenomena. But since excessive free-radical production can be so damaging, our body maintains a complex antioxidant system to keep free radicals in check. Unchecked free radicals can damage cell walls and structures, as well as the genetic material within cells. They may even speed up the aging process. Over time, free-radical damage becomes irreversible, leading to chronic diseases such as cancer. Oxidation's effect on the body has often been compared to the effect of rust on metal.

How Free Radicals Do Their Damage

Free radicals have a kind of biological "identity crisis": they are unstable molecules that need to become stable. These highly reactive compounds will "steal" an electron from another molecule in order to stabilize themselves. This process creates a new free radical, namely the molecule the electron was stolen from. The new free radical then steals an electron from another molecule, and thus a vicious cycle perpetuates itself.

Besides being a natural by-product of cellular activity, free radicals are created by exposure to various environmental factors, including tobacco smoke and radiation.

Antioxidants neutralize free radicals. While some antioxidants simply control free radicals, others transform them into less damaging compounds, and some actually repair damaged cells.

VEGETABLES

A clinical study at the Fred Hutchinson Institute in Seattle concluded that vegetable consumption may help reduce prostate cancer risk by an average of 45 percent. The more fruits and vegetables consumed, the lower the cancer risk. Cruciferous vegetables (cabbage, broccoli, cauliflower, Brussels sprouts) reduce cancer risk the most.

Researchers think that three separate compounds in the cruciferous vegetable family are most beneficial as anticancer agents: indole-3-carbinol, sulforaphane, and glucaric acid.

How cruciferous vegetables are prepared has a major effect on the

CRUCIFEROUS VEGETABLES: A POWERFUL ARSENAL OF PROSTATE HEALTH BENEFITS

Indoles are phytochemicals found in cruciferous vegetables, including broccoli, bok choy, cabbage, cauliflower, Brussels sprouts, collard greens, kale, and turnip greens. Indoles help maintain prostate health by blocking enzymes that produce changes in prostate cells that can lead to cancer. Isothiocyanates, also found in cruciferous vegetables, may lower prostate cancer risk by boosting the immune system and deactivating carcinogens. Lignans are another powerful phytochemical found in cruciferous vegetables, including broccoli and cauliflower (and also in berries, cereal bran, flaxseeds, sesame seeds, sunflower seeds, and legumes). Sulforaphane is an antioxidant found in broccoli, Brussels sprouts, cauliflower, and kale. It increases the synthesis of cancer-combating phase 2 enzymes.

Other vegetables, such as artichokes, contain silymarin, which may protect against prostate cancer: studies suggest that it inhibits tumor formation.

potency of their cancer-fighting nutrients. Instead of boiling cruciferous vegetables, they should be lightly steamed or microwaved.

SELENIUM SUPPLEMENTS

Selenium is a mineral that has been shown to suppress cancer cell proliferation and to enhance the immune response. Low selenium levels in the blood are observed in people with prostate and other cancers.

Researchers at the Arizona Cancer Center reported a 60 percent reduction in the incidence of prostate cancer among patients taking a selenium supplement, as opposed to a control group taking a placebo (sugar pill). Although the selenium dose used in the clinical trial was two to three times the Recommended Daily Allowance (RDA) of 50–100 mcg, there were no side effects or toxicity (1,000 mcg, or 1 mg, daily is considered toxic). Bear in mind that this is the finding of a single study and that, while impressive, it should not lead you to think that all you need to do is take a daily selenium supplement to protect against prostate cancer.

Good sources of selenium include fish, shellfish, and whole grains and cereals such as barley and bulgur. When it comes to grains, selenium content is greatly influenced by processing techniques and soil content. For example, brown rice contains higher amounts of selenium than white rice.

FOODS CONTAINING LYCOPENE

Lycopene is one of a group of antioxidant compounds known as carotenoids. Beta-carotene—the substance that gives carrots their orange color—remains perhaps the best known among the carotenoids.

Carotenoids also add pigment to other vegetables: lycopene, for example, gives tomatoes their vivid redness. Watermelon and pink grapefruit contain smaller quantities of lycopene. Scientists have discovered that lycopene is the most powerful antioxidant among the carotenoids. Researchers at Harvard Medical School followed the diets of more than 47,000 men over a six-year period. They found a strong inverse correlation between intake of tomato-based products—which contain abundant amounts of lycopene—and prostate cancer incidence. Researchers concluded that men who ate ten or more servings a week of tomato-based foods had a 45 percent lower likelihood of contracting prostate cancer. An even more recent Harvard follow-up study showed similar results.

Other studies have indicated that consumption of lycopene may help reduce the risk of colon, rectal, breast, lung, and stomach cancer, as well as the risk of heart attack.

According to the Harvard studies, the lycopene found in cooked tomato products—for example, spaghetti and pizza sauces and tomato soup—appears to provide even more cancer protection than that found in raw tomato products, such as whole tomatoes or tomato juice. It appears easier for the body to absorb lycopene after the tomatoes have been cooked, crushed, or chopped.

GREEN TEA

Next to water, green tea is the most commonly consumed beverage in the world—and that's a very good thing. If you have a problem with caffeine, decaffeinated green tea is readily available.

The Japanese adopted green tea from the Chinese around 800 A.D. In a book published in 1211 entitled *Maintaining Health by Drinking Green Tea*, a monk named Eisai wrote, "Tea is a miraculous medicine for the maintenance of health. Anywhere a person cultivates tea, long life will follow." It has become increasingly clear that the ancient monk was right.

Japanese men, who commonly drink four to six cups of green tea a day, have a significantly lower prostate cancer mortality rate than Americans. The incidence of prostate cancer in China—where the populace drinks more green tea than the Japanese—is the lowest on earth. While this doesn't prove that green tea prevents prostate cancer, and while many other factors are involved, mounting evidence from a number of clinical studies suggests that green tea may be protecting Asian men from developing or dying from prostate cancer.

Green tea harbors powerful antioxidants called polyphenols (flavonoids, isoflavones, and ellagic acid are examples of polyphenols). The specific polyphenol in green tea we're most interested in is EGCG (epigallocatechin gallate), similar to substances found in red wine and some vegetables. EGCG is present in green tea in a form called tannins (or catechins). These large polyphenol molecules have been shown in clinical trials to have anticarcinogenic and antiviral properties. Like other cancer-fighting chemicals, EGCG appears to inhibit the enzyme activity necessary for the growth of cancer cells.

GREEN TEA'S ANTIOXIDANT ACTIVITY

The antioxidant activity in green tea is 25 to 100 times more potent than that in vitamins C and E. A single cup of green tea has stronger antioxidant activity than a serving of broccoli, spinach, carrots, or strawberries.

Even small amounts of EGCG—as little as can be found in three cups of green tea—are enough to inhibit cancer growth. At high concentrations, EGCG has killed cancer cells in test tubes outright.

A Mayo Clinic study confirmed that EGCG inhibits the growth of prostate cancer cells and, in high concentrations, destroys them.

Although EGCG is the most potent cancer-fighting substance in green tea (containing 10 to 50 percent of polyphenol content), several other polyphenols are also present in significant quantities: epicatechin (EC), epigallocatechin (EGC), and epicatechin gallate (ECG).

There is some evidence that the black tea consumed in Western nations—such as orange pekoe, Darjeeling, and breakfast teas—may also have some cancer-preventive benefits. This seems logical, since

TEA AND THE IFCP

Institute for Cancer Prevention scientists have discovered that readily available green and black teas have similar health-promoting properties, although green tea is more potent. The IFCP has studied the underlying preventive mechanism of tea in a number of extensive studies.

IFCP studies confirmed that tea drinkers have a lower risk of prostate and other types of cancer, as well as heart disease. Populations that include large segments of avid tea drinkers live longer lives with less incidence of chronic disease.

IFCP researchers determined the following:

- Tea is an antioxidant, reducing the oxidation of cholesterol, the key mechanism of heart disease. Tea prevents damage to DNA, a key factor in the development of cancer.
- Tea stimulates enzymes that detoxify potentially harmful chemicals and enhances the excretion of toxic chemicals, including cancer-causing agents.
- Tea decreases tumor growth and cancer progression in animals.
- Regular tea consumption creates a healthier bacterial composition in the intestinal tract.

green and black teas both come from the same plant (*Camellia sinensis*). However, due to differences in the fermentation process, a portion of the active anticancer compounds in black tea are destroyed.

Getting the Most from Green Tea

• Try to drink at least two to four cups a day of freshly brewed green tea. Bottled "energy" and green tea flavored drinks do not count.

• Steep the tea longer for more flavonoids. If you steep it for just one minute, the average flavonoid content is 208 mg; if you steep it for four minutes, the flavonoid content rises to 300 mg.

• Supplement capsules of green tea extract (500 mg daily) containing at least 50 percent polyphenols may be a useful substitute for drinking tea.

• If you're taking aspirin or other anticoagulants on a daily basis, be aware that green tea might enhance the blood-thinning effect of those drugs (in some cases, green tea might somewhat prolong bleeding time).

Green Tea for Weight Loss

Current data from animal studies indicates that, in addition to its cancer-fighting properties, green tea increases caloric expenditure, promotes fat oxidation, and helps control body weight. In one animal study, female mice were fed differing levels of green tea for four months; control mice were fed the same diet without the green tea. The mice that consumed the green tea had a significant suppression of appetite, weight gain, and fat tissue accumulation. Their cholesterol, triglyceride, and leptin levels were lower, signifying that green tea may have a direct effect on weight regulation. (Leptin is the hormone produced by fat cells that signals the amount of body fat content and influences food intake.)

ZINC

Zinc is vital to the body. In addition to supporting a healthy immune system, it's needed to heal wounds, it's important for DNA synthesis, and it even helps maintain the senses of taste and smell. It also supports normal growth and development from infancy through adolescence.

While zinc is an important mineral found in virtually every cell, the prostate has about ten times as much zinc as any other part of the body. Men with prostate cancer have low zinc levels, leading many researchers to suspect that zinc is essential to prostate function and that it may even help prevent prostate cancer. A laboratory study reported in the journal *Prostate* suggests that zinc can trigger cancer cell destruction. Dietary zinc may also be helpful in treating prostate enlargement and chronic prostatitis.

Oysters contain more zinc than any other food. Maybe zinc's effects on the prostate help account for oysters' purported effect on virility! Pumpkin seeds and wheat germ are also high in zinc. Alternate healthy sources of zinc include beans, nuts, and whole grains. Unfortunately, it is from red meat and poultry that average Americans obtain the bulk of the zinc in their diet.

Excessive zinc intake can affect the balance of other nutrients in the body, including calcium, selenium, vitamins A, B1, and C, iron, phosphorus, and copper. Excessive intake can also lead to gastrointestinal problems, depressed immune function, and muscle spasms.

MAGNESIUM

Pumpkin seeds are the king of magnesium-rich foods. Peanuts, tofu, and broccoli are other foods with high magnesium content. Also high in magnesium are spinach, chard, soybeans, sweet potatoes, tomato paste, black beans, all types of nuts, and a variety of seeds.

Magnesium levels decline as we age. It is reasonable to think that there is a correlation between this and the higher incidence of prostate cancer in older men. Patients with enlarged prostates are commonly found to be deficient in magnesium.

Magnesium is the fourth most common mineral in the body. It is becoming increasingly recognized as a prostate cancer fighter and a prime element in overall prostate health. Magnesium plays a key role in more than three hundred enzymatic reactions involving fat, protein, glucose, and other nutrients. It contributes to cardiovascular health, helps turn food into energy, and helps transport electrical impulses across nerves and muscles, allowing muscles to flex (magnesium deficiency is often signaled by muscle cramps). Magnesium is also important in controlling blood sugar levels: it plays a very important role in the secretion and action of insulin. Magnesium supplementation is used to treat everything from asthma to chronic fatigue syndrome (CFS).

If you're physically active, you need even more magnesium than if you're sedentary, but adequate magnesium levels are important for everyone. Nutritionists from the National Health and Examination Survey (NHANES) find that many of us don't get enough magnesium in our daily diet. While many vegetables, peas, beans, lentils, and cereals are good sources of magnesium, mineral-depleted soil causes many of these ostensibly healthy foods to have less magnesium content than they normally would.

Even if we do consume magnesium-rich foods on a regular basis, there are factors within our body that may inhibit magnesium absorption. High amounts of calcium, oxalic acid, phytates, phosphates, and poorly digested fat can interfere with magnesium absorption. For example, a twelve-ounce can of soft drink, containing about 30 mg of phosphate, may inhibit a like amount of magnesium absorption and utilization.

Unless you take absorption into account—even while carefully following the Prostate Health Pyramid—you may still find your magnesium levels coming up short. Since magnesium levels are not easy to check, magnesium deficiency may not be evident to your doctor. Most magnesium is found within our cells, and only about 2 percent is found in bodily fluids, including blood serum.

How can you ensure that you're getting enough magnesium? Supplementation is one possibility. Another novel possibility is to soak in magnesium-rich bathwater. The water and magnesium will be absorbed through your skin and from there migrate to your bloodstream, which will channel it throughout your body.

SULFORAPHANE
Sulforaphane is an antioxidant that stimulates natural detoxifying enzymes.

Sulforaphane was identified in broccoli sprouts by scientists at the John Hopkins University School of Medicine. Researchers investigating the anticancer compounds in broccoli discovered that broccoli sprouts contain anywhere from thirty to fifty times the concentration of protective chemicals found in mature broccoli plants.

Researchers at Stanford University Medical Center studied the stimulative effects of sulforaphane on protective enzymes in human prostate cancer cells. Sulforaphane was shown to stimulate the production of phase 2 enzymes, considered biomarkers for protection against cancer.

In another study, feeding sulforaphane-rich broccoli sprout extracts to laboratory rats exposed to a carcinogen dramatically reduced the frequency, size, and number of tumors.

In addition to broccoli sprouts, sulforaphane is found in cauliflower, cabbage, and kale.

FOLATE

Folate (another name for folic acid) is a form of a water-soluble B vitamin.

Folate is necessary for the production and maintenance of new cells, needed to make cell building blocks DNA and RNA. Folate also helps prevent mutations to DNA that may lead to cancer. Diets low in folate have been linked to increased risk of breast, colon, and pancreatic cancer. To date, no linkage between folate blood level and prostate cancer has been established, but there is some evidence that a low level of folate in the blood is a biomarker for increased cancer risk.

Folate is found in leafy green vegetables such as spinach, dried beans and peas, fortified cereals and grains, and some fruits (cantaloupe, oranges, bananas). In 1998, the FDA established regulations requiring the addition of folic acid to breads, pastas, cereals, flours, rice, cornmeal, and other grain products. This was primarily to reduce the incidence of certain birth defects called neural tube defects, but it has also had the effect of significantly improving the folate status of the entire population.

Some medications, such as anticonvulsants, can interfere with folate utilization.

LECITHIN

Lecithin is a phospholipid (a fatty acid and its derivatives) needed by every cell in the body. Cell membranes are composed largely of lecithin, and lecithin makes up the bulk of the protective sheaths that surround nerve fibers in the brain and throughout the body. While lecithin is manufactured in the liver by the compounds choline and inositol, it still needs to be supplied by nutritional means.

Lecithin protects cells against oxidative free-radical cell damage. In a clinical study, subjects with enlarged prostates given doses of lecithin showed a reduction in their prostate size, as well as improved symptoms, such as a decreased need for nighttime urination (nocturia), less urine dribbling, and a stronger urine stream.

Lecithin also helps protect against atherosclerosis and other cardiovascular diseases; it increases energy levels; and it aids in the digestion of fat (though itself a fatty substance, it is also a fat emulsifier).

Lecithin can be found in abundance in pumpkin seeds, melon seeds, sunflower seeds, soybean oil, nuts, and wheat germ.

NATURAL ANTIOXIDANTS

Phase 2 Enzymes

Phase 2 enzymes are antioxidants that detoxify carcinogens, turning them into water-soluble substances that can be excreted by cells. They can be found in natural foods such as broccoli sprouts, cabbage, Brussels sprouts, kale, and mustard greens.

GSTP1 Enzyme

GSTP1 is an enzyme present in normal prostate tissue but often absent in prostate cancer cells. Thus, it is a significant biomarker for prostate cancer. GSTP1 detoxifies actual carcinogens, as well as free-radical oxidants. Natural sources of this enzyme include garlic, Chinese cabbage (brassica), and soy products.

Alpha-Lipoic Acid

This is one of the more recently discovered antioxidants. Found naturally in small amounts in the body, it helps cells convert sugars into energy and enhances the action of vitamins C and E. Potatoes, carrots, yams, sweet potatoes, and beets contain alpha-lipoic acid; it can also be found in small amounts in liver and yeast.

AMINO ACIDS

You've often heard amino acids referred to as the "building blocks" of life. The description is an apt one. Amino acids are the chemical units that make up protein, and protein is the base of all living tissue. Three amino acids in particular have a beneficial effect on conditions such as enlarged prostate (and its attendant urinary problems); they are glycine, alanine, and glutamic acid.

Glycine is found in significant amounts in prostate fluid. Reliable, consistent clinical studies report that glycine, combined with alanine and glutamic acid, reduces the symptoms of prostate enlargement. Glycine is found in many high-protein foods, including beans, fish, and dairy products. Very few people are glycine-deficient, since glycine is a nonessential amino acid (that is, the body makes its own supply). But that doesn't mean that glycine shouldn't be supplemented through nutritional intake.

Alanine is another nonessential amino acid that is present in prostate fluid and a clinically recognized element of prostate health. Like glycine, it should be an important part of the diet. Good alanine sources include fish, eggs, and poultry.

Glutamic acid (glutamate) is another significant component of prostate fluid that plays a role in normal prostate function, in addition to its salubrious effect on enlarged prostate and its symptoms. Glutamic acid is also the most common stimulating neurotransmitter in the central nervous system.

While some glutamic acid is made in the body, we can fulfill our necessary nutritional requirements with a protein-rich diet. Good dietary sources include vegetables, fish, eggs, and poultry. Monosodium glutamate (MSG) is a form of glutamic acid used widely as a flavor enhancer, but due to the addition of preservatives and other substances it does not qualify as a health food. Many people are allergic to it.

AMINO ACIDS AND BENIGN PROSTATIC HYPERPLASIA (BPH)

In a double-blind clinical study—where neither group of enlarged prostate sufferers knew if they were receiving a combination of glycine, alanine, and glutamic acid or a sugar pill (placebo)—the results were dramatic among those who received the amino acids:

- 92 percent experienced a reduction in prostate size.
- 95 percent experienced less need to urinate during the night.
- 81 percent had less of an urgency to urinate.
- 73 percent urinated less frequently.

SOY PRODUCTS

The soybean is a legume native to northern China, now commonly grown in the United States. A variety of soy products turn up in the amino acid–rich food groups, as well as in the zinc-rich and magnesium-rich food groups. When buying soy products, be sure to choose the low-sodium, low-fat kind.

Compounds called isoflavones are found in soybeans and soy by-products such as tofu, flavored soy milk, and soy nuts. Isoflavones exert anticarcinogenic properties in a variety of ways. Isoflavone compounds found in soy stimulate binding proteins called globulins that keep testosterone and estrogen levels in check. Because prostate cancer cells feed off testosterone, scientists theorize that the less elevated testosterone levels are, the less effect this hormone has on the body and the lower the risk of cancer development and progression. In a study, genistein, an isoflavone found in soy, reduced prostate tumors in mice.

Soy isoflavones tend to concentrate in prostate tissue. Since isoflavones are known to influence cell growth and regulation, there

THE BEST SOURCES OF SOY ISOFLAVONES
The following soy foods provide in the range of 30–50 mg of isoflavones per serving:

- Textured soy protein (½ cup)
- Black soybeans (½ cup)
- Roasted soy nuts (1 ounce)
- Soy flour (½ cup)
- Soy grits (¼ cup)
- Soy milk (1 cup)
- Tofu (½ cup)
- Tempeh (½ cup)

Soy oil does not contain isoflavones. Soy-based hot dogs and burgers contain widely varying amounts of isoflavones, depending on processing and other factors. Soy protein may or may not contain a high level of isoflavones, depending largely on how it is processed.

is strong laboratory evidence that they inhibit cancer growth during the initial onset of the disease.

Soy is said to block the action of the enzyme tyrosine kinase, whose increased activity has been linked to the growth of cancer cells. Soy products even appear to prevent the formation of blood vessels that tumors need in order to grow and spread.

PHYTOCHEMICALS

Phytochemicals increase resistance to disease and boost immunity. Whole foods containing phytochemicals have wonderful disease-fighting properties. Studies indicate that supplements derived from phytochemicals are not as effective.

GARLIC

Recent studies indicate that daily servings of garlic and other vegetables in the allium group (onions, scallions, leeks, chives) may have a preventive effect against prostate cancer. Garlic contains allicin, a remarkable anticancer agent.

Nothing could be easier than introducing more garlic into your daily diet. Fresh garlic is a superb flavor enhancer, and garlic is a

---

KEY PHYTOCHEMICALS AND THE FOODS RICHEST IN THEM

- **Genistein:** Soybeans, peas, lentils, cabbage
- **Indoles:** Cabbage, broccoli, kale, Brussels sprouts
- **Carotenoids:** Tomatoes, watermelon, grapefruit
- **Lycopene:** Cooked tomatoes (these have much more lycopene than uncooked), pink grapefruit, watermelon, strawberries
- **Phytosterols:** Alfalfa sprouts, yams
- **Isoflavones:** Soy products
- **Allium:** Garlic, leeks, onions
- **Flavonoids:** Onions, grapes, red wine, kale, citrus fruits, tomatoes, berries, peppers, carrots
- **Quercetin:** Citrus fruits
- **Capsaicin:** Hot peppers

must ingredient for tomato and other sauces. Baked garlic has a more mellow flavor and is less likely to linger on your breath.

A daily serving of allium vegetables may help prevent the development of prostate cancer. These vegetables are prime sources of flavonoids and active sulfur compounds that inhibit prostate tumors. They also inhibit the cell division and proliferation that are the hallmark of cancer, and they help keep cell DNA in good repair. Some research suggests that an ingredient in garlic may help modulate the effect of hormones on prostate cells.

Numerous scientific investigations support the claim that garlic prevents the formation and spread of certain cancers, improves the responsiveness of disease-fighting white blood cells, and lowers cholesterol formation.

In studies at the Institute for Cancer Prevention, garlic constituents have been shown to blunt the growth of human prostate cancer cells in the lab to a remarkable degree. IFCP researchers determined that garlic components prevent cancer cells from multiplying. Increased testosterone levels are linked to increased development of prostate cancer.

In a separate Institute study, allium derivatives from garlic showed great promise in controlling the incidence and spread of prostate cancer. Laboratory observation indicated that the proliferation rate of cancerous cells was markedly reduced, and the testosterone concentration in the cells decreased rapidly. The IFCP's results strongly suggest that allium-induced inhibition of cell proliferation and accelerated removal of testosterone are linked.

OBESITY AND PROSTATE CANCER

Researchers from the American Cancer Society examined the relationship between body mass index (BMI), height, and prostate cancer mortality rate among two large groups of men. There were more than 380,000 men in the first study group (1959–1972), and more than 430,000 in the second group (1982–1996). Researchers found that prostate cancer death rates were 27 percent higher in men who were obese—defined as having a BMI greater than 30—compared to men with a BMI of less than 25.

EXAMPLES OF ONE SERVING

Many food products tell you the number of servings they contain. The contents of the package does not equal one serving unless it says so. If the package indicates "two servings," half the contents equals one serving; if it indicates "four servings," one-fourth the contents equals one serving; and so on.

What if the serving size is not indicated? This list will give you a good working sense of what constitutes a typical serving size in the Prostate Health Pyramid:

- ½ cup of pasta
- 2–3 ounces of tofu
- ¼ cup of nuts or seeds
- ⅓ cup of cooked legumes
- 1 slice of whole-wheat bread
- 4 small multigrain crackers
- 1 tortilla
- 1 medium-size piece of fruit
- ¼ cup of dried fruit
- 3 ounces of fish, poultry, or lean meat
- ½ cup of cooked or chopped vegetables
- 1 cup salad greens or raw vegetables
- 1 cup of cold cereal
- ½ cup of cooked cereal
- ½ cup of rice

FAT

Fat acts as both a cancer promoter and an agent that stimulates the growth of existing cancer. The Institute for Cancer Prevention recommends that men focus on reducing fat in their diet and limiting total fat intake as much as possible, rather than concentrating on simply avoiding saturated fat.

While high cholesterol levels and "bad" fats are closely linked to cardiovascular disease, there is no clear understanding of the relationship between types of fat and the incidence and growth of cancer. The bottom line: you should limit all kinds of dietary fat, especially animal fats. The foods highest in fat include beef, pork, cheeses, cakes, pies, cookies, chocolate, and full-fat dairy products.

The foods lowest in fat include fruits and vegetables; dry cereals; and nonfatty seafood such as shrimp, crab, scallops, squid, light tuna, crayfish, perch, pollock, and mussels.

The most prostate-healthy alternative among fats is olive oil—the higher the grade, the better—and omega-3 fish oil. Olive oil is high in monounsaturated fat. Monounsaturated fats increase the level of high-density lipoproteins (HDL, the "good" fat) in the blood and reduce the level of LDL, the "bad" fat. Some population groups that consume relatively large amounts of mono- and polyunsaturated fats have a lower rate of heart disease than in the United States. On the Greek island of Crete, where fat constitutes as much as 40 percent of total calories, the rate of heart disease is actually lower even than in Japan, where fat constitutes only 8 to 10 percent of calories in the average diet.

THE INSTITUTE FOR CANCER PREVENTION'S DIETARY GUIDELINES FOR PROSTATE HEALTH

- **Maintain a low-fat diet,** with calories from fat constituting no more than 15 percent of daily calorie intake.
- **Stay away from red meat** as much as possible, or eliminate it from your diet altogether.
- **Eat at least ten to twelve servings of fruit and vegetables every day.**
- **Eat ten or more servings of lycopene every week,** in the form of tomatoes, tomato sauce, tomato products, and tomato juice.
- **Add plenty of soy products to your diet.**
- **Drink at least two to three cups of green tea, preferably decaffeinated, a day.**
- **Avoid processed, smoked, and salt-cured foods.**
- **Do not eat charred, charcoaled, charbroiled, blackened, burnt, or barbecued food.**
- **Choose whole-grain breads and baked goods, bran, and oat products.**
- **Stay away from ground meats and ground fish** such as fish cakes, fish "portions," and fish sticks.
- **Eat at least one raw food meal every several days**—such as a green salad or fresh fruit salad—or even every day if your palate is willing.
- **Consume sprouts,** long touted as a superb source of nutrients. Now scientists have discovered that they have important curative properties as well. Sprouts such as broccoli, alfalfa, clover, soybean, and radish contain highly concentrated amounts of phytochemicals that help protect against disease. Alfalfa sprouts are one of the primary sources of

saponins, which stimulate the immune system and increase activity against carcinogenic and other destructive substances.

- **Reduce your consumption of sugar and refined flour.**
- **Always choose olive oil,** the least processed of cooking oils; look for the words "extra-virgin" on the label (meaning minimally processed).
- **Eliminate fatty** foods such as poultry skin, chocolate, gravy, and creamy sauces and soups (substitute tomato sauce and soup).
- **Include beans in your soups and stews.**
- **Add peppers, tomatoes and onions to your omelets.**
- **Eat garlic.** Garlic is rich in allicin, which bolsters immune function and reduces cancer risk.

5. Negative Nutrition

The Fats and Calcium Controversies

While many nutrients and foods protect the prostate, there are also many substances that are potentially damaging to and even cancer-promoting for the prostate.

Fats

Fats have been studied more closely and linked to cancer more often than any other element in the diet. Vast national differences in prostate cancer incidence and mortality rates have led scientists to the conclusion that total fat intake is directly linked to prostate cancer and other chronic diseases.

The Lowdown on Fats

Saturated Fats. These are found in meat, dairy products, palm and coconut oils, butter, lard, eggs, and milk. Saturated fats are definitely bad for you. A high intake of saturated fat has been linked to prostate cancer. Saturated fats are easily identified: they become solid at room temperature. Of the saturated fats, simple butter may be your best choice.

Trans–Fatty Acids (Hydrogenated Fats). These are present in fried foods, red meat, dairy products, margarine, cakes, cookies, and biscuits. Avoid these the same way you do saturated fats.

Polyunsaturated Fats. These are found in margarine; sunflower, safflower, soybean, and corn oil; and oily fish. Omega-3 and omega-6 are the two main types of polyunsaturated fats. Polyunsaturates may bring down the total blood cholesterol level, both the good (HDL) and the bad (LDL). Omega-3 polyunsaturates are found in oily fish (salmon, halibut, sardines, herring, mackerel, trout, etc.), walnuts, sesame and pumpkin seeds, flaxseed oil, and leafy green vegetables. Omega-3 fats are said to have an anti-inflammatory effect. There is some speculation that fatty fish high in omega-3 fatty acids can reduce the incidence of prostate cancer (see below) and alleviate enlarged prostate symptoms, including frequent urgency to urinate.

Omega-6 polyunsaturates are found in polyunsaturated margarine and sunflower, corn, and soybean oils. Essential fatty acids are polyunsaturates important to metabolic processes such as the manufacture of cell membranes. These fatty acids are referred to as "essential" because your body can't make them—they have to be supplied from food intake. Linoleic acid (an omega-6 fat) and alpha-linoleic acid (an omega-3 fat) are the major essential fatty acids. Polyunsaturates are less "sticky" than saturated fat and remain fluid-like in the blood, but that does not make them healthy. Under extreme heat, even good polyunsaturates are destroyed, transforming them into unhealthy *trans*-polyunsaturates.

Monounsaturated fats. These are derived mainly from plants. These are the fats men should emphasize in their prostate health diets—always remembering that the real goal is to minimize overall fat intake. Processed monounsaturates are not good for prostate health. Olive oil (extra-virgin, minimally processed), canola oil, peanut oil, rapeseed oil, blended vegetable oil, avocados, and nuts are good sources of monounsaturated fat. Monounsaturated fats maintain or slightly increase good cholesterol levels, while aiding in reducing bad cholesterol levels. Monounsaturates can also help protect against cell damage.

STARCHES AND SUGARS
Clinical studies have looked at the potential relationship between high insulin levels and prostate cancer growth. We know that elevated insulin levels go hand in hand with high blood sugar levels and elevated blood lipid levels, and that cutting down on sugars and starches is a good way to control insulin levels.

CAN EATING FATTY FISH REDUCE THE RISK OF PROSTATE CANCER?

A controversial Swedish study published in 2001 in the medical journal *The Lancet* concluded that consumption of fatty fish high in omega-3 fatty acids (salmon, herring, mackerel, halibut) can reduce the risk of prostate cancer by as much as 50 percent.

The study tracked the diet of more than 6,000 twins for thirty years. The study concluded that subjects who didn't include fatty fish in their diet had two to three times the frequency of prostate cancer of subjects who consumed moderate-to-large quantities of such fish.

The Institute for Cancer Prevention considers the study provocative but not definitive. Many questions remain. Was fish consumption really the primary factor associated with the decreased incidence of prostate cancer? What specific kinds of fish were consumed, and in what quantities? How reliable was the dietary information provided by the subjects?

The diets of men who eat the most fish—such as the Japanese—also tend to contain the most soy. Since fish and soy products both contain omega-3 fatty acids, many Asian studies attribute the inhibition of tumor growth to soy consumption or to a combination of dietary factors, rather than to the consumption of fatty fish per se. More studies are needed to confirm or refute the link between fatty fish and prostate health.

Another study to take into consideration is a recent one by the Environmental Working Group, which found that seven of ten farm-raised salmon purchased in grocery stores in Washington, D.C., Portland, and San Francisco contained concentrations of PCBs (polychlorinated biphenyls, chemical contaminants) sixteen times as high as those found in wild salmon and four times as high as those found in other seafood or in beef. Most of the salmon sold today is farm-raised.

Although federal Food and Drug Administration tests also show higher levels of PCBs in farm-raised salmon than in wild salmon, FDA officials say the levels are far below the agency's threshold. On the other hand, the Environmental Protection Agency recommends restricting the consumption of fish with much lower PCB levels than those set by FDA standards. Consider moderating your salmon consumption until this issue is definitively resolved.

Simple carbohydrates are sugars such as the ones found in candy, baked goods, and fruit. Complex carbohydrates are starches found in vegetables, whole grains, beans, and nuts. Concentrate on including unrefined complex carbs such as whole grains in your diet.

SODIUM

You should minimize your intake of sodium, which is found in salt and, in the form of additives, in highly processed foods. Check your food labels and look for the low-salt alternatives, which are becoming easier and easier to find. Also, many salt substitutes contain additives that make them a less-than-healthy alternative to regular salt. Furthermore, highly processed foods, such as processed ham, bacon, and hot dogs, may also be high in carcinogenic nitrosamines and should be limited as much as possible.

CALCIUM

Some recent studies indicate that an increased risk of full-blown prostate cancer may be associated with a high dietary calcium intake. Men at higher risk for prostate cancer—for example, those with "red flag" PSA levels—should consider monitoring their dietary calcium intake.

However, there are conflicting studies that actually link dairy products to a *lower* cancer risk. The Institute for Cancer Prevention, in collaboration with Rockefeller University Hospital, is working on a research project aimed at determining the effects of calcium in this regard.

In a clinical study, researchers found the risk of advanced prostate cancer was 112 percent as high among men who consumed the most calcium (more than 1,200 mg, equivalent to four or more glasses of milk) as among those who consumed the least calcium (less than 500 mg a day). It didn't matter whether the calcium came from natural foods or supplementation.

The underlying mechanism of calcium's effect on prostate cancer risk isn't clear, but some scientists theorize that a high calcium intake suppresses blood levels of the active form of vitamin D, which may protect against prostate cancer by preventing the development of cancerous cells. Vitamin D plays a number of other health key roles. It is an important element in regulating calcium balance, aiding the body's absorption of dietary calcium. Vitamin D is essential to maintenance of healthy bones.

The recommended daily calcium intake for men over fifty is 1,200 mg. Dietary sources of calcium include milk, dairy products, salmon, and dark, leafy greens. There is also considerable calcium content in fortified foods, including breakfast cereals and juices. A serving of fortified cereal can contain up to 1,000 mg of calcium.

According to the American Dietary Association, vegetarians can obtain all the calcium they need from plant foods alone. Studies have shown that vegetarians have lower rates of osteoporosis, and can absorb and retain more calcium from foods, than nonvegetarians.

Vitamin D is produced by skin cells in response to exposure to ultraviolet rays. Given sufficient sun exposure, the body will make all the vitamin D it needs. Some oncologists have pointed out that there is a higher incidence of prostate cancer in northern latitudes, where there is less exposure to sunlight. Is there a relationship among exposure to ultraviolet rays, vitamin D production, and the incidence of prostate cancer? Researchers at Boston University's School of Medicine studied this phenomenon, focusing on regions of the country where there is less sunlight and where there may not be enough UV radiation to stimulate adequate vitamin D production.

THE WORST FOODS FOR YOUR PROSTATE

Red Meat. This is the number one food to avoid in any prostate-healthy diet. Because of its fat content and the carcinogenic toxins generated during the cooking of red meat, it is best to avoid red meat altogether. Eat fish and white meat instead.

Barbecued, Smoked, Pickled, and Salt-Cured Foods. As meat is barbecued, charcoal-broiled, or grilled, fat oozes off of it onto the burning coals and forms a carcinogen called benzopyrene, which is then reabsorbed on the surface of the meat. Additional mutagens, toxins, and carcinogens are formed when barbecued, charcoal-broiled, or grilled meat is cooked at a temperature exceeding 300 degrees.

The high nitrate and nitrite content of pickled and salt-cured foods is converted into carcinogenic compounds.

Whole-Fat Dairy Products (Ice Cream, Cheese, Cream, Whipped Cream, Cakes, and Pastries). Their high fat content is detrimental to prostate health, and many of these foods are highly processed and contain harmful additives.

Gravies and High-Fat Sauces. Gravies and sauces (with the exception, of course, of tomato sauce) are anathema to prostate health.

THE CALCIUM CONTROVERSY: DOES TOO MUCH CALCIUM INCREASE THE RISK OF PROSTATE CANCER?

Some recent clinical studies suggest that higher milk intake may increase the risk for prostate cancer, but a review of all the scientific literature shows that other studies do not reach the same conclusion. A study published in *The American Journal of Clinical Nutrition* noted that the risk of prostate cancer may increase with calcium intake, especially from dairy products.

Researchers at the Fred Hutchinson Cancer Research Center in Seattle, in conjunction with the National Cancer Institute, investigated the connection among dairy products, calcium consumption, and prostate cancer in a large group of physicians. Men with the highest levels of dairy product consumption had a significantly (34 percent) greater risk of getting prostate cancer than those with the lowest levels of consumption.

The researchers stated, "Our findings clearly show decreased risk for late-stage prostate cancer in men with diets that are low in fat and moderate in calcium, possibly because these diets slow progression of prostate cancer. For men diagnosed with early-stage prostate cancer, this is important because it suggests that moderating fat and calcium consumption may reduce the risk of cancer recurrence following treatment."

The Institute for Cancer Prevention recommends *moderating* your intake of dairy-based products, given their relatively high fat content and in light of the ongoing controversy over excessive dietary calcium intake and its possible inhibition of the body's production of vitamin D. Consult with your physician or nutritionist.

THE IRRITANTS

Certain foods and substances can irritate the prostate. One thing you can do to help ensure prostate health immediately is drink lots of water. Less concentrated urine—urine that has a lighter shade of yellow—contains fewer toxins and has an easier effect on the prostate and the urinary tract.

How can a man determine what does and does not irritate his prostate, since this can vary from one man to another? There is no simple answer. The most effective path for most men is simply a process of elimination, or general avoidance, of some of the prime prostate irritants, such as caffeine, alcohol, and spicy foods.

In many cases of prostatitis, a specific diet may be recommended to avoid foods and beverages that are irritants to the urinary system.

Spices (Red Pepper). Spicy foods cause prostate irritation in some men and not in others. However, though commonly considered prostate irritants, chili peppers and jalapeños also contain the chemical capsaicin, which neutralizes cancer-causing substances called nitrosamines.

Alcohol. Alcohol is a suspected risk factor for prostate cancer. It has also been linked to other cancers, specifically colon cancer. Although only a relatively slight risk of prostate cancer has been associated with alcohol consumption in clinical studies, even a small risk must be factored against other risk factors, both modifiable ones (diet) and unavoidable ones (a family history of prostate cancer).

In a study reported in the *American Journal of Epidemiology,* nine hundred men (evenly divided between African Americans and Caucasians) who were diagnosed with prostate cancer between 1986 and 1989 were questioned about their alcohol consumption. Any man who had consumed at least one drink per month for six months was defined as an alcohol drinker. Seven to eight drinks per week constituted light consumption; eight to twenty-one drinks per week constituted moderate consumption; twenty-two to fifty-six drinks per week was considered heavy consumption; and fifty-seven or more drinks per week was considered extremely heavy consumption.

The increased risk of prostate cancer associated with drinking in general was found to be slight for both blacks and whites. There was, however, a significant increase in the risk for men who were heavy or very heavy drinkers, whatever their age or race. No difference in risk was found between men who had stopped drinking and who were still drinkers, leading researchers to suspect that alcohol consumption is related to early-stage development of prostate cancer.

Coffee (Even Decaffeinated Coffee) and Products That Contain Caffeine. Caffeine is notorious for causing bladder irritation. Decaffeinated coffee can also be an irritant. Decaffeinated coffee also contains known carcinogens. In addition, coffee is a diuretic that aggravates conditions associated with frequent urination, such as enlarged prostate. Eliminating coffee and caffeine-rich products (soda, chocolate, and tea) can help relieve a number of symptoms of BPH.

Hydrogenated Oils (Margarine) and Polyunsaturated Vegetable Oils. Researchers at the University of Athens Medical Center in Greece stated that margarine may increase the risk of enlarged prostate and irritate the lower urinary tract. Polyunsaturated vegetable oils can also irritate the prostate, especially when they are converted to *trans*-polyunsaturates under extreme heat.

Fried Foods. A simple rule for prostate health: If it's fried, don't eat it. Fried foods are a prime prostate irritant for many men. Several carcinogens are by-products in fried foods. Deep-fried foods soak up oil like a sponge, increasing their calorie content. French fries, to cite a common example, get more than 50 percent of their calories from absorbed fat.

Medications. A wide variety of medications can irritate the prostate, especially for prostatitis sufferers, or men who are in early or prestage development of the condition. Diuretics, tranquilizers, decongestants, and antidepressants can irritate the urinary tract and worsen the symptoms associated with common prostate problems.

ADDITIVES

Maintaining prostate health depends not only on what foods you consume. It's also a matter of the damaging effects of additives contained in those foods. Additives, in one way or another, disrupt the natural chemical balance of the body.

That is why natural whole foods are preferable to highly processed foods. Even though natural foods may in some instances contain pesticides and chemical or environmental toxins, the vast array of additives in commercial foods staggers the imagination.

Food additives—including artificial colorings, preservatives, flavor enhancers, and artificial sweeteners—can irritate the prostate. These substances aren't readily absorbed by the body and wind up in high concentrations in the kidneys and urine.

Resistance to numerous diseases and chronic health conditions can diminish due to lifelong consumption of additives, some of which are linked to cancer-causing agents. Chemicals with the ability to produce mutations through chromosomal damage are called mutagens. The most sophisticated toxicology testing cannot predict the combined, synergistic effect of the more than three thousand additives and environmental toxins present in most common supermarket foods.

ARTIFICIAL COLORINGS

Artificial colorings include caramel; blue Nos. 1 and 2; red Nos. 3 and 40; citrus red No. 1; and yellow Nos. 5 and 6. You'll note that these generic names don't tell you anything about the chemicals that are in these colorings.

These mysterious substances are used to color everything from candy and soft drinks to baked goods and frostings to jams and processed meats. American food manufacturers add more than 3,000 tons of food coloring to processed foods each year.

Before you consider living off of only what you can grow in your own garden, you'll be encouraged to know that only 10 percent of the food consumed in the United States contains synthetic food colors made from molecules derived from petroleum or coal tar (no wonder the manufacturers don't tell you what's in them). The remaining food products use natural colors.

Tests have indicated that high doses of most FDA-certified synthetic food dyes can cause cancer when injected into laboratory animals. (The FDA points out that these food dyes have been shown to cause cancer only when injected into animals, not when consumed by them.)

Every synthetic food coloring has its own toxicological properties. Green No. 3 has been linked to bladder tumors; red No. 3 to thyroid tumors; red No. 40 to lymphatic tumors; yellow No. 6 to kidney tumors; and blue No. 2 to brain tumors.

If an artificial coloring is clinically shown to cause cancer at high doses, who can say that it will not cause cancer at lower doses over a prolonged period of time?

PRESERVATIVES

Nitrates and nitrites are two ingredients used extensively in cured meats: "cold cuts," hot dogs, and ham, among others. These preservatives combine in the body to form nitrosamines, known to be carcinogenic. Nitrates and nitrites are also used as flavor enhancers and food colorings. While preservatives have been clinically linked to increased cancer risk in laboratory animals, the FDA and the food industry continue to claim that the risk is slight. Consuming these substances in your breakfast sausage or in your salami sandwich at lunchtime is an invitation to increased risk of prostate and other cancers.

Sulfites occur naturally as a result of the fermentation of alcoholic beverages, including beer and wine. Sulfites are also used to prevent food spoilage and discoloration. In 1984, their use was banned by the FDA on foods that are consumed raw, such as fruits and vegetables. However, sulfites can still be used legally in processed foods and all too often continue to turn up illegally in restaurant salad bars. The American Institute for Cancer Research notes that the primary danger of sulfites is to people with asthma or serious allergies, who may have trouble breathing, become dizzy, or develop severe headaches as a result of consuming them.

Good Preservatives
Preservatives considered safe include benzoic acid and sodium benzoate (found in soft drinks, beer, fruit products, margarine, olives, and many other foodstuffs) and the sorbate family of compounds, including sorbic acid, potassium sorbate, sodium sorbate, and calcium sorbate.

FLAVOR ENHANCERS
Flavor enhancers such as monosodium glutamate (MSG) are often "hidden" on food labels under names such as textured vegetable protein (TVP) or plant protein extract. The word "hydrolyzed" on a food's label is a tip-off that it contains MSG. Amazingly, MSG was once added even to baby food, until it was discovered that the enzymes that help metabolize MSG in adults are not present in infants. Too much glutamate or aspartame (see next section) can trigger excessive free-radical production, which is why these substances are sometimes referred to as "excitotoxins."

Other common flavor enhancers have tongue-tripping names such as dioctyl sodiumsulfosuccinate and disodium guanylate. Many of them are considered potential risk factors for cancer.

ARTIFICIAL SWEETENERS
Aspartame is widely used in sugar substitutes (NutraSweet and Equal among them) and in many chewing gums. What some of us may not be aware of is that aspartame is also present in gelatin and

other frozen desserts; some multivitamins, pharmaceuticals, and supplements; some yogurt; and instant tea and coffee. Aspartame accounts for more than 75 percent of the adverse reactions to food additives reported to the FDA.

Saccharine has been long suspected of being linked to bladder cancer, but there is no clinical evidence that consumption of this artificial sweetener is related to prostate cancer.

Supplements: Good and Bad

Supplements are intended to augment the food we eat, not to replace it. The Institute for Cancer Prevention emphasizes that men should get the vitamins and minerals they need from a variety of natural foods in a nutritious, well-balanced, prostate-healthy diet. A study published in the journal *Nature* found that the natural antioxidants in fresh fruits were far more effective than the antioxidants found in dietary supplements. For example, the antioxidant benefit of a medium-sized apple equaled that of a 1,500 mg supplement dose of vitamin C. That's enough to make you think twice about the need for supplements.

Some men feel more comfortable "covering the bases" by taking a one-a-day-type multivitamin. Doing so is unlikely to have any negative effects and may in fact provide some health benefits. Supplements contain one or more of the following ingredients: vitamins, minerals, amino acids, herbs, or other botanicals. There are also specific supplements intended to bolster or help ensure prostate health.

However, the nutritional supplement industry is relatively unregulated by the Food and Drug Administration (FDA), and there is no

WHO SHOULD TAKE SUPPLEMENTS?

There are some men who should seriously consider supplementation:

- Dieters whose calorie intake is restricted
- Individuals with food allergies
- Strict vegetarians, who may not be getting enough zinc, vitamins B12 and D, or even protein in their diet

accurate way to tell what a supplement contains, other than to have it lab-tested yourself.

LABELS CAN LIE

Many nutritional supplements simply do not supply what is listed on the label. A Canadian analysis reported in *The Journal of Urology* of supplements promoted for prostate health turned up some disturbing, if unsurprising, results. While the quantity of vitamin D in the products tested was close to what the label claimed, the vitamin E content varied from −41% to +57%. Lycopene content varied from −38% to +143% from the notation on the label. Saw palmetto supplements varied from −97% to +140%. Some products had as little as 3% of the saw palmetto content claimed on the label.

A key question in terms of prostate health is whether supplementation with antioxidants or other phytochemicals will have appreciable benefits even if the amounts listed on the label are actually delivered. In many cases, the answer is still very much open to debate.

One thing you should never do is take megadoses of supplements under the misguided conception that massive doses will work wonders for your prostate health. Quite the opposite may happen. Generally speaking, any dose above ten times the daily values (DV) from all sources—listed on the supplement label as "1,000% of the DV"—is considered a megadose. Excessive supplementation can result in serious side effects, chronic health problems, or even a toxic reaction. Since many supplements include more than one ingredient and many foods we eat have already been "enriched" with vitamins, men need to keep careful track of what nutrients are duplicated in their whole-food and supplemental intake.

INSTITUTE FOR CANCER PREVENTION RECOMMENDATIONS

SUPPLEMENTS THAT MAY PROMOTE PROSTATE HEALTH
SELENIUM
A supplement with 200 mcg of selenium a day can be considered. Use a natural source of this essential trace mineral, such as yeast, when supplementing, as the nonorganic forms (selenite, selenate) can be toxic at high levels.

Selenium blood levels should be monitored regularly by a physician if you're taking
(continued on next page)

more than 400 mcg a day. Symptoms of selenium toxicity include loss of appetite, weight loss, bad breath, and hair loss.

Avoid supplementing with selenium if you live in certain regions of the country. The soils in the high plains of northern Nebraska and the Dakotas have very high selenium levels. People living in those regions have the highest selenium intake in the country.

VITAMIN E

This important antioxidant helps protect against the damaging effects of free radicals. According to epidemiological studies, higher vitamin E intake has been shown to promote prostate health, including latent conditions that may not be clinically detectable. Vitamin E can interfere with blood clotting. Always consult with your doctor, especially if you are on blood thinner (anti-coagulation) drugs.

ISOFLAVONES (GENISTEIN, DAIDZEIN)

Preliminary studies indicate that regular consumption of soy-derived isoflavone supplements may help protect against prostate cancer, as well as cancers of the breast and endometrium, but that supplemental isoflavones are simply not as effective as those derived from whole foods. However, good-quality soy extract does contain a high concentration of isoflavones, as well as many of the other nutrients found in soy.

Since the long-term effects of isolated isoflavone supplementation are not yet known—especially at megadose levels—it is best to limit supplemental isoflavone intake to no more than 200 mg a day (the estimated high-end amount found in the Japanese diet, which is more typically 50–100 mg a day).

Soy contains a compound called phytic acid, which can interfere with mineral absorption.

A ongoing clinical research project by the Institute for Cancer Prevention on the effects of soy supplementation is being conducted at St. Luke's–Roosevelt Hospital Center in New York. This three-pronged project is looking at:

- The effect of soy isoflavones on estrogen metabolism
- Cosupplementation with lactobacillus to determine whether altering the balance of colonic bacteria enhances the beneficial effects of soy, by making the isoflavones more readily available to the body
- Analysis of soy-induced changes in gene expression

VITAMIN D AND CALCIUM CITRATE

Current research linking excess calcium consumption to a higher risk of prostate cancer suggests that calcium supplements should be avoided by prostate cancer patients and men with elevated PSA levels.

Vitamin D and calcium citrate are frequently combined in supplement form (vitamin D is necessary for calcium absorption). If your doctor recommends a calcium supplement, take no more than 1,000 mg a day. Calcium supplements are available in a variety of forms: calcium citrate, carbonate, lactate, gluconate, and phosphate. Calcium citrate is well absorbed by the body and is especially recommended for men with lower gastric acid levels. Calcium supplements are best taken with meals—but not with high-fiber meals, which may interfere with the mineral's absorption. Alcohol, caffeine, carbonated beverages, and smoking may also interfere with calcium absorption.

If you're homebound, don't get out in the sun much, or live in a region where sunlight is limited for much of the year, you may want to supplement with vitamin D.

LYCOPENE

A synthetic lycopene supplement has been introduced that is considerably cheaper than natural lycopene supplements. But is it any good? There is growing clinical evidence that lycopene supplements are not as effective as lycopene derived from whole foods. Regular consumption of tomato-based products is the best and by far the most pleasant way to ensure adequate lycopene intake. Furthermore, lycopene supplements generally lack the other important nutrients found in tomatoes. But given the importance of lycopene in relation to prostate health, you might want to supplement with 20–40 mg a day for additional support.

SUPPLEMENTS THAT MAY DAMAGE PROSTATE HEALTH OR CAUSE OTHER SERIOUS HEALTH EFFECTS
BETA-CAROTENE

Beta-carotene supplements were quite popular until the mid-1990s, when several prominent studies concluded that they provided no discernible health benefits. Two of the studies even indicated that synthetic beta-carotene supplements might prove harmful to smokers, increasing the incidence of lung cancer. On the other hand, a study conducted in Finland stated that synthetic beta-carotene supplements created no appreciable risk of lung cancer when subjects smoked less than twenty cigarettes a day and drank little or no alcohol.

The Institute for Cancer Prevention emphasizes that if you are considering a beta-carotene supplement, you should stick to natural supplements.

(continued on next page)

CHONDROITIN AND GLUCOSAMINE

A report published in *The Prostate Forum* states that several studies have linked consumption of chondroitin sulfate to the development of metastatic prostate cancer. This supplement is often used to treat osteoarthritis and should not be taken by men with prostate cancer or with a high risk factor for prostate cancer, such as an elevated PSA level or family history of the disease.

Glucosamine, a substance frequently added to chondroitin sulfate for treatment of joint problems, has not been linked to prostate cancer.

BORON

Boron supplementation has been touted as a method of increasing testosterone or estrogen levels, although there is no clinical evidence to confirm this. Boron supplementation should be avoided in terms of prostate health, especially by men with existing prostate conditions.

There is some scientific basis for the claim that boron prevents calcium loss. However, the consumer has little guarantee of the safety, strength, or purity of products containing (or alleging to contain) boron.

WHAT ARE NUTRACEUTICALS AND FUNCTIONAL FOODS?

The food and agriculture industries and the American consumer have begun to look at food not only for its nutritional value but also for its health benefits, blurring the conventional line between food and medicine.

A nutraceutical is a food-derived substance, generally sold as a supplement in dosage form, that provides health benefits, including the prevention and treatment of disease, above and beyond the food's established nutritional value. There are thousands of nutraceuticals in the worldwide marketplace, including those derived from fish oils, garlic, green and black tea, rice, and bran oil, to name but a few.

A functional food—also known as designer food, pharmafood, or therapeutic food—is a whole food or combination of whole foods with beneficial health properties beyond the purely nutritional. Like supplement manufacturers, producers of functional foods are not allowed to claim that these foods prevent, treat, or cure any disease. For example, a calcium-fortified fruit drink cannot be marketed as preventing, treating, or curing osteoporosis.

6. THE TRANSITION DIET

A GRADUAL APPROACH

Getting people to eat healthfully is one of the major challenges that modern health care and society at large face. Consuming the kind of diet we present in Chapters 4 and 5 would reduce the risk of developing prostate cancer; and the best way to prevent prostate cancer turns out to be a useful way of *treating* prostate cancer when detected early. The interventionist therapies that we examine (surgery,

---

THE DANGERS OF FAD DIETS

A low-carbohydrate, high-fat, and high-protein diet (the basis of several bestselling diet books) can be hazardous to your health. Whatever other harm such a diet can do, there is significant research that indicates that some fad diets—particularly those high in fat—may accelerate the growth of cancerous tissue and promote the spread of cancer through the body. According to the American Cancer Society, "Men who eat high-fat diets, particularly saturated fat, may have a greater chance of developing prostate cancer."

Moreover, the eating habits promoted by such fad diets are unhealthy and, for many people, dangerous. In addition to recommending fats, which increase the risk of prostate cancer, many such diets pay scant attention to the *amount* of food consumed. Being mindful and in control of one's food intake is so difficult and important that any regimen that leads away from those goals and values should be regarded with suspicion.

radiation treatments, chemotherapy, etc.) all have their uses, but they are not without risks and side effects, some quite serious and long-lasting. It is far preferable for men to eat and conduct their lives so as to minimize the risk of contracting prostate cancer or developing other prostate problems, to have timely tests and checkups, and to treat their problems without resorting to the more radical treatments. It would then be possible—as it is in many countries where the diet is more like the one we describe in Chapter 5—for men to live to a ripe old age and succumb to something else while any cancerous lesions they may have developed in their prostate stay dormant, localized, and under control. Unfortunately, many of us don't consume a prostate-healthy diet.

A BETTER WAY

We call our approach the Transition Diet, but it's not a diet in the traditional sense. Yes, it does prescribe a regimen of eating—meals,

KNOW WHAT YOU'RE EATING

We cannot overemphasize that you need to know exactly *what* you're eating, which turns out to be harder than it sounds. You can't always tell by the taste, looks, or name of a food whether it has any real nutritional value or is the dietary equivalent of a neutron bomb.

Granted, if you're eating a handful of buttery, chewy chocolate chip cookies, you can probably guess that you're not doing your heart, waist, and prostate any favors, but many, many foods are not as obviously detrimental—they're stealth junk foods, if you will.

That's why we emphasize reading labels so much. Even though the current version of food labels isn't perfect (the FDA will soon require foods' *trans*–fatty acid content to be included on labels, for example), they can give you a decent idea of what you're eating.

By the way, reading a label means more than just looking at the name on the label. I have friends who thought they were doing something good by eating oat bran muffins. All they looked at was the name on the label. Further reading would have revealed an artery-busting amount of fat that far overwhelmed the tiny amount of oat bran in the muffin.

Which brings up the point: If a muffin or bagel or pastry doesn't have a label on it (it doesn't have to unless it's "packaged"), then you really have to be careful—or, better yet, avoid it altogether. There's no telling how much fat lurks in that belly bomb.

menus, do's and don'ts, and the like. But it has one element that distinguishes it from most other diets: at no time during the thirty days—we call it a thirty-day plan, but, as you'll see, we've built in some time to let the lessons and habits developed during the diet "take," so that the plan may actually require three months to complete—of the Transition Diet are you eating the way you should (except, perhaps at the very end of that period). You are, in fact, eating as you should only *after you're off* the diet. That's the point. The Transition Diet takes you from where you are now—a place where you are not eating healthfully—through a thirty-day program—during which you will change your eating habits one at a time, until you are eating in a healthful way, a way that minimizes your risk of developing prostate cancer.

There are two elements in this approach that are special. One is that we address one "food setting" at a time. We devote one period to breakfast; another to lunch; a third to the afternoon (when snacking becomes a problem); another to dinner; a fifth to late-night eating; and a sixth to eating out. We stay on a particular Food Setting until we've satisfactorily changed the way we eat into one that manages weight and promotes good health—and we won't leave that setting until our work is done and the transition (to healthy eating) has taken place!

Then, in each case—and here is the second element of the Transition Diet—we spend some time going through a series of steps—we call them "passageways"—that are aimed at understanding and evaluating our eating profile in that setting; dismantling the unhealthy elements of that profile; substituting healthy foods in place of the foods we should be avoiding; and then spending some time reinforcing the lessons learned and the new habits we have developed. For each of the Food Settings, there are five Passageways—each one of which is a transition from where we are to where we want to be—and while we propose that each step ideally take a single day, the plan allows for some Passageways to take longer than a single day. In fact, we recommend that once you have completed the transition in one food setting by going through all five Passageways, you spend a week sticking to that diet before going on to the next food setting.

Much of what you will see in this chapter draws from the nutritional information and the Prostate Health Pyramid in Chapters 4 and 5. We provide some menu ideas and recipes for dishes that will keep you healthy without having you feel deprived in Chapter 7. And you'll find guidance and helpful exercise routines in Chapter 8.

This diet is directed at prostate health and aimed at reducing the risk of prostate problems for men in the high-risk category: men over fifty who are overweight, who have a history of prostate cancer, other forms of cancer, or prostate problems in their family history, and who have been consuming a fat-rich diet of more than 30 grams of fat per day. Though following the principles of the Transition Diet will probably also result in weight loss, that is not our immediate goal.

GETTING READY—SUITING UP

There are several basic principles that apply to the six food settings.

- **One key to eating right is knowing *what* you're eating.** The easy availability of food in our society makes it vital that you become aware of the contents of the food you are eating. Fortunately, laws have been passed in the United States that require food manufacturers to list "nutritional facts" on the packaging of the foods they manufacture. Below we'll offer a short course in reading and interpreting these labels, but for now, let's make it a rule: We're not going to buy any food that doesn't have a label, and we're not going to buy anything without looking at the label and asking ourselves, "Is this food good for me or not?"

- **Another key to eating right is knowing *that* you're eating.** So much of our eating (and especially overeating and binge eating) occurs during moments of extreme stress and anxiety. In many instances, we are not even aware that we are eating. Eating should be reserved for those times that are designated as mealtimes. In between you may take an afternoon or late-night snack.

By the same token, don't skip a meal if you can help it. You will only gorge yourself at the next one. *In order to focus more attention on what and when you eat, we ask you to buy a small notebook and maintain a food diary by recording all of your food intake.*

- **If someone else prepares your food, even if they know what you're eating, you don't.** Eating out, even for routine meals (as opposed to special occasions), is one of the major sources of nutritional problems in America today. Restaurants typically prepare food to appeal to a diner's palate rather than to his or her health, and portions are frequently much larger than what we would prepare for ourselves in our own home.

Preparing food for yourself gives you control over what and how much you eat and results in a healthier meal. Remember to record whatever you eat in your food Journal (see page 95).

- **Food provides energy for movement and work, so if you're not also exercising a regular and effective amount, you're wasting time (yours, ours, and everybody's).** We are just beginning to appreciate the important role exercise plays in human physiology and health. Not unlike with a car, extended periods of dormancy and inactivity are as harmful as overwork and overuse. That's why we have included a chapter on exercise (Chapter 8) in this book.

- **There is no law that says you have to clean your plate.** For a variety of reasons—guilt (something about starving children in India); habit (there's one third of the potatoes on the plate and ten more minutes left in the TV program we're watching); frugality (I paid for it, and by golly, I'm going to eat it); etiquette (we wouldn't want to insult the cook by leaving anything on our plate, would we?); compulsiveness (once I start something, I finish it)—we tend to finish every morsel of food on our plate whether we're hungry

PORTION CONTROL

As we have said, you don't *have* to be a member of the clean plate (or empty bag of chips) club. You *can* leave food on your plate or eat just half that bag of chips you bought in a weak moment. Personally, I have a lot of trouble leaving food on the plate; maybe it was the way I was brought up. That's especially true when I eat "family style" at home. I find that when there's food in big serving dishes on the table, I just keep picking at the dishes until I've had the equivalent of seconds or even thirds.

I've found that a good strategy for portion control is to serve yourself one reasonable plateful of food and then put the leftovers away so you won't be tempted to go back for more.

And when you're eating out, remember, it's okay to take some home. Most restaurants serve such large portions that I routinely make a couple (or three!) meals out of one restaurant meal. It's better for your diet and saves money, too!

or not, whether we're enjoying the food or not, even whether or not we are aware that eating is what we are doing. One habit we would recommend highly is learning to leave some food on the plate. This will remind us to maintain control over what and how much we eat, and it will result in our eating less, even if only a single mouthful.

THE SIX FOOD SETTINGS

Let's first look briefly at the six situations we will be attacking. Each presents its own problems and challenges.

FOOD SETTING ONE: BREAKFAST

Breakfast is often called the most important meal of the day, and it is for a variety of reasons. But the typical American breakfast is, to put it plainly, a disaster loaded with fat. Because it is often eaten on the run or picked up at a drive-in window, healthy choices are hard to find. **Get your breakfast under control, and you will have gone a long way to getting your diet under control.**

One important recommendation is to have breakfast at home. Having breakfast at home puts you in control.

FOOD SETTING TWO: LUNCH

Here the ideal is to make your own lunch and take it with you. You can control the bread used in the sandwich you pack, as well as the kind of tuna used (packed in water as opposed to packed in oil) and how much and which kind of mayonnaise you use. If you do eat out, search out a healthy source of prepared food. If you choose foods from a salad bar, avoid dressing or take only salad oil and vinegar. It is also a good idea to do something to "depressurize" before you sit down to eat. We highly recommend a fifteen-minute walk.

FOOD SETTING THREE: AFTERNOON SNACK

The between-meal snack is one of the major sources of fat in the American diet. For many Americans, *one fourth of caloric intake and even a greater percentage of daily fat intake occurs as a result of between-meal snacking,* and the most persistent kind of snacking is during the six- or seven-hour stretch between lunch and dinner.

FOOD SETTING FOUR: DINNER

Of the main meals of the day, only dinner has a psychological element. People often feel that a huge dinner is a reward for a day of hard work and that to deprive oneself of a huge hunk of beef at the end of the day is an aspersion on one's worthiness (or one's manhood). Remember to plan what and where you eat, record all foods in your Food Journal (see p. 95), and leave some food on your plate.

FOOD SETTING FIVE: LATE-NIGHT SNACK

That late-night craving—is it the result of not getting enough nourishment in the course of the day? Who are we kidding? Late-night food cravings are more often the accumulated effect of a day with too much caffeine or a day with too much stress and anxiety. If you are a late-night binger, take control by preparing a healthy snack ahead of time and storing it in the refrigerator.

FOOD SETTING SIX: EATING OUT

A lunch or dinner out is likely to be a social situation, perhaps celebrating an event. There is a preoccupation with something other than the meal (namely, the reason for gathering), and this makes it difficult to concentrate on the quality and quantity of the food. Consuming wine and/or liquor can also make it difficult to focus on what one is eating.

It is especially important in this setting to plan what kind of dish you will choose ahead of time and to ask important questions. Remember to ask for all dressing on the side, and request foods that are broiled, not fried. Find out if a soup or pasta sauce is made with cream *before* you order it.

THE FIVE PASSAGEWAYS

Let's look at the five "Passageways" for each of the food settings. They are Orientation, Demarcation, Substitution, Mindfulness, and Reinforcement.

PASSAGEWAY ONE: ORIENTATION

Proper orientation begins with reading labels and becoming adept at identifying and selecting foods that are nutritious and healthful and avoiding those that are not. There's no great mystery here: foods high in fat are not good; foods high in saturated fat are particularly harmful. On page 93 you will find a typical "nutrition facts" food label as currently mandated by the U.S. government on all foods. Several things are worth noticing about this label, from a pack of potato chips.

• A serving size is a highly subjective measure, and what is a serving to you may not be what the manufacturer considers a single serving. A bag of potato chips may contain two cups of food and will likely be considered two servings, yet an ordinary consumer would look upon the bag as a single serving. All the information on the label is per serving, which means that all the numbers have to be doubled if you eat an entire bag of chips.

• We recommend the following as a hard-and-fast rule: **If there's no nutritional information on the label, you shouldn't be eating it.**

• The value of nutritional information appearing on the package depends on what you *do* with that information. Not all the information on the label is easily decipherable, so here are some general guidelines:

1. A food in which more than 30 percent of the calories come from fat (as is the case here) is not a very efficient deliverer of nutrition and thus should be avoided.
2. A food in which 20 percent or less of the calories come from fat is usually a desirable food; it depends on what else is in there.
3. Another way of keeping track of the fat you are getting from the foods you eat is as follows: If you set a goal of following a diet of 2,000 calories per day (which is reasonable for most men; for people seeking to lose weight, a daily caloric allowance, subject to consultation with their physician, is more likely to be in the neighborhood of 1,500 calories), you will want optimally about 300 calories coming from fat. Since one gram of fat contains 9 calories, you will want optimally 33 grams of fat per day or less, and you will want to have less than one third of that in saturated fat. If you have a serving of the food represented by the label shown here, a single serving will provide you with 13 grams of fat, which is nearly 39 percent of your daily allowance. (The label reproduced here says that those 13 grams of fat represent only 20 percent of the daily allowance, but that assumes a larger

daily allowance—as you can see at the bottom of the label—of 65 grams for a 2,000-calorie-a-day diet. We think that's too high even for people not in a high-risk group for prostate cancer and prostate problems. If you *are* in a high-risk group—overweight, over 50, with a family history of prostate problems or prostate cancer—then you should certainly be taking in no more than 15 percent, or 33 grams, of fat, no more than a third of which should be saturated fat.)

Nutrition Facts

Serving Size 1 cup (228g)
Servings Per Container 2

Amount Per Serving

Calories 260   Calories from Fat 120

	% Daily Value*
Total Fat 13g	**20%**
Saturated Fat 5g	**25%**
Cholesterol 30mg	**10%**
Sodium 660mg	**28%**
Total Carbohydrate 31g	**10%**
Dietary Fiber 0g	**0%**
Sugars 5g	
Protein 5g	

Vitamin A 4%	•	Vitamin C 2%
Calcium 15%	•	Iron 4%

* Percent Daily Values are based on a 2,000 calorie diet. Your daily values may be higher or lower depending on your calorie needs:

	Calories:	2,000	2,500
Total Fat	Less than	65g	80g
Sat Fat	Less than	20g	25g
Cholesterol	Less than	300mg	300mg
Sodium	Less than	2,400mg	2,400mg
Total Carbohydrate		300g	375g
Dietary Fiber		25g	30g

Calories per gram:
Fat 9 • Carbohydrate 4 • Protein 4

- The nutritional information on foods keeps changing (because ingredients are revised or serving sizes change), so what you knew about a food yesterday may not be true today. Always read the label, no matter how often you buy the same food.

PASSAGEWAY TWO: DEMARCATION

For each of the Food Settings, it is important for you to learn to avoid foods that are not good for you.

The most important elements of a diet are recognizing which foods you should avoid; determining that you will avoid those foods; and taking the steps necessary to avoid those foods and eliminate them from your diet. Here's how to accomplish that:

- **Clean house.** Get rid of the foods you need to avoid—get them out of your refrigerator, out of your cupboard, out of your house. Sure, you paid good money for them. But they're no good for you—so throw them out.

Cleaning house also applies to your workplace—your desk, your office, the refrigerator in the lunchroom, your vacation house, and anywhere else you spend a great deal of time and have access to the refrigerator and the cupboards. During the Breakfast Setting, we'll eliminate the forbidden breakfast foods; during the Lunch Setting, the forbidden lunch foods; and so on. Taking it one step at a time and taking that step fully, deliberately and exclusively—those are the keys to the Transition Diet.

- **Establish your "off-limits" places.** In addition to physically removing *foods* you should not be eating, you also need to identify and eliminate the *places* at which you shop and dine that promote poor food choices: crowded lunch counters; places where food automatically comes with a side order of chips or French fries and they frown upon substituting salad; restaurants that tempt you with whipped cream–topped desserts.

PASSAGEWAY THREE: SUBSTITUTION

Now it's time to restock, only this time with healthy foods. In each of the six Food Settings, you will substitute healthy foods to replace the foods you have eliminated, and you will find better places to eat and shop.

THE CANCER PREVENTION FOOD JOURNAL

The Institute for Cancer Prevention has produced a Cancer Prevention Food Journal that is designed to be consistent with the Transition Diet and that contains important nutritional information as well as space for recording your food purchases and consumption. The IFCP Cancer Prevention Food Journal is free for the asking (see box below).

Passageway Four: Mindfulness

Keep a Food Journal—a small notebook in which you record everything you eat and in which you keep notes on your progress in the Transition Diet, nutritional information on foods that are good and not good for you, and places to eat that are more healthful or at least more conducive to healthy eating.

Before embarking on the Transition Diet, we recommend that you eat normally for a full week, Sunday to Saturday, and record everything—and we mean *everything*—you eat during that week in your Food Journal. You should then review the Food Journal and embark on each Food Setting, going through each of the Passageways in turn—and recording that process in your journal.

Passageway Five: Reinforcement

As with any diet, there has to be a mechanism for staying on the diet and continuing to eat healthfully even after the first rush of resolve and enthusiasm has passed—after you have transitioned to a healthy food regimen. We believe this can be accomplished in two ways:

1. Keep a careful record of your eating during earlier Food Settings to compare with what you eat during the five Passageways for

AN OFFER YOU CAN'T REFUSE

Here is the second half of the IFCP offer: Send your "Starting Point Food Profile"—recorded in the IFCP Cancer Prevention Food Journal, in a notebook of your own, or simply on sheets of paper—to the Institute for Cancer Prevention (or simply IFCP), 390 Fifth Avenue, Third Floor, New York, NY 10018, and we will analyze what you send us, indicate how we recommend you transition from where you are now to where you should be, and send along an IFCP Cancer Prevention Food Journal—all at no cost.

KEEPING A JOURNAL

I've never been a big fan of record or journal keeping (or any paper-work, for that matter) and I was never a big believer in the value of such things. Then I actually kept a Food Journal for a week, and was it an eye-opener! There's an amazing amount of fat and calories that somehow sneaks into our mouths without us even realizing it. By keeping a Food Journal, you'll see where your calories—and the extra inches on your waistline—are really coming from.

And those cute sayings such as "If you eat standing up at the sink, it doesn't count as calories" or "If you're picking off someone else's plate, that doesn't count" don't hold up under the cold, cruel light of a Food Journal analysis.

But if you're going to make the transition to a healthy eating lifestyle, it's vital you count everything you put into your mouth—even the stuff you eat standing up.

later Food Settings. Maintain notes on food options—substitute foods and good places to eat and shop.

2. When you are done—when you have transitioned through all six Food Settings by going through all five Passageways—start again from the beginning! Go through the Transition Diet again; only this time go through the Food Settings one at a time, looking for ways to improve your eating—fat that can be cut; places where you can add fiber—and to improve the taste of what you are eating. We call this the **Second Transition,** and many people will find this a very enjoy-able experience once they reach it. It is during the Second Transi-tion that we learn new things about the foods we eat, reinforce our newly formed healthful eating habits, and find ways to improve the nutrition in our eating and enhance our eating experience through tastier recipes and more varied menus. If you initially cut down your total daily intake of fat to 20 grams, during the Second Transition, you'll aim to cut it down further, to 15 grams—which should be your ultimate goal. The dishes and menus that appear in Chapter 7 will prove even more valuable during the Second Transition.

Now we turn to each Food Setting in turn and apply the five Pas-sageways to each one. Food Journals at the ready . . . let's begin.

STAYING THE COURSE

When you talk to people who have an addiction of any sort (drugs, alcohol, gambling—and, yes, food can be an addiction for some people), they often speak of how they were doing so well controlling their urges until they fell off the wagon "just once." That one time began a
spiral of loss of control, and before they knew it, they were right back where they'd started.

That often happens to people who are trying to change their eating habits, or go on a diet if you must. They binge at a wedding or some other celebration, and their thoughts, maybe subconsciously, are "Well, it's over. I've ruined it now, clearly I've got no self-control. I'm a failure at this; I might as well keep on eating." Next stop: OBESITY!

That's *not* the way to look at it. We're all human, and we're bound to falter now and then. In fact, an occasional, small "cheat treat" may make it easier to stay on the wagon for life. The key words here are "small" and "occasional," *not* "often" and "binge"!

In any case, don't give up or despair when you falter, even if it's a big misstep. Confront your sins and resolve to do better. It's not the end of the world; you're in this for the long haul, so get right back on the horse that threw you and move on. Soon your new, healthy ways will become easier to stick to and your transgressions fewer.

FOOD SETTING ONE: BREAKFAST

PASSAGEWAY ONE: ORIENTATION

It should come as no great surprise that the Great American Breakfast—eggs and bacon with a side of grits or hash browns, or maybe a short stack of pancakes covered with maple syrup, buttered white toast, pastry (Danish or muffin), and coffee with whole milk or cream and sugar—is unhealthy. This breakfast is laden with fat and short on fiber; we're going to have to reverse that; the goal should be to reduce your daily breakfast fat intake to 7 grams and take in more fiber.

Let's look at a typical breakfast and count up the grams of fat consumed:

2 eggs = 10 grams of fat
2 strips of bacon = 7 grams of fat
Side order of hash browns = 6 grams of fat
Buttered white toast (2 slices) = 10 grams of fat
1 ounce of whole milk and sugar in coffee = 4 grams of fat
1 pastry = 5 grams of fat (at least)

That's a whopping 43 grams of fat at a minimum—almost one and a half times the amount of fat you should be consuming in an entire day! If those eggs are a three-egg cheese omelet instead, that breakfast climbs to 52 grams of fat; if instead of the hash browns there's a short stack of pancakes covered with maple syrup, you're over 60 grams of fat. If you eat cereal for breakfast instead of eggs but use whole milk on that cereal, you have gained nothing, at least as far as fat goes—a typical bowl of cereal with a cup of whole milk contains about 10 to 12 grams of fat, depending on the cereal.

For men who are determined to lose weight and who are in the high-risk group for prostate problems, these foods simply have to be eliminated from the diet. So here is the first step, Passageway One: Identify the foods you normally eat for breakfast that are high in fat content; note them in your Food Journal. On the first day of your Transition Diet, simply list the foods you habitually eat for breakfast (or cull them from the week of normal eating that you have recorded, if that is your preference).

On this first day, you'll begin to stock up on foods that are low in fat so that you will be ready for Passageway Three, two days down the road. Also on this day, buy yourself a measuring cup, preferably one that measures both cups and liquid measure (ounces).

PASSAGEWAY TWO: DEMARCATION

Now you're ready for Passageway Two: On the second day, throw the foods high in fat out—simply discard them. The whole milk— down the drain; the butter; the white bread; the pancake mix; the box of Danish pastry—into the trash. Go through all the places in your home where food is kept: the refrigerator; the cupboard; the pantry; the countertop.

Apply the same to your place of work: clean your desk of any foods that are high in fat. If you are keeping high-fat food in a lunchroom refrigerator, throw it out.

Once you have identified the places outside your home where you habitually have breakfast and determined that they are places that provide the kind of breakfast we want to avoid, then "demarcate" them—place them on the off-limits list (write them down in the Food Journal you are keeping) and simply don't set foot in those establishments.

PASSAGEWAY THREE: SUBSTITUTION

Once the forbidden foods have been identified and tossed, you're ready to substitute more healthful food that is lower in fat and higher in fiber—the all-important Passageway Three for breakfast. Here are some shopping tips to help you:

- **Have cereal for breakfast at least 4 days a week.** Make sure you buy a cereal low in fat; some cereals are high in fat, in some cases higher in fat than eggs. Even cereals such as granola and bran, which sounds very healthy, can have more than 4 grams of fat. Buy three or four kinds of cereal—setting a limit of 3 grams of fat per serving— first, to determine which you like best, and second, to alternate and introduce some variety into breakfast. Make certain that at least two of the cereals you select contain more than 4 grams of fiber per serving.

- **Get a container of 2% milk.** Naturally, it would be preferable to switch to skim milk or 1% milk, but people accustomed to whole milk find this substitution too difficult. Unless you have no objection to skim milk or 1% milk, start with 2% milk; you can go on to lower-fat milk in the Second Transition.

- **Get some whole-wheat bread.** Be careful not to get whole-wheat bread with nuts and raisins—that can be as fat-filled as white bread. Look for whole-wheat bread that contains less than one gram of fat per slice—and never have more than a single slice of bread for breakfast. Also look for whole-wheat bread with high fiber—many companies list it right on the front of the package.

- **Find a suitable substitute for butter.** That might be low-fat margarine, but be sure it has no *trans*-fats (make sure that it's really low-fat: less than 1 gram per teaspoon serving), a low-fat jam or preserve, or low-fat cream cheese.

- **Introduce fruit into your breakfast.** The best fruits to include are those high in vitamin C: strawberries, oranges, and grapefruit. (These are also high in many other phytochemicals, such as ellagic acid.) Fruit juice may be looked upon as a suitable substitute for fruit, but juices do not contain nearly as much fiber and can add many sugar calories to a meal.

- **No yolking around.** We're introducing foods to replace the egg-based breakfast at least four days a week, but on those other three days, we'll allow eggs. They have to be either egg whites—the whites contain zero fat—or a nonfat egg substitute, which is also likely to have virtually no fat.

• **Go light on the sides.** On two, and certainly no more than three, days of the week, allow yourself a breakfast side dish to replace the bacon that was a routine part of your pretransition breakfast. Substitute 1 ounce of low-fat processed meat, such as lean Canadian bacon or baked (cooked) ham, but be aware that they are likely to contain high amounts of salt. You might also look for other substitutes in the supermarket. A variety of breakfast patties and products low in fat have been produced that can replace bacon. You may also consider other foods to add to your breakfast as a side dish on the mornings you have eggs. Such foods could include vegetables—spinach, asparagus, eggplant, cucumbers, tomatoes, or carrots, all at less than one gram of fat per serving; fish—3 ounces of fresh fish poached or baked (and properly seasoned) will add no more than 3 grams of fat to breakfast, but beware of salted and cured fish, which generally has oils added to it in processing and far too much salt; and cheese—many low-fat cheeses are available on the market, including low-fat cottage cheese, and these are suitable side dishes as long as you are careful about portion size.

The following mnemonic may be helpful in your transition:

Margarine Monday: Change from butter and high-fat cream cheese to low-fat margarine, preserves, and extra-virgin olive oil.

Two Percent Tuesday: Change from whole milk to 2% milk.

Whole-Wheat Wednesday: Change from white bread to whole-wheat bread that is high in fiber.

Cereal Thursday: Make cereal your main course for breakfast at least four days a week.

Fruity Friday: Add fruit to breakfast, either on cereal or as a side dish.

Egg Substitute Saturday: On those few days a week you'll be having eggs, make it egg substitutes or two egg whites.

Side Dish Sunday: Add a side dish (other than fruit, which you will add to every breakfast) on no more than three days a week. Make it low-fat breakfast meat, fish, or cheese.

A Word About Coffee

Coffee is something that Americans have become so used to that it seems pointless to recommend giving it up (in favor of coffee substitutes, decaffeinated coffee, or tea). Caffeine is a stimulant (that's why it's so useful in getting us up to speed in the morning), but that means it also stimulates our appetite. There are ample opportunities to turn a fat-free cup of coffee into a fat fest by adding milk, sugar, and pastry. So if coffee is a must for breakfast, try to adopt the following practices:

• Use 2% or fat-free milk only; never whole milk or cream (not even a little). Milk in cereal is a greater taste challenge than in coffee, and you'll find it easier to take the change in coffee lightener. Also, many people use milk or cream to cool the coffee, but it would cool by itself after just a minute or two.

• A number of sugar substitutes are available. Some pose health risks of their own, and we are loath to recommend them. Some are natural, made with such substances as maltodextrin and sucralose, both derived from sugar (such as the product sold as Splenda), but most people find it difficult to accept their taste. Our best advice is to reduce your use of sweetener in coffee—gradually, if you like, cutting it in half every two days. You might also keep your intake of coffee low—no more than a cup in the morning, and if you get it to go, make it a small. Make an effort during this Transition to have no fewer than three breakfasts of the workweek at home (and, of course, all weekend and nonworkday breakfasts). Then systematically go to having all breakfasts at home.

PASSAGEWAY FOUR: MINDFULNESS

The essence of Passageway Four is keeping track of your progress and documenting your eating regime, one Food Setting at a time.

PASSAGEWAY FIVE: REINFORCEMENT

Once you have spent a week transitioning (either all at once or piecemeal) your breakfast, you may want to take another week to let the routine become established. In Passageway Five, you will want to fine-tune the Transition; try various acceptable foods (different cereals, egg substitutes, side dishes); explore different food markets; examine different eateries or breakfast options; even experiment with changing your sleep and commuting patterns so that you can more easily have breakfast at home.

It is also important to resolve to **get breakfast in order before going on to the next Food Setting.** For most people, we think this will require one extra week, possibly two, so that the Transition for the first Food Setting—breakfast—could well take three weeks. Record everything carefully in your Food Journal and note your progress; even note your failures.

FOOD SETTING TWO: LUNCH

We next come to lunch. We need to distinguish between the lunch you make for yourself—either at home or one that you prepare ahead of time (the night before or in the morning) and take to work—and the lunch you eat out. In many urban settings, a very high percentage of people (in some areas as many as 80 percent) eat lunch in a restaurant or at a lunch counter—or worse, in a fast-food outlet.

PASSAGEWAY ONE: ORIENTATION

Eating out: Delis and lunch counters are notorious for providing large portions and sandwiches that are drenched with mayonnaise and laden with fat. A typical tuna fish sandwich can average about 30 grams of fat—almost your entire daily fat allotment! Beef sandwiches are even worse, since inexpensive restaurants routinely seek out the fattier cuts of beef. Restaurants often fill the plate with potato chips or mayonnaise-rich coleslaw—both very high in fat.

For this Passageway, it may be necessary to do a bit of scouting: explore the area for a radius of several blocks. You are looking for grocery stores where you can buy fresh food and fruits and vegetables or establishments that make the nutritional content (especially the fat content) of their prepared foods clear.

It is also important to set up your workplace to accommodate healthier eating with a refrigerator for storing food brought from home and a microwave for heating food.

PASSAGEWAY TWO: DEMARCATION
Avoid:

• **The classic sandwich.** The classic tuna salad, egg salad, or chicken salad sandwich has to become a thing of the past. The same is true of the classic hamburger, especially in a fast-food outlet, and most especially if a slice of cheese is added.

• **The deadly salad.** Just because a dish is called a salad doesn't mean it's healthy and low in fat or calories. Salads typically include high-fat dressings, eggs, cheese, oil-soaked croutons, bacon or meat strips, and possibly an edible pastry shell.

• **Ethnic foods.** These can be very dangerous and unhealthy. Duck—a staple in Chinese cuisine—is quite fatty, and many dishes are deep-fried (particularly breaded chicken and meat as well as lo mein, noodle, and sweet-and-sour dishes). Mexican food can also be very high in fat, especially refried beans, nacho chips (even dipped in salsa, which, because of its low fat content and tomato base, can be good for you), fried meats (used in fajitas, enchiladas, etc.), and the particularly misleading "taco salad," which can pack more than 50 grams of fat and more than a thousand calories. Delis are also great sources of fat: the complimentary dish of coleslaw that is placed on the table before you even order is likely to contain an entire day's al-lotment of fat. Cold cuts are almost always very high in fat and sodium (even when advertised as lean and low-salt), and there are very few side dishes on any delicatessen menu we've ever seen that aren't brimming with fat, salt, and calories.

• **Side dishes.** The foods that are typically placed alongside the sandwich, the omelette, or the piece of fish you are having for lunch constitute one of the chief sources of fat in the lunch menu. French fries, refried beans, onion rings, potato salad, coleslaw—these are all laden with fat. And if we (in a burst of health-consciousness) substi-tute a salad for the fried side dish, we are apt to add a heavy salad dressing that adds even more fat to the meal.

• **Dessert.** If you have had a decent lunch, there should be no earthly reason to add a pastry or pudding for desert. Dessert should be relegated to special occasions and then thoughtfully planned and created.

PASSAGEWAY THREE: SUBSTITUTION

Once the forbidden foods have been identified and tossed, you are going to have to reconstruct your lunch, do a little experimenta-tion, and find the foods you like and that satisfy you. Here are some of the food areas in which to look:

• **Sandwiches.** If you like having a sandwich for lunch (some people are simply used to it), try to make the sandwich yourself and "brown-bag" it to work. Use high-fiber whole-wheat bread; a wide variety of whole-wheat breads—pitas, English muffins, French and Italian breads, fruit-flavored loaves, etc.—is now available.

If you are having meat for dinner, try to avoid meat at lunch that day. The daily intake of meat should not exceed 6 ounces—about the size of two decks of playing cards. Trim away all fat visible on the edge and inside the meat, and try broiling or microwaving it instead of frying it. You might also like to experiment with stir-fries and casseroles, which use meat to flavor vegetables, but beware of casserole recipes that rely on butter and rich sauces. Many good low-fat casseroles use vegetables and grains in a three-to-one ratio (three parts vegetables to one part meat) for a tasty and satisfying meal.

Here are some specific guidelines for adding healthier meat to your diet:

• **Beef, veal, or pork.** Top round cuts, at 5.5 grams of fat per 3 ounce serving, are preferable to bottom round, eye of round, sirloin, or tenderloin, all of which contain 7.5 to 8.5 grams per 3 ounces. Veal and pork are generally less fatty—a pork tenderloin (cut lean, meaning with all fat removed) has about 4 grams of fat per 3 ounces; veal cutlet and veal chop have about the same; veal loin chops are higher at 7.5 grams per 3 ounces.

• **Chicken, turkey, or duck.** Chicken and turkey are good choices for meat dishes; duck is not. Duck without the skin still has 9.5 grams of fat per 3 ounces, and with the skin, the fat content per 3 ounces balloons to a whopping 24 grams. As for chicken and turkey: turkey is lower in fat than chicken for comparable cuts—turkey white meat without skin has about 2.5 grams of fat per 3 ounces, while chicken white meat comes in at about 4 grams per 3 ounces. Add skin to either, and you add 5 grams of fat. The dark meat of both chicken and turkey has double the fat content of white meat, so that 3 ounces of chicken dark meat with skin can contain 13.5 grams of fat.

• **Seafood.** Not all seafood is equal when it comes to fat: there is high-fat seafood and low-fat seafood. In the United States, people are often under the misapprehension that all fish tastes the same—like fish. That's not true if it's fresh and prepared properly. Learning to eat fish and find it tasty is an important health skill; it may require some testing and experimentation until you find the kind of seafood you like best.

In the low-fat category—all with about 1 gram of fat per 3-ounce serving—are bass, bream, cod, crappie, flounder, grouper, haddock, halibut, mahimahi, perch, pike, red snapper, rockfish, scrod, speckled trout, sunfish, sole, and fresh tuna. Shellfish—clams, crayfish, lobsters, scallops, and shrimp—generally have 2 grams of fat per 3 ounces; oysters are a bit fattier, coming in at 4 grams per 3 ounces. In the medium-fat category—fish containing about 5 grams of fat per 3 ounces, so it is not too bad—are angelfish, bluefish, catfish, croaker, fresh sardines, kingfish, mackerel, orange roughy, shark, swordfish, trout, whitefish, and yellowtail. High in fat—8 to 10 grams of fat per 3 ounces—are pompano, salmon, and wahoo. However, the fat in these fish is high in omega-3's and other unsaturated fats that are actually beneficial. For seafood, the no-skin rule applies just as it does for fowl: skin adds fat, nearly doubling what is contained in the meat of the seafood.

• **Salads.** One of the (few) encouraging developments in American cuisine is the comeback salads are making, but we still have a long way to go. The key to making salads enjoyable and satisfying is variety: use a mix of ingredients, combining classic vegetable fare—lettuce, tomato, cucumber, green pepper—with other vegetables—asparagus, artichokes, broccoli, carrots, cauliflower, green beans, parsnips, peas, radishes, squash—along with beans and nuts (measured carefully), fruits, mushrooms, and some spices—basil, ginger, mint, oregano, rosemary. Dressings on salads are a source of trouble: we tend to use too much. Many low-fat salad dressings are available, but for all dressings, the basic rule is: Less is more. Add it with a spoon instead of pouring it out of a bottle or a carafe.

• **Fruits and vegetables.** It is ironic that in a country as bountiful as ours, people are virtual strangers to fruits and vegetables. This is in part due to the fact that we are so far removed from the sources of fresh fruits and vegetables. Become reacquainted with the many varieties of apples there are on the market, many with very different tastes and textures, and the many fruits in the orange, plum, berry, and melon families. Spend time with your greengrocer.

Having Lunch Out

We have been urging you to prepare your lunch at home and bring it to work as often as possible. But there are going to be situations that make that impossible and you are going to have to eat out. Here are some tips on ordering a nutritious meal that will keep the fat down.

• **Stay away from fast food.** Fast-food establishments are unhealthy not simply because of the content of their food and the way they prepare it but because eating food fast promotes undisciplined, unmindful eating.

• **Be precise in your order.** A "number two" from virtually any menu will almost certainly arrive with fatty side dishes and elements. Instead, order exactly what you want and no more.

• **Take your time while eating.** The bustle of a restaurant at lunchtime can get you caught up in the frenzied way people eat, and before you know it, you're paying the check and leaving a tip and you're not even aware of what you ate or even *that* you ate.

PASSAGEWAY FOUR: MINDFULNESS

The kind of record keeping that you applied to breakfast has to be applied to lunch as well, even though in the middle of the workday you may be rushed and preoccupied.

PASSAGEWAY FIVE: REINFORCEMENT

One of the great challenges of this Food Setting is all the ways you can fall off track. You're away from home; you're at work; you're involved in the work of the day; you're meeting people for a business lunch; you're pressed for time. That's why transitioning lunch may be difficult. We can only advise that you keep at it: don't give up—and *don't go on to the next Food Setting until you have a solid week of healthy lunches under your belt.*

FOOD SETTING THREE: AFTERNOON SNACK

You may have noticed that we have not included a midmorning snack in this scheme. A decent breakfast and a nutritious lunch should get most people to the afternoon sufficiently satisfied and energized. *If* a snack is necessary, it should be eaten in the afternoon. If a morning snack is preferable, apply what we say here to that snack—but don't have both. Afternoon snack or morning snack—take your pick.

As with other Food Settings, you may have to go through a Transition here as well: start with a morning snack *and* an afternoon snack *and* a late-night snack, and slowly cut one of them out entirely.

PASSAGEWAY ONE: ORIENTATION

Studies have shown that many Americans consume a quarter of their day's fat during a snacking episode in the afternoon or late at night, and that this will often contain more than 15 grams in a single sitting. Clearly, this kind of snacking has to go.

The first step is to note (in your Food Journal) what you are eating now, then eliminate the foods that are high in fat and substitute healthy foods that are low in fat.

PASSAGEWAY TWO: DEMARCATION

Read labels and take note of the fat content of foods and how much fat you ingest every day.

SNACK SUBSTITUTIONS

INSTEAD OF	*HAVE ONE SERVING OF*
½ cup chocolate pudding (4.5 grams of fat)	Fat-free chocolate pudding (0.2 gram of fat)
½ cup ice cream (16 grams of fat)	Fat-free ice cream or yogurt (0.2 gram of fat)
½-inch slice pound cake (6 grams of fat)	Angel food cake (0 gram of fat)
1 oatmeal raisin cookie (8 grams of fat)	1 fat-free cookie (0 gram of fat)
1 cream puff filled with custard (9 grams of fat)	1 fat-free pastry (0 gram of fat)
1 ounce of potato chips (12–14 grams of fat)	1 ounce of fat-free potato chips (0 gram of fat)
1 ounce tortilla chips (8 grams of fat)	1 ounce of fat-free tortilla chips (0.5 gram of fat)
Cake icing (15 grams of fat)	No-fat frosting (0 gram of fat)

PASSAGEWAY THREE: SUBSTITUTION

Once the forbidden foods have been identified and tossed, it's time to replace the snacks you've been eating with less fatty, more healthful foods. Most of us have little trouble identifying the snack foods that are high in fat, such as potato chips, cookies, and the like. Fortunately, there are now many low-fat snack foods on the market, so you needn't feel deprived (at least not as deprived).

Here are some things to watch out for and think about when you plan your snacking regimen:

- **First, *have* a snacking regimen.** Never buy a snack food impulsively. Plan your snack for any given day no later than the previous meal. Even better, plan the entire week of snacking ahead of time.
- **Variety is critical.** Planning makes it easier to introduce variety into snacking—alternate fruit and fat-free baked snacks during the week.
- **Make it fruit.** Fruit is by far the healthiest choice you can make for a snack. But try to be selective here as well. An avocado is quite high in fat—an average whole avocado contains 27 grams of fat.
- **Make it "zero."** Whichever snack food you choose, try to limit your snack to a food with less than a full gram of fat—a food that has 0.9 gram of fat or less.
- **Sit and eat.** Don't eat "on the run" or while you are working.

PASSAGEWAY FOUR: MINDFULNESS

As with other Food Settings, it is vital that you record your eating habits. Being mindful is particularly important in this Food Setting, since so much snacking is unplanned and unscheduled—and that leads to eating without being aware of what you are eating or even *that* you are eating. Record not only *what* you eat as a snack, but *when you eat it—the exact time of day.*

PASSAGEWAY FIVE: REINFORCEMENT

It is likely that some exploration of the neighborhood and experimentation with different foods will be necessary until you find snacks that satisfy both your hunger and your taste buds. Don't leave this Food Setting until you have gone through an entire week—

QUICK NOTES ON ADDED FATS
Here are some points about fat to bear in mind when preparing food:

- 1 teaspoon of butter adds **4 grams of fat** to a slice of bread.
- 2 teaspoons of butter to grill a sandwich add **8 grams of fat.**
- 1 tablespoon of oil and vinegar dressing adds **7 grams of fat** to salad.
- Pan-frying meat, poultry, or fish adds **11 grams of fat** to a 3-ounce serving.
- Deep-frying adds **15 grams of fat** to a 3-ounce serving of breaded meat, poultry, or fish.
- 3 tablespoons of gravy add **2 grams of fat** to a 3-ounce serving of meat or poultry.
- 2 tablespoons of cream or cream sauce add **10 grams of fat** to potatoes.
- Marinating or stir-frying adds **4 grams of fat** to vegetables.
- Deep-frying adds **8 grams of fat** to ½ cup of vegetables or potatoes.

seven full days—of healthy snacking; that is, eating only snacks that are low in fat.

FOOD SETTING FOUR: DINNER

In most American homes, dinner is the big meal of the day. Let's go through the five Passageways for the transitioning of this Food Setting.

PASSAGEWAY ONE: ORIENTATION

More than in any other Food Setting, taste is important at dinner. Yet many people "chow down" at dinner the way they do during the rest of the day, when they are just looking for sustenance to get through the day. Paying attention to the environment in which we have dinner will pay dividends in making the dining experience more pleasurable—and that will help keep the menu healthy, which is, after all, our ultimate goal.

• **Set the setting.** Try to make the area where you have dinner as neat and as pleasant as possible. Get the papers off the table; put on a tablecloth, placemats, napkins (even if they are paper ones), and place settings.

• **Conduct the meal.** Don't slap together a meal from what happens to be in the cupboard or refrigerator at the moment. Plan all dinners, if possible, at the beginning of the week.

ON FOOD PREPARATION

We've already seen how important it is to prepare food properly if it is to be truly healthy and nutritious. Here are some further tips on healthy food preparation:

- Braise food in flavored liquid, never in fat or oil.
- Use yogurt for sauces instead of cream.
- Stir-frying in a wok (or even in a standard nonstick frying pan) provides the flavor of frying without as much grease and fat.
- Consider alternatives to frying, such as broiling, poaching (particularly fish), and boiling (such as for pasta dishes).

- **Put down the paper, turn the TV off; turn yourself on.** Concentrate on the tastes and textures of the food in front of you.

PASSAGEWAY TWO: DEMARCATION

We have to learn not to add side dishes impulsively to a main dish. And we have to learn that it's no crime to leave some food on the plate.

Here are some other dinnertime suggestions:

- **Cut the meat—especially red meat—and you'll cut the fat.** By now, this message should be well known to you: meat is a major source of fat in the American diet, and we would all do well to cut down on the amount we consume. Start out by limiting the number of meals per week in which you consume meat to three, and then cut that down by one or two more meals, so that you transition to having only one meat meal per week.
- **Getting there is half the battle (and a lot of the fun).** The preparation of dinner ought to be an important part of the enjoyment of the dinner experience. Devoting some effort to preparing dinner—even if it's only popping something into the microwave—will give you a greater sense of control over your dinner eating.

PASSAGEWAY THREE: SUBSTITUTION

Although the next chapter contains menus and recipes for all Food Settings, the material on Dinner is probably the part you'll find most useful. Chef Mark Erickson from the Culinary Institute of

America has prepared these recipes with taste uppermost in mind, and we think you'll find it *is* possible to eat well and feel satisfied while consuming no more than 20 grams of fat a day.

• **Quality trumps quantity.** Replacing large quantities of food (and getting one's satisfaction from the sheer bulk of what we are eating) with food that is well made, tasty, and modest in size while still being satisfying—that's the essence of good eating.

• **Fresh trumps canned.** As much as possible, opt for fresh ingredients over canned, packaged, or prepared foods. In addition to giving you control over the amount and content of the food you eat, you will avoid the high salt and other flavor additives that food manufacturers (even of low-fat products) add to their food.

• **Taste it!** *Really* **taste it!** Zen masters teach the importance of concentrating on the taste of each mouthful when eating. In addition to allowing a meal to last longer and thus requiring less food to satisfy your hunger, you will also enjoy the eating experience more. During the rest of the day, we are rushed and preoccupied, but at dinner, we often have more time.

PASSAGEWAY FOUR: MINDFULNESS
Plan your meals—preferably well in advance—and focus on the eating experience—the taste; the environment; the company—during the meal. Once the meal is over, we recommend that you not only record what you ate but that you also:

• **Record the occasion.** Add a note of the same kind—where you sat; who was at the table; what was discussed; what the weather outside was like—anything that can be routinely repeated that will separate the dinner experience from the other eating experiences of the day.

PASSAGEWAY FIVE: REINFORCEMENT
If you are in this Food Setting of the Transition Diet, your eating habits have already undergone quite a change. This would be a good time to take stock of how you are doing. Once you have adjusted the dinner Food Setting, start recording full days where you have adhered to the Transition Diet for the first four Food Settings. If you spend a solid week transitioning the breakfast, lunch, afternoon

snack, and dinner, then you are well along in transitioning to a healthy diet. You'll then be ready to tackle two Food Settings that often are the undoing of the best-planned diets—late-night snacks and eating out.

• **Watch out for "portion creep."** One thing you have to be vigilant against is "portion creep"—the tendency of the portions in each meal to get larger and larger as the day goes on. This is especially dangerous at dinner, where you are more likely to be designing the plate, than in other settings (where someone else is preparing the food or else it comes in discrete portions). Try to use the same plates for dinner meals as for lunch and breakfast.

FOOD SETTING FIVE: LATE-NIGHT SNACK

More diets and eating plans come apart late at night than at any other time. It is when we are tired and when we have time to brood about any problems we might be having in our lives. The nexus between emotion and hunger is a complicated one that we are just beginning to understand.

We recommend that you apply the same technique to this Food Setting as you have to the others. That way, even if it hasn't been "planned" like the other meals, it will never get out of control.

PASSAGEWAY ONE: ORIENTATION

Late as it is, record what you eat and evaluate it over the course of a week or two.

• **Make sure sleep isn't the problem.** Many people who eat late at night do so because they are having trouble sleeping; conversely, eating late at night can interfere with sleeping. It's a vicious circle. If you have a problem sleeping, try reading a book. If you still consistently have trouble sleeping, you might want to get a sleep evaluation or study to find the problem, certainly before you resort to sleep medications.

PASSAGEWAY TWO: DEMARCATION

A late-night snack is so decidedly a "snack of opportunity" that not having unhealthy foods easily available is essential to preventing late-night binge eating.

PASSAGEWAY THREE: SUBSTITUTION

Once the forbidden foods have been identified and tossed, replace them with some healthy foods. You can refer to what we have said about afternoon snacks and make those the basis for this Food Setting, but we think it is more advisable to set aside particular foods that are this Food Setting's alone. That will make the late-night snack a treat instead of more of the same. Here are two recommendations; alternate and introduce lots of variety into this as you have tried to do with the Food Settings:

- **Fruit and cheese.** Berries (strawberries, blueberries, or raspberries) and a half cup of low-fat cottage cheese or a soft cheese such as low-fat ricotta or mozzarella.
- **Green tea with toast and jam.** Now's an excellent time to enjoy the soothing qualities of green tea. Drink half a cup with the berries and cheese or with a fat-free whole-wheat cracker or a single slice of whole-wheat toast (or fat-free Melba toast) with a smear of jam or preserve.

PASSAGEWAY FOUR: MINDFULNESS

Record a thought or two, but set yourself a limit: one or two lines; ten to fifteen words; a single sentence, or two at the most—and stick to it.

PASSAGEWAY FIVE: REINFORCEMENT

You may need a few days of experimentation to find the kind of late-night snack that's right for you—give yourself a week to find those foods and stock up on them. Don't consider the Transition for this Food Setting complete until you have completed a solid week of low-fat late-night snacking.

FOOD SETTING SIX: EATING OUT

Now we come to the last Food Setting. There will surely be times when you feel you have to go out for a meal in order to satisfy your hunger, celebrate an occasion, and/or socialize with family and friends.

PASSAGEWAY ONE: ORIENTATION

If you are going out to a restaurant, it is important for you to evaluate what kinds of foods will be available and how they will be prepared. Clearly, whenever you have a choice, you will want to choose a restaurant that will give you the opportunity to select a healthy meal.

PASSAGEWAY TWO: DEMARCATION
Stay away from fast-food outlets and steak houses that serve food—especially meat—in gargantuan portions.

• **Watch out for appetizers, hors d'oeuvres—and cocktails.** If you do choose an appetizer, you might want to skip the main course. In many fine restaurants, one or two appetizers can be an entire meal—tasty and filling without going off the scale nutritionally.

• **Stay out of the bread basket.** If the bread proves too tempting, don't hesitate to ask the waiter to remove it from the table.

• **Watch those desserts.** If you absolutely have to have dessert, go for fresh fruit or at least share a dessert with someone. You might also apply what we call "the rule of 10": take a bite from the dessert and rate it on a scale of 1 to 10. If the dessert rates a 10, take another spoonful (or forkful) and rate it again: if it still gets a 10, continue— but stop the instant the dessert no longer rates that 10. In most cases, you will find the dessert has lost its special flavor after the first three or four mouthfuls. Leave the rest.

• **Take your time.** No matter how many glares you get from the waiter or the maître d', take your time with dinner, eat slowly.

PASSAGEWAY THREE: SUBSTITUTION
• **Don't be bashful—ask!** Don't be afraid to ask about what is in the dishes that are on the menu, and don't be hesitant to ask for a substitution: vegetables for a starchy side dish; poaching instead of frying. Most restaurants will be happy to prepare your food the way you prefer—you are, after all, the customer.

PASSAGEWAY FOUR: MINDFULNESS
Here, record keeping can be very important. Some people find a restaurant they like and keep going there; others prefer to try new ones and not to eat at the same place twice. Either way, keeping a record of the eating-out experience is important.

PASSAGEWAY FIVE: REINFORCEMENT
Because we are trying to cut down the eating-out episodes to no more than one per week, don't consider this Food Setting complete

or yourself transitioned until you can point to thirty consecutive days during which you have eaten out—and done so healthfully—only four times.

A PARTING WORD

The program we have just gone through is not an easy one: no truly effective diet can be all that easy. We have taken the approach that you are trying to alter the way you eat so that you eat less fat and more fiber, and eat more healthfully. Transitioning to a healthier eating lifestyle will have a positive influence over many other aspects of your life. The important thing to remember is that this is a one-step-at-a-time program. Each step may have fits and starts, victories and defeats, progress and backsliding, but staying with it over thirty days, sixty days, or even six months—however long it takes to complete the Transition—will result in a healthier you.

7. MENUS AND RECIPES: PROSTATE HEALTH, THE DELICIOUS WAY!

CHOOSING THE RIGHT MEALS

Good nutrition is the foundation of prostate cancer prevention. However, nutritious meals don't have to be bland or taste awful. Pizza . . . pasta . . . corn and crab chowder . . . tortilla pie . . . citrus baked snapper . . . veal and eggplant casserole . . . yogurt and berry parfait . . . all these can help keep your prostate healthy.

Prostate-healthy meals *can* taste great! Master Chef Mark Erickson of the Culinary Institute of America has developed these unique recipes in conjunction with the Institute for Cancer Prevention. We've provided you with a varied, nutritious Seven-Day Menu Plan, as well as a sampling of recipes for many of the scrumptious meals contained in the plan. Everything else is simple enough to find in any ordinary household cookbook—or you can access *all* the recipes on the Institute for Cancer Prevention website (www.ifcp.us)—or look for the IFCP cookbook now being produced by the IFCP volunteer action group with Chef Erickson and the Culinary Institute of America.

But suppose you're the kind of guy who hasn't cooked anything since he broke out the hot plate during college? Don't panic. These recipes are *easy* to prepare and quick. You'll have fun making them. Getting involved in the cooking of your meals is part of the satisfaction and joy of eating—a joy that we often substitute for simply by eating more.

Then again, the person reading this may be the one who does the cooking in the house and not the person who needs a prostate health plan! All right, then, ladies—these recipes are ones your guy will love and they will keep him healthy (and he will more than likely lose weight in the bargain). While prostate health counts most in these unique recipes, the pleasure is in the eating! Enjoy!

THE SEVEN-DAY MENU PLAN

Refer to the individual recipes for one serving size. (Dishes for which recipes appear in the recipe section below are indicated by page number—but recipes for the entire menu are on the IFCP website: www.ifcp.us.)

Day One

Breakfast
Bran cereal (1 cup) with skim milk (1 cup) and strawberries (½ cup)
Half grapefruit
Green tea (decaffeinated, if preferred)

A.M. *Snack*
(All snacks are optional; too much snacking can throw you off track if you're on a weight-loss diet. All the snacks that appear here are low-fat and prostate-friendly.)
Low-fat fruit yogurt (1 cup)

Lunch
Barley Risotto (page 133)
Fresh-squeezed fruit juice

P.M. *Snack*
Apple

Dinner
Pinto bean soup
Tossed Salad (2 cups lettuce) with Creamy Herb Salad Dressing (page 138)
New England Shore Dinner (page 127)

Cherry Rice Pudding Brûlée (page 144)
Green tea

Day Two
Breakfast
Apple and raisin bran muffin with fruit preserves (2 tablespoons)
Orange
Soy milk (1 cup)

A.M. *Snack*
Banana

Lunch
Curried chicken salad pita sandwich
Carrot sticks (2 ounces)
Green tea

P.M. *Snack*
Air-popped popcorn (2 cups)
Low-fat fruit yogurt (1 cup)

Dinner
Tossed salad (2 cups) with low-fat Italian dressing
Tomato, Mozzarella, and Basil Pizzas (page 128)
Fresh steamed zucchini (⅔ cup)
Fresh cherries
Green tea

Day Three
Breakfast
Swiss muesli
Cranberry juice cocktail (½ cup)
Honey whole-wheat bread with preserves (2 tablespoons)
Soy milk (1 cup)

A.M. *Snack*
Orange

Lunch
Pasta and Shrimp Salad (page 131)
Green tea

P.M. Snack
Oven-baked tortilla chips with low-fat salsa

Dinner
Pinto bean soup
Grain burgers
Mashed Sweet Potatoes with Ginger (page 135)
Fresh steamed broccoli (⅔ cup)
Carrot Custard (page 143)
Green tea

Day Four
Breakfast
Peach and ricotta pancakes
Orange
Soy milk (1 cup)

A.M. Snack
Apple and raisin bran muffin

Lunch
Mexican tortilla pie
Fresh-squeezed fruit juice (2 cups)

P.M. Snack
Air-popped popcorn (2 cups)

Dinner
Hearty Lentil Soup (page 130)
Country-Style Pasta (page 122)
Tapioca pudding with figs and basil
Green tea

Day Five

Breakfast
Apple, raisin, and cheese blintzes
Half grapefruit
Soy milk (1 cup)

A.M. *Snack*
Apple and raisin bran muffin
Banana

Lunch
Tuna fish sandwich (6 ounces tuna, water-packed) on honey
　whole-wheat bread
Jicama Slaw (page 134)
Fresh-squeezed fruit juice (2 cups)

P.M. *Snack*
Soy nuts (½ cup)

Dinner
Lettuce salad (2 cups) with low-fat creamy herb salad dressing
Fusilli Pasta with Pan-Grilled Chicken and Red Pepper Sauce
　(page 123)
Fresh Potato Salad (page 129)
Bran bread (2 slices)
Burgundy Poached Peach with Its Sherbet (page 142)
Green tea

Day Six

Breakfast
Mix of Total (½ cup) and All-Bran (½ cup) cereals with strawberries
　(½ cup) and skim milk (1 cup)
Orange
Whole wheat toast
Green tea

A.M. *Snack*
Apple

Lunch
New England clam chowder
Honey whole-wheat bread
Soy milk (1 cup)

P.M. Snack
Oven-Dried Tomatoes (page 140)

Dinner
Black bean and cornmeal loaf (appetizer)
Veal and Eggplant Casserole (page 125)
Brown rice pilaf
Fresh steamed lima beans (⅔ cup)
Warm apricot pudding
Green tea

Day Seven

Breakfast
Whole-wheat apricot and cheese crêpes with Berry and Amaretto
    Breakfast Syrup (page 137)
Apple and raisin bran muffin
Green tea

A.M. Snack
Nonfat yogurt (1 cup)
Banana

Lunch
Grain burger
Fresh-squeezed fruit juice (2 cups)

P.M. Snack
Orange

Dinner
Summer Gazpacho (page 132)
Seven-Vegetable Couscous with Harissa Sauce (page 136)
Yogurt and Berry Parfait Americana (page 145)
Green tea

RECIPES

MAIN DISHES

The main dishes in the menu and the sampling we provide here have an underlying theme: "main" doesn't mean "only." American main dishes are so central to the meal that all the other elements of the meal are just not treated with respect. Think in terms of the whole meal, and don't demand that the main dish carry the entire burden of providing a satisfying meal.

COUNTRY-STYLE PASTA

Yield: 2 servings

Pasta meals can be quite hearty and easy to prepare, and this dish contains a generous helping of nature's own bounty—fresh vegetables. Getting to like pasta and center meals around it is an important step toward lowering fat and increasing fiber in your diet.

1 cup dry pasta (bowtie, fusilli, penne, or rigatoni)
2 teaspoons olive oil
¼ cup diced prosciutto
¼ cup chopped onion
2 cloves garlic, chopped
2 cups packed coarsely shredded escarole

1 cup drained, cooked white beans (canned)
1 tomato, seeded and chopped
1 cup chicken broth
¼ teaspoon black pepper
2 tablespoons chopped fresh basil
¼ cup grated Parmesan cheese

1. Cook the pasta in a large quantity of boiling water until tender. Drain, rinse, and reserve.

2. Heat the olive oil in a 2-quart saucepan over moderate heat. Add the prosciutto and fry for 1 minute. Add the onions and garlic and cook until the onions become translucent, about 4 minutes. Add the escarole and cook until it wilts, about 2 minutes.

3. Add the beans, tomato, cooked pasta, and chicken broth and bring to a simmer. Cook for about 5 minutes, until the flavors are well incorporated.

4. Remove from the heat and add the pepper and basil.

5. Divide into 2 servings and top each with Parmesan cheese.

Per serving:
Fat grams 11   Protein grams 29
Fiber grams 12   Carbohydrate grams 73
Calories 504   Sodium milligrams 714

FUSILLI PASTA WITH PAN-GRILLED CHICKEN AND RED PEPPER SAUCE

Yield: 4 servings

Avoid traditionally grilled foods, since there is evidence that foods grilled directly over burning fuels such as charcoal and wood produce nasty carcinogens. Unfortunately, there's a price to pay, as grilling is an excellent low-fat cooking technique.

We can simulate some of the appeal of grilled foods by using a pan grill, which is a cast-iron skillet with a ribbed cooking surface. As the meat cooks, excess fat drains away along the ribs while the pan's surface gives the meat the "scored" appearance of food grilled over a flame.

Lightly coat the pan grill with nonstick vegetable spray before using to keep the food from sticking, and never scrub it with anything more abrasive than a soapy sponge or dishcloth. (Also, store the pan grill with a light film of vegetable oil rubbed on its surface to prevent rusting.)

½ teaspoon salt
⅛ teaspoon white pepper
1 tablespoon lemon juice
2 cloves garlic, minced
12 ounces chicken breasts, boneless and skinless
3 cups fusilli pasta
1 cup Red Pepper Sauce (see IFCP website)

2 tablespoons chopped fresh basil
3 tablespoons ripe olives (preferably Kalamata), pitted and coarsely chopped
¼ cup grated Parmesan cheese (or crumbled mild chèvre [goat] cheese)

1. Combine the salt, pepper, lemon juice, and garlic in a shallow bowl to make a marinade. Add the chicken breasts and coat well. Allow to marinate for at least 1 hour. Preheat the broiler or grill.

2. Cook the pasta in a large quantity of boiling water until tender. Drain but do not rinse, and keep hot.

3. Heat the Red Pepper Sauce in a large saucepan. Add the basil and olives. Combine the sauce and cooked pasta and toss until well coated.

4. Remove the chicken breasts from the marinade and pat dry. Pan-broil for 4 to 5 minutes on each side, or until the outside is golden brown and the pink color in the center is almost gone.

5. Divide the pasta among 4 serving plates and sprinkle with cheese. Slice the cooked chicken breasts into finger-sized pieces, arrange them over the pasta, and serve.

Per serving:

Fat grams 6	*Protein grams 35*
Fiber grams 3	*Carbohydrate grams 47*
Calories 392	*Sodium milligrams 426*

VEAL AND EGGPLANT CASSEROLE

Yield: 6 servings

There are few dishes as delicious as a traditional Greek moussaka, and here is a healthy variation on that theme.

What is different here is that we broil the eggplant instead of frying it in oil. We have also revised the ingredients of the rich custard topping. As a result, this dish remains low-fat without losing any flavor.

This is a great dish to cook in advance and keep in the fridge. A few tricks will help you so it looks and tastes just right. Cut it when it's chilled, reheat it in the microwave, and then slip it under the broiler to make the top crisp. The recipe looks long, but it's really very simple.

1 large eggplant (about 2 pounds)	1 bay leaf
1 pound lean ground veal	1 teaspoon dried oregano
1 onion, diced	1/4 teaspoon salt
4 cloves garlic, minced	1/4 teaspoon black pepper
1 red bell pepper, diced	1/4 cup all-purpose flour
1 green bell pepper, diced	1 1/2 cups skim milk
1 cup tomato sauce (canned or	1/2 cup grated Parmesan cheese
fresh)	1/2 cup chopped basil
1/4 teaspoon cinnamon	3 egg whites
1/8 teaspoon allspice	

1. Preheat the broiler to high. Slice the eggplant lengthwise so it's about 3/8 inch thick. Place the eggplant slices on the broiler rack and brown on both sides. Remove from heat and set aside.

2. Lightly coat a skillet with nonstick vegetable spray and add the veal. When the meat is first added, it will give off a great deal of moisture. As it cooks, the moisture will evaporate and the meat will begin to brown. As the meat browns, break it into clumps with a fork.

3. When the veal is lightly browned, add the onions, garlic, and peppers. Sauté until the onions are translucent. Add the tomato sauce, cinnamon, allspice, bay leaf, oregano, salt, and pepper. Bring to a simmer and cook for 15 minutes, stirring often to prevent scorching. Remove from heat, discard the bay leaf, and set the meat aside.

4. Combine the flour and skim milk in a small saucepan and place over medium heat. Stir constantly until the contents thicken and

come to a boil. Simmer lightly for 10 minutes and remove from heat. Add the Parmesan cheese and basil and mix well. Place the egg whites in a small bowl and beat lightly. Pour the hot liquid over the eggs while whisking. Set this aside.

5. Preheat oven to 350 degrees.

6. Lightly coat a 9-by-9-inch pan with nonstick vegetable spray. Line the bottom of the pan with one third of the browned eggplant as you would pasta for lasagna. Run the slices up the sides so they hang slightly over the edge of the pan. Place half of the meat sauce in the pan and spread evenly. Layer another third of the eggplant so that it just covers the meat sauce. Add the remaining meat sauce and repeat with the eggplant. Flap over any eggplant that hangs over the edge of the pan so that it completely seals the layers. Pour the cheese sauce over the top.

7. Bake for 1 hour, or until the cheese sauce is well browned. Remove from the oven and allow to cool slightly before cutting into 6 servings.

Per serving:
Fat grams 6   *Protein grams 25*
Fiber grams 8   *Carbohydrate grams 27*
Calories 249   *Sodium milligrams 618*

NEW ENGLAND SHORE DINNER

Yield: 4 servings

Is that a waft of sea breeze coming out of the kitchen or just an over-active imagination on your part? No matter. Nothing can beat devouring a deliciously prepared fresh catch on a midsummer New England evening—but this recipe comes close!

1 teaspoon vegetable oil
1 small onion, minced
1 garlic clove, minced
1½ cups reduced-sodium chicken or vegetable broth
1 bay leaf
1 sprig fresh thyme
3–4 whole black peppercorns

2 ears of corn, shucked and halved
4 small red bliss potatoes, parcooked
8 boiling onions, parcooked
2 lobster tails, split lengthwise
4 (2-ounce) pieces of scrod fillet
16 mussels, scrubbed and debearded

1. Heat a steamer over a large pot over medium heat. Swirl in the oil and add the onion and garlic. Saute until the onion is translucent.

2. Add the broth, bay leaf, thyme, and peppercorns to the onions and bring them to a simmer.

3. Arrange the remaining ingredients in a steamer insert in the following sequence: the corn, potatoes, boiling onions, and lobster tail as the first layer; the scrod and mussels on the second layer.

4. Place the steamer insert over the simmering broth, cover tightly, and steam for about 20 minutes over a low heat. Remove the cover and serve the vegetables, fish, and shellfish with a cup of the flavorful broth.

Per serving (¾ cup):
Fat grams 6
Calories 270
Cholesterol milligrams 120

Protein grams 30
Carbohydrate grams 9
Sodium milligrams 195

TOMATO, MOZZARELLA, AND BASIL PIZZAS

Yield: 4 servings

Instead of four smaller pies, you can make one big pizza (or two)—especially if the guys are coming over on a Sunday afternoon for football and fun.

4 uncooked 7-inch thin-crust
   pizza shells
¼ cup tomato sauce
2 cups oven-dried tomatoes or
   4 fresh ripe tomatoes

¼ cup chopped fresh basil
4 ounces grated low-moisture skim
   milk mozzarella cheese
¼ cup grated Parmesan cheese

1. Place a pizza stone in the oven and preheat to 450 degrees.

2. Set each pizza shell onto a dinner plate lightly dusted with cornmeal. Spread the tomato sauce onto the top of each shell. Arrange the tomatoes on sauce. Scatter the basil, mozzarella, and Parmesan cheese over all.

3. Carefully slide the pizzas onto the hot stone and bake for 12 to 15 minutes, or until the cheese is browned and the dough is crisp. Lift off stone with a metal spatula and place on a cutting surface. Cut into wedges and serve.

Per serving (1 pizza):
Fat grams 8   Protein grams 21
Fiber grams 9   Carbohydrate grams 70
Calories 431   Sodium milligrams 756*

* Higher in sodium than ideal. Do not eat if fluid retention or hypertension is a problem.

SOUPS AND SALADS

What you have to be careful about in soups and salads are the "add-ons"—the bread you have with the soup and the croutons you put on the salad. Try to remember—it's the soup or the salad, not the add-ons, that's the dish.

FRESH POTATO SALAD

Yield: 6 servings

Potato salad doesn't have to be heavy. It's a delicious dish when it isn't just filler. In fact, when it's fresh and light, it's delicious, and you can enjoy one of life's "indulgences" without guilt or worry.

2 pounds red-skinned potatoes (scrubbed)
1 tablespoon olive oil
1 tablespoon red wine vinegar
½ cup chicken broth
½ teaspoon salt
½ teaspoon white pepper
1 tablespoon chopped fresh tarragon
or parsley (If fresh tarragon is not available, don't put any tarragon in. Do not use dry tarragon.)
1 tablespoon Dijon mustard
¼ cup shallots, peeled and halved
2 cloves garlic, minced
2 tablespoons minced fresh chives
2 tablespoons chopped fresh parsley

1. In a medium saucepan, cover the potatoes with cold water. Bring to a boil and cook 15 to 20 minutes or until tender. Remove from the heat and drain and set aside.

2. Meanwhile, combine the remaining ingredients in a bowl and mix.

3. When the potatoes are just cool enough to handle, slice them into ¼-inch slices and add them to the bowl. Toss carefully to prevent breaking the potato slices excessively.

4. Serve the salad while it's still slightly warm, or refrigerate it until used.

Per serving (¾ cup):
Fat grams 2   Protein grams 4
Fiber grams 2   Carbohydrate grams 32
Calories 162   Sodium milligrams 203

HEARTY LENTIL SOUP

Yield: 10 servings

Hearty lentil soup is filling, satisfying, nutritious, flavorful, and prostate-healthy. Store it in small freezer containers for quick lunches. If you have a microwave at work, pack it in microwave-safe individual serving containers to take along with you.

1 teaspoon oil	2 tablespoons cider vinegar
½ cup diced lean ham	1 cup uncooked lentils
½ cup diced onion	6 cups chicken broth
½ cup diced carrots	1 bay leaf
½ cup diced celery	Pinch of thyme
1 clove garlic, minced	¼ teaspoon black pepper
1 tablespoon tomato paste	1 teaspoon dry mustard

1. Heat the oil in a medium saucepan over low heat and add the ham, onion, carrots, celery, and garlic. Sauté until the onions become translucent, about 2 minutes.

2. Add the tomato paste and vinegar and continue to cook for 3 minutes.

3. Add the lentils, broth, bay leaf, and thyme. Raise heat and bring to a boil. Reduce heat and simmer for 20 minutes.

4. Remove from heat, discard the bay leaf, and season with pepper and mustard.

Per serving (¾ cup)

Fat grams 2	Protein grams 11
Fiber grams 3	Carbohydrate grams 14
Calories 111	Sodium milligrams 299

PASTA AND SHRIMP SALAD

Yield: 8 servings

Summer meals of chilled pasta salads—what could be more enjoyable? Not only are they healthy, they're easy to make too. In the summer, there's no reason to spend more time in the kitchen than you have to. Toss this salad with your hands and serve it on a bed of lettuce.

2 cups snow peas
4 cups penne or shell pasta, cooked
1 teaspoon salt
1 cup small cooked shrimp (if you like, you can buy them already cooked in the fish section of your local supermarket)

½ cup Creamy Herb Salad Dressing (page 138)
¼ cup chopped fresh parsley
¼ teaspoon white pepper
1 red bell pepper, sliced

1. Place the snow peas in a microwavable container and sprinkle with 1 teaspoon water. Cover and cook over high heat for 1 minute. Drain and cool. Or place in a steamer on the stove over boiling water for 1 minute.

2. Combine all of the rest of the ingredients in a mixing bowl and toss carefully.

3. Chill in the refrigerator before serving. *Wasn't that easy?*

Per serving (1 cup):
Fat grams 1
Fiber grams 2
Calories 158
Protein grams 11
Carbohydrate grams 25
Sodium milligrams 340

SUMMER GAZPACHO

Yield: 6 servings

Gazpacho is a delightfully refreshing dish, just perfect for a hot summer day or evening. Although our recipe is specific, it's a long-standing tradition that people feel free to improvise and substitute their own favorite ingredients and vegetables. Just make sure you're using really ripe tomatoes, or you'd be better off using canned tomatoes instead.

This is the kind of soup to which you can also add cooked shrimp, crab meat, or crayfish.

1½ pounds very ripe tomatoes, peeled and seeded (or 3 cups drained, diced, canned tomatoes)
3 scallions, chopped
½ green bell pepper, seeded and chopped
1 Italian long hot pepper
½ cucumber, peeled, seeded, and chopped
¼ red onion, chopped
4 cloves garlic, peeled
¼ cup chopped parsley
¼ cup chopped basil
1½ teaspoons olive oil
2 tablespoons red wine vinegar
1 cup tomato juice
1 teaspoon salt
2 slices Italian bread, cubed and baked in the oven until brown and crisp

1. Place the tomatoes, scallions, peppers, cucumber, onion, garlic, parsley, and basil in a food processor and chop until quite smooth but still retaining some texture.

2. Pour the vegetables into a bowl and add the remaining ingredients, except the croutons. Mix well and refrigerate for several hours. Garnish with the croutons when serving.

Per serving (1 cup):
Fat grams 2   Protein grams 3
Fiber grams 3   Carbohydrate grams 17
Calories 87   Sodium milligrams 221

SIDE DISHES

Develop a "philosophy of side dishes." They're meant to be eaten in small bites along with the main dish. Most Americans load up on side dishes (they "supersize" them) instead of using them to complement the flavor of the main dish. Getting to this point may take some time and effort, but the culinary benefit is well worth it.

BARLEY RISOTTO

Yield: 6 servings

Risotto is an Italian vegetable rice stew prepared by cooking a special high-starch rice called arborio in a rich broth with butter and Parmesan cheese; many Italian families have their own risotto recipe (often closely guarded and handed down from generation to generation). There are many grains that can be used, but barley produces great results. This is a great stand-alone meal if you want an easy lunch, but it also goes with nearly any meat dish or can be served as a base for baked or broiled fish.

1 teaspoon olive oil
¼ cup diced onion
¼ cup diced carrots
¼ cup diced celery
½ cup pearl barley
2 cups chicken broth
1 bay leaf

¼ cup evaporated skim milk
½ teaspoon salt
Pinch of white pepper
1 teaspoon chopped fresh rosemary and/or parsley
2 tablespoons grated Parmesan cheese

1. Heat the oil in a small saucepan and add the onion, carrots, and celery over moderate heat. Sauté a few minutes until the onion becomes translucent.

2. Add in the barley and stir well.

3. Add ¼ cup of the broth and the bay leaf, and bring to a simmer. Stir thoroughly to keep the barley from sticking together. When all the liquid is absorbed, add another ¼ cup of the broth and continue to stir over the heat. Repeat until all of the liquid is added and continue to cook until the barley is tender. This should take about 15 minutes.

4. Add the evaporated skim milk, salt, and pepper. When the contents of the pan take on the consistency of porridge, remove from the heat. Remove the bay leaf and add the rosemary and/or parsley and Parmesan cheese. Serve hot.

Per serving (½ cup):
Fat grams 2   *Protein grams 5*
Fiber grams 3   *Carbohydrate grams 16*
Calories 96   *Sodium milligrams 295*

JICAMA SLAW

Yield: 4 servings

The vegetable known as jicama is usually referred to as a "Mexican potato." It tastes like a cross between an apple and a potato—firm and a little bit sweet. It is brown on the outside and white on the inside with a flesh that has the texture of potato. This dish responds well to the addition of strips of sweet red and green bell peppers. The slaw will keep for several days in the refrigerator. (Technically, "cole" refers to the cabbage that is the usual ingredient in coleslaw, but standard coleslaw that does not have a lot of fatty ingredients doesn't taste right to our palate, so this is a tasty substitute. You get the idea.)

2 cups peeled and grated jicama   *2 tablespoons chopped cilantro*
½ cup non-fat yogurt cheese   *½ cup grated carrot*
1 tablespoon sugar   *2 tablespoons fresh lime juice*
¼ teaspoon salt

Mix all the ingredients together. Allow to marinate for ½ hour before serving.

Per serving (½ cup):
Fat grams 0   *Protein grams 4*
Fiber grams 1   *Carbohydrate grams 14*
Calories 70   *Sodium milligrams 184*

MASHED SWEET POTATOES WITH GINGER

Yield: 6 servings

Ginger adds a delicious flavor accent to sweet potatoes. Try this tasty, healthy alternative to the traditional mashed potato side dish. It's the perfect accompaniment to meat, poultry, or any sweet-and-sour main dish.

2 medium sweet potatoes	1 tablespoon chopped fresh ginger-
1 medium white potato	root
½ cup canned evaporated	¼ teaspoon salt
skim milk	¼ teaspoon white pepper

1. Wash the potatoes and place them in a medium saucepan with enough cold water to cover by at least 1 inch. Bring to a boil and reduce to a simmer. Cook until the potatoes are fork-tender (you can stick a fork in them and then pull it out without the potato sticking to the fork). This should take about 20 minutes. Then drain and set it aside.

2. In a small saucepan over low heat, combine the evaporated skim milk with the ginger. Allow these to steep together for approximately 10 minutes. Strain and discard the ginger.

3. Peel the potatoes while they are still quite hot and mash with a sturdy whisk or a potato masher. Once the potatoes are free of lumps, add the strained milk and the remaining ingredients and whip until smooth.

Per serving (½ cup):

Fat grams 0	Protein grams 3
Fiber grams 2	Carbohydrate grams 21
Calories 95	Sodium milligrams 120

Seven-Vegetable Couscous with Harissa Sauce

Yield: 5 servings

If you've never tried couscous, you'll be addicted once you do. This flavorful, vegetable-rich bonanza is enough to turn anyone into a practicing vegetarian. Even those of us who don't turn vegan as a result of sampling gazpacho will appreciate the delicious blend of carrots, onions, artichoke hearts, tomatoes, zucchini, spinach, and so much more.

4 cups low-sodium vegetable broth
3 cloves of garlic, bruised
1 teaspoon curry powder
½ teaspoon ground turmeric
½ teaspoon salt
⅛ teaspoon freshly grated nutmeg
1 cinnamon stick
2 carrots, sliced on the diagonal ½-inch thick
½ cup peeled pearl onions
3 artichoke hearts
½ cup canned chickpeas, drained and rinsed

3 tablespoons raisins, blanched for 12 minutes, drained, and cooled
1 medium zucchini, cubed
1 peeled, seeded and cubed tomato
1 10-oz. bag triple-washed spinach, rinsed and torn
1 cup couscous
2 tablespoons chopped, toasted peanuts
1 tablespoon drained capers (optional)
4 lemon wedges
Harissa Sauce (page 139)

1. To 2 cups of the vegetable stock, add the garlic, curry powder, tumeric, salt, nutmeg, and cinnamon stick and bring to a boil. Reduce the heat, and add the carrots and onions; simmer until the carrots are barely tender, about 12 minutes.

2. Add the artichoke hearts, chickpeas, and raisins and simmer until the artichoke hearts are very hot, about 5 minutes. Add the zucchini and tomato and simmer until the zucchini is tender and translucent, about 5 minutes more. Add the spinach and simmer until it is green and wilted, about 5 minutes. Discard the cinnamon stick.

3. To prepare the couscous, bring the remaining 2 cups of stock to a boil and add the couscous. Return to a boil, cover the pot tightly, and remove it from the heat. Let the couscous sit for 5 minutes. Remove the cover and gently fluff the couscous with a fork.

4. To serve, place the couscous in the center of a platter or plate.

Encircle it with vegetables, and sprinkle a little of the broth over everything. Garnish with peanuts, capers, and lemon wedges. Drizzle with a little Harissa Sauce.

Per serving (½ cup vegetables with ½ cup couscous):

Fat grams 3	*Protein grams 10*
Fiber grams 8	*Carbohydrate grams 46*
Calories 230	*Sodium milligrams 0*

DRESSINGS (INCLUDING OVEN-DRIED TOMATOES) AND SAUCES

Dressings are not a standard part of our cuisine, but the array of dressings and salads available is astounding. Many of the concoctions we have presented here can be used in a wide variety of settings.

BERRY AND AMARETTO BREAKFAST SYRUP

Yield: 2 cups

You can serve this cold if you prefer, but you can also heat it up in the microwave before serving with low-fat waffles, French toast, or hotcakes. Unlike maple syrup, this syrup is filled with fiber, vitamins, and minerals—and it doesn't have the additives or chemicals that the store-bought stuff has. It's easy to cook up in large batches and store it in the refrigerator.

3 cups fresh or frozen unsweetened berries (blueberries, strawberries, or raspberries)
1 tablespoon lemon juice
1 teaspoon lemon peel, grated

¼ cup light corn syrup
½ cup sugar
2 tablespoons Amaretto liqueur (optional)

1. If you're using fresh berries, wash and hull them if necessary. Place half of the berries in a blender or food processor and puree. Strain the puree into a medium saucepan and add the lemon juice, lemon peel, corn syrup, sugar, and remaining berries. Place over high heat and bring to a boil. Reduce heat to a simmer and cook, stirring

frequently, until reduced by half. Remove from heat and allow to cool.

2. If desired, stir in the Amaretto.

3. Cover and refrigerate until needed.

Per serving (¼ cup):
Fat grams 0.4   Protein grams 0.3
Fiber grams 1   Carbohydrate grams 29
Calories 115   Sodium milligrams 5

CREAMY HERB SALAD DRESSING

Yield: 2½ cups

Now that you're watching what you eat, you'll be eating a lot of salads. You should develop some dressings you really enjoy, so experiment with this recipe and add other herbs you like. In any case, a nice trick is to fold capers into the finished dressing; but don't forget to rinse and chop them first. Always stick to the proper serving size.

1¼ cup part-skim ricotta
1 tablespoon shallots, peeled
1 clove garlic, peeled
1¼ cup parsley
¼ cup basil

1½ cups nonfat yogurt
¼ cup red wine vinegar
1¼ cup chives
3 tablespoons Dijon mustard

1. Place the ricotta, shallots, garlic, chives, parsley, and basil in a blender or food processor and process to a silky smooth consistency. Stop the machine several times and scrape down the sides of the bowl to ensure that all of the cheese is processed.

2. Add the yogurt, vinegar, and mustard and process to incorporate.

3. Strain the mixture. Cover and refrigerate until used.

Per serving (1 tablespoon):
Fat grams 0.4   Protein grams 2
Fiber grams 0   Carbohydrate grams 2
Calories 17   Sodium milligrams 47

HARISSA SAUCE

Yield: 12 servings

Harissa Sauce is a versatile concoction used in many different recipes. Once you get the hang of it, you'll be able to put it on almost anything that comes out of your fridge.

4 ounces dried New Mexico chilis   *¾ teaspoon ground caraway*
2 garlic cloves, mashed to a paste   *½ teaspoon ground coriander*
1 teaspoon fresh lemon juice   *1 tablespoon olive oil*

1. Soak the chilis for 15 minutes in just enough cold water to cover them and then drain well, being sure to press out any excess water. Chop the chilis coarsely.

2. Transfer the chilis to a food processor, add the garlic, lemon juice, caraway, and coriander, and puree to a fine paste. Add the olive oil through the feed tube with the machine running until completely incorporated. Transfer the Harissa Sauce to a jar or carafe and refrigerate (covered, to preserve the spiciness) until ready to serve.

Per serving (1 teaspoon):
Fat grams 1   *Protein grams 1*
Fiber grams 5   *Carbohydrate grams 4*
Calories 35   *Sodium milligrams 0*

OVEN-DRIED TOMATOES

Yield: 2 cups

Slow roasting has the power to add great flavor to your cooking by focusing and intensifying all flavors. These slow-roasted tomatoes taste fresher and tangier and have a more pleasing texture than store-bought dried tomatoes. On pizza or chopped up and put into any pasta sauce or added to any salad, they enhance any dish they're added to. Make a large batch and store them in a covered container in the refrigerator. They should keep for more than a month, but you won't be able to resist snacking on them like jerky.

12 ripe tomatoes (preferably Roma
    or plum)
3 cloves garlic, minced

½ cup chopped fresh basil
½ teaspoon salt
1 teaspoon black pepper

1. Preheat oven to 200 degrees.
2. Cut the tomatoes into quarters.
3. Combine the garlic, basil, salt, and pepper in a large bowl.
4. Toss the tomatoes with seasoning mixture and place skin side down on a cake rack over a sheet tray.
5. Place in a very low oven (or use just a pilot light) for 4 to 8 hours or until the tomatoes take on a dried and leathery texture.
6. Remove from rack and store covered in refrigerator until needed.

Per serving (¼ cup):
Fat grams 0.6   Protein grams 2
Fiber grams 3   Carbohydrate grams 9
Calories 43   Sodium milligrams 151

YOGURT CREAM

Yield: ½ cup

This dish is one of the foundations of a low-fat kitchen. Nonfat yogurt takes on the consistency of sour cream. The flavor is better and fresher than that of store-bought sour cream—and, of course, it's healthier and lower in fat. (It also has less of the additives we like to avoid.) It's simple but versatile, a great ingredient in any recipe that calls for sour cream. You can make a large amount and store it in the refrigerator; it keeps for several weeks and is useful in so many recipes, you're likely to run out well before it loses its freshness. It's great on top of a baked potato and in Mexican dishes that call for sour cream. (You'll also notice: it has one ingredient and one step—what could be simpler?)

1 cup nonfat yogurt

Place a paper coffee filter in a funnel or a coffee filter holder and set over a small container or canning jar that holds at least ½ cup. Pour the yogurt in the coffee filter and put the filter-and-jar assembly in the refrigerator overnight. The process is complete when about ½ cup of water has been drained from the yogurt. Pour out the water, put the yogurt in the jar, and refrigerate.

Per serving (1 tablespoon):

Fat grams 0	*Protein grams 2*
Fiber grams 0	*Carbohydrate grams 2*
Calories 16	*Sodium milligrams 22*

DESSERTS

Let's face it: most people eat dessert when they are already stuffed from the earlier part of the meal. That's not the way it's supposed to be. Dessert should be eaten when we are still a bit hungry, since the dessert dish is likely to end that right away. Remember, the purpose of dessert is not to leave you so full you're gasping for air—it's to end the meal leaving a sweet and pleasant taste in your mouth. These recipes are guaranteed to do just that. We're including a few dessert recipes because dessert is where many low-fat diets fail (and because, for some reason, desserts are more fun to make yourself). Store-bought desserts are almost all very high in fat.

BURGUNDY POACHED PEACH WITH ITS SHERBET

Yield: 8 servings

This dessert is both elegant and low in fat. You'll use the liquid to make the sherbet to be served alongside the fruit. Vary the fruit with cherries and pears, depending on the season; that makes the dish look even fancier.

4 large fresh peaches	*4 cloves*
2 cups red Burgundy wine	*15 black peppercorns*
½ cup plus 2 tablespoons sugar	*1 cup Yogurt Cream (page 141)*
1 cinnamon stick	*8 sprigs fresh mint*

1. Bring a large pot of water to a boil. Set up a bowl of ice water. Plunge the peaches into the boiling water for 20 seconds, then quickly remove them (with a spoon or a ladle) and drop into the ice water. Use a paring knife to pull the peel away from the flesh of the peach. Split the peaches in half and remove the pit.

2. Combine the wine with the sugar, cinnamon stick, cloves, and peppercorns in a medium saucepan. Add the peach halves, place over medium heat, and bring to a very slow simmer. Poach for 8 to 10 minutes. Remove from heat and allow to cool to room temperature in the liquid. Remove the peaches from the poaching liquid and refrigerate.

3. Strain the poaching liquid and place in a shallow baking dish. Place the baking dish in the freezer. Stir the poaching liquid every 15 minutes as it begins to freeze. When the mixture becomes firm enough, scrape it with the edge of a spoon to create a smooth but slushy texture.

4. Combine the Yogurt Cream with the remaining 2 tablespoons sugar.

5. Place a scoop of the frozen wine sherbet in the bowls of 8 cham-

pagne glasses or goblets. Place a peach half over the top of each and garnish with a tablespoon of sweetened yogurt and a sprig of fresh mint.

Per serving:
Fat grams 0.5   Protein grams 2
Fiber grams 1   Carbohydrate grams 23
Calories 139   Sodium milligrams 23

CARROT CUSTARD

Yield: 10 servings

People who are served this dessert usually can't believe it's made of carrots. An alternate presentation of this dessert is to bake the custards in small individual cups—for example, in a cupcake tin—and turn them out onto the plates when you are ready to serve. (If you go this route, bake the cups for 45 minutes at 275 degrees.)

1½ pounds carrots, peeled and   4 ounces evaporated skim milk
   coarsely chopped   1 tablespoon sugar
½ teaspoon salt   ⅛ teaspoon white pepper
4 egg whites

1. Boil the carrots in lightly salted water until they are very tender, about 15 minutes. Allow them to cool slightly.

2. Preheat oven to 325 degrees.

3. Transfer the carrots to a blender or food processor and add the remaining ingredients. Puree to a very smooth consistency.

4. Pour into a lightly oiled 2-quart baking dish.

5. Place the baking dish in a larger pan and add boiling water to the larger pan to a depth of 1 inch. Place the pans in the oven and bake for 30 minutes or until a knife inserted in the custard comes out clean.

6. Spoon onto plates and serve.

Per serving (3 ounces, or about 6 tablespoons):
Fat grams 0   Protein grams 3
Fiber grams 2   Carbohydrate grams 10
Calories 50   Sodium milligrams 112

CHERRY RICE PUDDING BRÛLÉE

Yield: 6 servings

This cross between rice pudding and crème brûlée is another of those desserts people can't believe is low-fat. You can substitute other dried fruits for kiln-dried cherries—whatever is available in your neck of the woods—blueberries, cranberries, apricots, and just plain old raisins are all great if you can't get (or don't like) cherries.

¼ cup nonconverted rice	½ cup kiln-dried cherries
1 quart skim milk	1 tablespoon grated orange peel
¾ cup sugar	1 teaspoon vanilla extract
⅛ teaspoon nutmeg	¼ cup brown sugar

1. Preheat oven to 300 degrees.

2. Combine the rice, milk, ½ cup of the sugar, and nutmeg in a 1-quart casserole. Place over high heat and bring to a boil. Bake, uncovered, for 2 hours, stirring every 15 minutes.

3. Stir in the cherries, grated orange peel, and vanilla extract and bake without stirring for another half hour.

4. Remove from the oven and allow to cool to room temperature.

5. Preheat the broiler at the highest setting. Rub together the brown sugar and the remaining cup of white sugar and scatter evenly over the surface of the rice pudding.

6. Place the casserole under the broiler and allow the sugars to melt and caramelize, producing a rich brown crust over the entire surface of the pan. Refrigerate. Serve chilled.

Per serving:
Fat grams 0.5   Protein grams 7
Fiber grams 1   Carbohydrate grams 59
Calories 260   Sodium milligrams 91

YOGURT AND BERRY PARFAIT AMERICANA

Yield: 4 servings

We'll end with this one. It's an ambitious recipe but one you and your guests are certain to enjoy. In this dessert, yogurt is transformed into a fluffy, light mousse! This is an exciting dish and easy to put together. It's equally exciting to watch your guests eat it up. Don't count on there being any leftovers!

1 cup fresh blueberries, washed
1 cup fresh strawberries, hulled,
    washed, and quartered
4 tablespoons sugar
¼ cup white wine

½ tablespoon unflavored gelatin
1 ½ cups plain nonfat yogurt
1 teaspoon vanilla extract
2 egg whites

1. Place the blueberries and strawberries in 2 separate small bowls. Sprinkle 1 tablespoon of the sugar over the strawberries only and mix. Set aside.

2. Place the wine in a soup cup and scatter gelatin over the surface. Place in a microwave and heat on high just until it starts to steam, 30 to 45 seconds. Do not boil. Or place in a small saucepan on the stove over high heat, heat to just before boiling, and then remove from heat.

3. Place the yogurt and vanilla extract in a bowl. Add the wine and gelatin mixture in a slow, steady stream, stirring constantly.

4. Combine the egg whites and remaining 3 tablespoons sugar in a 1-quart stainless-steel bowl. Beat well. Place the bowl over a lightly simmering pan of water and continue to beat with an electric beater until the meringue is light and thick, about 7 to 10 minutes. Remove the bowl from the simmering water and allow to set at room temperature until cool.

5. Fold the meringue into the yogurt, being careful not to overmix.

6. Place a spoonful of the yogurt mixture in the bottom of each of 4 tall clear parfait (or pilsner beer) glasses. Into each glass, spoon a layer of strawberries, a portion of half the remaining yogurt, the blueberries, and the remaining yogurt mixture. Place in the refrigerator to chill for at least 2 hours before serving.

Per serving:
Fat grams 0   Protein grams 6
Fiber grams 2   Carbohydrate grams 27
Calories 149   Sodium milligrams 64

III.

PROSTATE HEALTH AND FERTILITY

8. THE HEALTHY PROSTATE FITNESS REGIMEN

THE LINK BETWEEN EXERCISE AND PROSTATE HEALTH

Nutrition and exercise are closely linked to prostate health. Exercise is a key way to help ensure overall health, improve cardiovascular conditioning, lose weight, and guard against prostate cancer (and other hormone-linked cancers), as well as conditions such as enlarged prostate.

Exercise has several major anticancer effects, including boosting the immune system, enhancing the body's defense against free radicals, and temporarily lowering testosterone levels. Exercise decreases body fat, increases lean body mass, and facilitates digestion. Exercise also improves joint and muscle movement, builds strength and endurance, stimulates oxygen delivery, helps regulate blood sugar levels, and increases the efficiency of numerous metabolic processes.

Any man who initiates an exercise program after age fifty will achieve excellent health benefits. This is also precisely the age when prostate health becomes a special consideration. If you have already had prostate surgery, refer to the section on page 163.

A key to attaining and sustaining physical fitness is to find activities that are challenging, fun, and part of the fabric of your daily routine. A simple behavioral change such as taking the stairs instead of the elevator can contribute to weight control and cardiovascular health, as well as stimulating blood flow in the lower body.

The two main categories of exercise are aerobic exercise (examples include swimming, jogging, treadmills, stair climbers) and anaerobic exercise (weight training with free weights [dumbbells, barbells] and machines).

Aerobic literally means "with oxygen," while anaerobic means "without oxygen." In aerobic exercise, the intensity of the activity is low enough that you can take in enough oxygen to perform it for a relatively long time. In anaerobic exercise, the intensity is simply too high to breathe in enough oxygen to do the activity for very long. To compensate, your body uses stored energy, and your muscles become fatigued quickly. So the essential difference between aerobic and anaerobic activity is not so much the activity itself as how intensely the activity is performed. Jogging slowly around the block is aerobic; sprinting around the block is anaerobic.

An excellent way to determine if the activity is aerobic or anaerobic is to use the "talk test." If you're able to carry on a normal conversation while performing the exercise—using complete sentences and not gasping for breath—it's an aerobic activity. If the intensity is so high that you can't converse comfortably (you're short of breath), it's an anaerobic activity. If you're unable to talk during supposedly aerobic activity, you are using way too much intensity and are outside what we call your aerobic training zone (more about that later).

A balanced exercise program is divided into cardiovascular, strength, and flexibility training. A healthy prostate fitness regimen is one that focuses on increasing blood flow to the prostate region and building pelvic floor muscles and other muscles in the genital-urinary system.

CAN EXERCISE PREVENT PROSTATE CANCER?

General exercise and physical activity—most particularly aerobic exercise—appear to protect against prostate cancer. Although the specific cause of prostate cancer is unknown, it is becoming evident that a sedentary lifestyle is a risk factor. There is a strong scientific basis for this belief.

The Institute for Cancer Prevention's prostate-specific health regimen shows you exercises you can do to help stave off prostate cancer and ensure prostate health.

Prostate cancer is believed to be linked to elevated testosterone levels. Reduced testosterone levels are associated with a decreased risk of prostate cancer. Anything that stimulates excess testosterone production—such as injecting anabolic steroids—can lead to the genesis and growth of prostate cancer cells.

The rationale for the prostate cancer/exercise connection is that physical activity reduces the male sex hormone testosterone. It is known that men who exercise have lower testosterone levels immediately following exercise activity. However, this lower postexercise testosterone level is only temporary, returning to pre-exercise levels within approximately twenty-four hours.

Several research studies have discovered a correlation between exercise (especially aerobic exercise) and less risk of prostate cancer. In one study, it was shown that men who burned 4,000 calories or more a week above and beyond their basal metabolism rate—the equivalent of approximately an hour of vigorous daily exercise—had a substantially lower risk of prostate cancer than relatively sedentary men who burned fewer than 1,000 calories a week. A consistent, substantial exercise regimen was clinically proven to result in temporarily lower testosterone levels and lower levels of other prostate-stimulating androgens.

One of the largest studies of increased exercise activity and decreased risk of prostate cancer was conducted at the Cooper Clinic in Dallas, Texas. Approximately 13,000 men were observed over an eighteen-year period. The study concluded that "moderate to high levels of cardiorespiratory fitness may protect against the incidence of prostate cancer." In addition, the study showed that even men who expended as little as 1,000 calories a week in physical activity consistently had a lower prostate cancer risk compared to those who were less active. It doesn't take a tremendous amount of activity to burn 1,000 calories. Walking about thirty minutes a day five days a week will burn about that amount.

The bottom line is that regular aerobic exercise, with its stimulating cardiovascular effects, performed for at least twenty to thirty minutes, three to five days a week, lowers the level of circulating testosterone. Aerobic exercise includes walking, joggling, cycling, and swimming. It is not known whether lower levels of circulating testosterone are a result of diminished production or increased metabolic effect. Whatever the case, it's a good thing.

It seems to be a case not only of whether or not you exercise, but of *how much* you exercise as well. A Harvard doctor examined the relationship between physical activity and prostate cancer among male health professionals. He found that men who exercised very frequently were only about half as likely to be diagnosed with metastatic prostate cancer as men who exercised often, but less frequently.

The Institute for Cancer Prevention believes there is enough clinical evidence to suggest a connection between exercise and a decreased risk of prostate cancer.

CONSULT YOUR PHYSICIAN BEFORE STARTING AN EXERCISE PROGRAM

You should always consult your physician before starting an exercise program.

Your physician will tell you that you don't need to run a ten-mile marathon or hoist fifty-pound weights to achieve serious physical benefits from an exercise regimen.

You will have to do enough exercise to burn at least 1,000 calories a week to obtain significant health benefits and reduce your risk of disease. Your doctor will likely advise you to start slowly and build up the duration and intensity of your exercise activity.

THE HEALTHY PROSTATE FITNESS REGIMEN

For the first time anywhere, the Institute for Cancer Prevention is pleased to offer this research-based prostate fitness regimen.

There are five groundbreaking elements to the program:

1. The exercises represent practical ways to stimulate blood flow to the prostate.
2. They help decrease testosterone production.
3. They strengthen the pelvic floor muscles and a variety of other muscles in the genital/urinary system.
4. They are simple, natural, and easy to do.
5. They can easily be done by men of any age.

Before you embark on this regimen:

- Set achievable goals; add variety to your routine; keep a journal of your progress.
- Don't eat for two hours prior to working out.
- Drink plenty of water before, during, and after your workout.
- Avoid aerobic activity that jars or irritates the prostate (such as cycling, horseback riding, or sprinting). There are bicycle seats that are ergonomically designed (that is, designed to fit the body) to be gentle on the prostate. These seats have a deep groove or cutout in the middle of the seat and are gel-padded. Such seats may be especially useful for those with an enlarged prostate. Prostate-friendly aerobic activities include walking, swimming, tennis and other racquet sports, stair climbing, and step aerobics.
- Some aerobic activities require equipment and skills that may be outside the realm of your budget or expertise. Try to keep your aerobic program simple. Always remember to do whatever it is you enjoy most.

REDUCING RISK AND INJURY: WARM-UPS, COOLDOWNS, AND STRETCHES

If you get a headache or start feeling exhausted, nauseous, or dizzy when working out, stop immediately; your body is telling you that something is wrong. Inappropriate form is probably the number one cause of exercise injury. If you're not sure how to perform an exercise or if you encounter a piece of gym equipment you're not familiar with, consult a qualified personal trainer or an experienced fellow exerciser.

WARM-UPS AND COOLDOWNS

Warm-ups and cooldowns are an essential part of any exercise program. Never work out without warming up first. Always be sure to cool your body down after a workout. Warm-ups and cooldowns help the body make the transition from rest to activity and back to rest again. They also help prevent muscle soreness.

Your warm-up should last about five to ten minutes. Older men may need a few more minutes to warm up. Low-level aerobic exercise is the best way to warm up. This can consist simply of gently running in place or riding a stationary bike at very low resistance, followed by a few minutes of swinging your arms. Stretching should be done only after you've warmed up, since stretching can injure cold muscles.

To cool down, walk around slowly or do some stretches (stretching is fine for cooldowns, since your muscles are already warmed up), until your heartbeat is ten to fifteen beats above its resting rate. Stopping exercise too suddenly can sharply reduce your blood pressure level and cause muscle cramping. If you've been doing lower-body exercises, cool down with appropriate lower-body stretches, emphasizing the groin, glutes, and leg muscles, such as the hamstrings, calves, and quads.

STRETCHING ROUTINES

There are some basic rules for stretching:

• Always stretch on an empty stomach. Wait until at least two hours after a meal before you stretch. Stretching on a full stomach can lead to stomach acid reflux.

• Always wear loose-fitting clothing.

• Never hold your breath while stretching; breathe evenly throughout the stretch.

• Always use proper form for even the most basic stretch.

• Never "bounce" a muscle that you're trying to stretch—you'll pull or tear it. A firm, constant stretch held for five to thirty seconds is the ticket.

A STRETCHING SAMPLER

There are many excellent stretches. However, some of them can put stress on your back. Consult with your physician to determine the best stretching regimen for you.

Standing Quad Stretch

This fundamental quadriceps stretch is simple and highly effective. Stand with one hand against the wall. Grasp one foot with your free hand and lift it behind you. Using a comfortable·range of motion, lift your ankle and touch your buttock with the heel of your foot (or at least bring your foot toward your buttocks). Be careful not to twist the knee. Hold for 15 to 20 seconds. Repeat with the opposite foot.

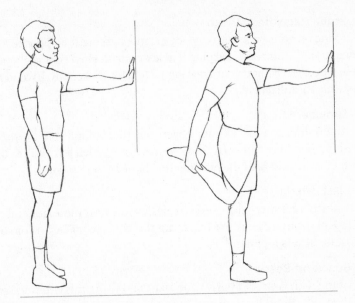

Lying Quad Stretch

Lying on your side, balance yourself on one arm and leg. Grasp the other leg and pull it in the direction of your buttocks. Hold for 15 seconds. Repeat from the opposite side.

Inner Thigh (Groin) Stretch

Sit on the floor with your hands on your ankles and the soles of your feet touching. Without pulling your feet apart, use your elbows to push your knees as far apart as is comfortable. Hold the stretch for about 20 seconds, then release it slowly.

Inner Thigh (Groin) Stretch II

Sit on the floor with the soles of your feet touching and your hands grasping your toes. Slowly pull yourself forward, stretching from the hips. Hold for 15 seconds. Avoid this stretch if you have lower back problems.

Inner Thigh (Groin) Stretch III

Sit on the floor with your legs extended and spread apart. Stretch forward until you feel tension in your groin area. Hold for 15 to 20 seconds. Avoid this stretch if you have back problems.

Prone Hamstring Stretch

Lying on your back with one leg extended, bring the opposite leg's knee toward your chest, keeping that leg straight. Hold your leg behind your thigh, not behind your knee joint. Hold for 15 seconds. Extend the opposite leg and repeat.

Shoulder Stretch

Stand straight and lock your fingers together behind your buttocks. Without bending your body, raise your arms as far back as you're comfortable with and hold the position for about 10 to 15 seconds.

CALISTHENICS

Calisthenics are light exercises designed to promote general fitness and strength. Here are two examples you can make part of your prostate fitness regimen:

Bend-and-Reach

Stand with your feet fairly wide apart and your arms extended out to the sides. Bend forward and twist your torso to the left, reaching the right hand toward the left ankle. The free arm remains straightened and in line with the upper body, lifting up and to the rear. Immediately straighten up and repeat to the opposite side. A touch to both ankles equals one repetition.

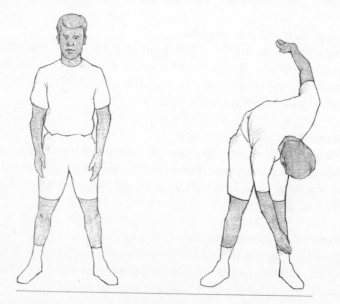

Toe Touches

Stand upright with your arms by your sides, feet approximately shoulder width apart. Keep the knees straightened or just slightly bent. Bend forward at the waist, reaching both hands toward your toes, touching them if you can. Bend in a smooth, controlled fashion. Straighten to the starting position. Repeat for the desired number of repetitions.

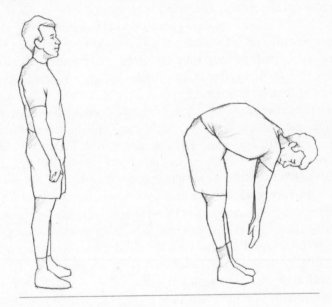

AEROBICS: A KEY TO PROSTATE HEALTH

Also known as cardiovascular exercise, low-impact aerobic exercise is a must element in any prostate health program. Unlike anaerobic exercise, which is done at high intensity, aerobic exercise is performed at low to moderate intensity for an extended period of time.

Aerobic exercise provides excellent benefit for your heart and cardiovascular system. Its stimulating effect on circulation makes aerobic activity really good for your prostate too. It's also a great way to lose weight or control weight. When you're working aerobically, the body first uses glycogen stored in muscles, then uses fat as its primary fuel source. And you burn more calories because you're able to do the activity for a relatively prolonged period of time.

YOUR AEROBIC TRAINING ZONE/TARGET HEART RATE ZONE

If you're unable to talk comfortably when performing an aerobic exercise, you're pushing too hard and are outside your aerobic training zone, also known as your target heart rate zone. Aerobic exercise that sustains your heart rate at 70 to 85% of maximum is considered optimal. To determine your heart rate, use two fingers to measure your pulse at the carotid artery on your neck or on the inside of your wrist. Count the pulse beats for ten seconds, then multiply by six for the per minute total. Your maximum heart rate per minute can be calculated by subtracting your age from the number 220. Older adults can exercise as often as anyone else but should aim for 60 to 73 percent of their peak heart rate.

The time spent in aerobic activity should decrease if your exercise intensity increases and vice versa (the time should increase if your aerobic intensity decreases). Let's say you're running on a treadmill and your heart rate is at the upper end of your aerobic training zone. You should stay on the treadmill for only about twenty minutes, at least until you build up endurance. If you're just walking on the treadmill and your heart rate is at the lower end of your aerobic training zone, you should continue for forty-five minutes or longer to achieve similar results. Adjust intensity and duration to keep within your target heart rate zone. Aerobics is about reaching and then staying comfortably in your training zone.

Popular aerobic activities include hiking, sports (volleyball, tennis, skiing, basketball), and dancing (this is a good one because you can achieve aerobic benefit and enhance your social life at the same time).

AMERICAN COLLEGE OF SPORTS MEDICINE RECOMMENDATIONS FOR AEROBIC ACTIVITY
- Train three to five days per week.
- Intensity should be 55 or 65 percent to 90 percent of your maximum heart rate.
- The duration of each session should be twenty to sixty minutes of continuous or intermittent aerobic activity. The ideal balance is thirty minutes or more of moderate-intensity aerobic activity.
- Choose an activity that works large muscle groups and is rhythmical in nature.

WALKING IS GOOD EXERCISE

Walking is serious exercise. As with all exercise, it is most effective when done with proper form. Walk with your shoulders back, your head up, and your arms swinging freely from your side. Use your entire body when walking.

Walking is a great activity for increasing blood flow to the prostate. You can expend 400 to 500 calories an hour while walking. Not bad for an activity many men don't even think of as exercise!

Choose comfortable, well-made walking shoes that allow your feet to "breathe." Combine chores or social activity with exercise: Walk to and from a specific destination, such as the store or a friend's house; walk with a companion; take a nature walk. Park your car a distance from your destination and walk the rest of the way; get off the bus or train a stop further from your destination and walk the rest of the way. A healthy prostate workout can be as simple as a good, aerobically effective brisk walk.

EXERCISES FOR IMPROVING BLOOD FLOW TO THE PROSTATE
Deep Knee Bends/Squats

If you have a problem with your knees, have ever suffered a major knee injury, or have suffered a minor knee injury in the recent past,

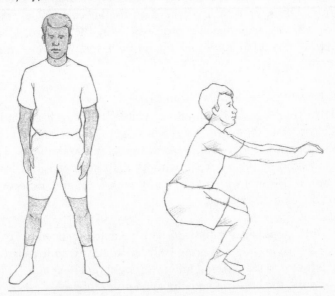

modify the exercise to half squats or carefully work through whatever range of motion you are comfortable with. Never bounce out of a knee bend.

Stand erect with your feet six inches apart, toes pointed slightly outward, arms straight and parallel to the floor. Hold your chin up and keep your spine vertical. Lower your body by bending the knees, your heels raised slightly off the floor. Keeping your arms up, return to the upright position, without bouncing at the bottom of the movement. Move in a smooth motion, maintaining good posture and balance throughout. This exercise strengthens the groin area and the front of the thighs. Repeat for the desired number of repetitions without resting.

Lunges

Stand up straight. Keeping the back straight, step forward with your right foot about 30 inches, or whatever length is comfortable while still maintaining balance. Push the front knee just out past the toe, keeping the back leg only partially bent and not allowing the rear knee to touch the ground. Push off the forward foot and return to the upright position. Repeat with the opposite foot. This constitutes one repetition. This exercise develops the quadriceps, hamstrings, and glutes. Beginners or older men might want to drop the knee only slightly. This exercise may be hard on the knees for older men or those who are experiencing problems with their knees. Consult with your physician before incorporating lunges into your training program.

A LOWER-BODY WATER WORKOUT

Turn your backyard pool into a gym! Water provides great resistance for simple lower-body exercises. Your body should be sufficiently immersed that your legs don't break the water level. These exercises can be done with or without light ankle weights. Have a partner in the pool with you to check your form and, if necessary, help you maintain balance.

• **Side steps.** Facing forward with your feet aligned, step your right foot to the side and bring your left foot next to it. Then step your left foot to the side and bring your right foot next to it. This exercise works the buttocks and inner and outer thighs.

- **Water walking.** With your feet shoulder width apart, move forward with small steps. Take longer strides as you become more comfortable. Take about six steps, then reverse your direction. This exercise works the buttocks, thighs, and legs.
- **Modified Knee Lifts.** With your feet shoulder width apart and your arms relaxed and comfortably bent at the elbows, alternately raise your knees, bringing them slightly out to the side. Raise them only to a level that does not compromise your balance. This exercise works the buttocks, thighs and legs.

KEGEL EXERCISES (PELVIC FLOOR EXERCISES) FOR MEN

The floor of the pelvis is made up of muscle layers and other tissues stretching from side to side like a hammock. It is attached to the tailbone (coccyx) at the back end and the pubic bone in front. This ham-

WORKOUT TIPS FOR OLDER MEN

Exercise can be of great benefit at any age! It is estimated that 32 percent of adults sixty-five and older are already following a regular exercise plan. Join them! Here are some simple tips that can help older men get the maximum benefit out of their exercise regimen. (Note that the first three tips are just as important for younger guys.)

- You should discuss any exercise plan with your primary care physician.
- It's best to have a qualified professional instruct you in the proper use of weights and machines.
- You should increase your training intensity slowly to maximize health benefits and avoid overexertion.
- Walking is a good aerobic activity for the older man. It helps build new bone and tissue and helps ward off or slow the progress of osteoporosis.
- Swimming is a good aerobic exercise if you suffer from arthritis or other mobility and joint-impeding conditions. Unlike some other aerobic activities, swimming does not put undue stress on joints.
- Resistance training has been shown to be beneficial for older adults with cardiovascular disease, as well as those with pulmonary disease, cancer, and osteoarthritis.
- You might check with the senior center or community center in your area to see if it has exercise classes or if it can recommend a facility that does.

mock of muscle supports the bladder and the bowel, playing a key role in bowel and bladder control.

The pelvic floor muscles have been traditionally ignored by most men. Strengthening the pelvic floor muscles through physical exercise isn't even on the radar screen! Because little attention is paid to them, they become weak and atrophied. Activating and toning these muscles increases the stimulation and circulation in the prostate, the bladder, and the rest of the genitourinary system.

Kegel (KEE-gul) exercises have traditionally been thought of as exclusively an exercise for women (given the connection among pregnancy, incontinence, and the pelvic floor muscles). But the pelvic floor muscles can be substantially weakened by an operation for enlarged prostate or prostate removal related to cancer. Pelvic floor exercises for men have shown to be especially effective following prostate surgery (although not immediately after). They are a superb general exercise for men of any age who care about the health of their prostate.

A variety of urinary system conditions are due to weakness of the pelvic floor muscles. Kegel exercises strengthen the pelvic floor muscles that help control bladder flow, combating incontinence and minor urinary leakage.

Kegel exercises are also great for improving virility and achieving greater ejaculation and arousal control. This impacts very favorably on the prostate, since a healthy sex life often equals a healthy prostate. Kegel exercises also reduce and eliminate problems associated with noncancerous and nonbacterial prostate inflammation.

Kegel exercises have a simple basis: repeatedly tensing the same muscles you use to keep from urinating or having a bowel movement. Kegel exercises strengthen and tone the pubococcygeus (PC) muscle. The PC muscle (or, more accurately, the PC muscle group) is located between the testicles and the anus. The PC muscle stops urine flow and is the muscle that contracts during ejaculation. It is easy to see why strengthening this key muscle could be of substantial benefit in urine control.

When performed properly, Kegel exercises force nutrient-rich blood into your penis and genital area, benefiting both the prostate and the urinary tract. In addition, Kegel exercises indirectly massage the prostate.

Fewer but more intense Kegel repetitions may benefit you more than a greater number of less intense repetitions, but it's really up to the individual to determine what combination of intensity/duration works best for him.

Intense Kegel exercise method: 10 to 30 repetitions a day
Moderate Kegel exercise method: 20 to 40 repetitions twice a day

Concentrate on focus and proper form. Contract only the PC muscle; do not flex your abdominals or any other muscle groups. Kegels can be done sitting (even on the toilet), standing, or lying down. If you're doing the exercise lying on the floor, tilt your pelvis toward the ceiling.

To perform Kegel exercises:

Tighten the muscles you would tighten to prevent a bowel movement and the muscles at the base of your penis you'd contract to keep from urinating. When both sets of muscles are properly tightened, you will feel a compression of all muscles in the area between your penis and anus. A good way to get a feel for this is to start and stop your urine stream a couple of times. That's your PC muscle at work! Hold both sets of muscles as firmly as you can for five seconds. Release and repeat.

You may want to slowly increase the total number of daily repetitions up to 40 total at strong intensity, or 60 total at moderate intensity.

EXERCISE AFTER PROSTATE SURGERY

How much exercise you can do after prostate surgery depends on your general health and the nature and extent of your surgery. It will be at least six to eight weeks before you are back to your presurgical stamina and strength. Basic aerobic exercises such as walking are recommended, but you must avoid exercises with jarring motions (running) and exercises that put pressure on the affected area (bike or horseback riding). There are a number of activities you should refrain from doing for the first month or two after surgery as they are too high-impact, stressing, or irritating to the prostate region. But if you love to do any or all of these things, rest assured you'll begin doing them again very soon, pending your physician's approval. They include cycling; tennis or racquetball; competitive running and other track events; bowling; baseball, basketball, football, and other competitive or team sports; and lifting weights of more than twenty pounds.

All men should consult with their physician before starting an exercise program, but for men who have just had prostate surgery, consulting with a physician is overwhelmingly important.

No matter how active and fit you were prior to surgery, you will experience reduced strength and a limited activity level following prostate removal. To return to normal activity, you will need to follow a sensible, circumscribed exercise regimen adapted to your level of health and fitness. Realistically, it will be six to eight weeks before you are back to your presurgical stamina and strength.

The good news is that you can begin some physical activity shortly after prostate surgery. While it may involve nothing more than getting out of bed (with assistance) and sitting on a chair, this simple movement is as relatively important to the recovering patient as a vigorous aerobic workout.

Do your legs feel strong enough to support you? When you do feel strong enough to stand up, make sure someone from the hospital staff is there to provide support.

Taking a few steps is your next goal. We often see hospital patients who have undergone extensive surgical procedures walking with assistance down the corridor within a day after surgery. Walking is the key postsurgical exercise. It's a wonderful way to keep fit without taxing yourself. When you're home from the hospital and beginning to get up and around, start taking daily walks of five to ten minutes' duration in your immediate neighborhood, building up over the course of a month to forty-five minutes. Slow or moderate walking on a treadmill is another fine postsurgical aerobic activity. **Not only does walking help regain fitness, it stimulates healing blood flow, and, perhaps most important, by keeping the blood moving in the legs, it helps prevent blood clots from forming there, which are the main source of clots that travel to, and lodge in, the lungs. That's how walking reduces the risk of pulmonary embolism (blood clots in the lungs), a potentially lethal complication after prostate surgery.**

STRETCHING

These are very gentle, modified, limited-range-of-motion stretches. It is important to start conservatively and sensibly. If you feel pulling or pain, stop immediately. Limited-range-of-motion stretches are permissible fairly soon after surgery, but you should stretch for only about five minutes. Continue to add stretches with greater range of motion over the course of a few weeks, slowly building the time up to fifteen minutes.

The first stretch is the wall stretch. Stand with your buttocks, shoulders, and the back of your head pressed against the wall. Straighten your back and legs. Breathe. Gently tighten your stomach muscles by pulling them in to the wall. Remember, stop if you feel any discomfort. Do this stretch several times, for a couple of minutes each time. As you feel able, you can do the same stretch on the rug or floor.

A modified toe touch is performed by starting in the standing position without slumping and gently bending your neck, then shoulders, forward. The object is to bend and loosen your back and shoulders, not touch your toes. But if toe touches are done correctly, your lower body and legs will feel the stretch.

Swimming is great exercise, but don't go into the water until your surgeon okays it. Up until a month after surgery, stick to the shallow end of the pool and do nothing more than wade in the water. After a month, try a little movement in the water, but stay on a flotation device at all times. Then gradually work your way back into a swimming regimen, relying on upper-body strokes and avoiding kicking motions.

Anaerobic activity should consist of little more than upper-body strength building exercises with very light weights (2–3 lb.) or elastic bands.

Pelvic floor exercises are especially effective following prostate surgery, but consult with your physician as to how much time should go by before you attempt them.

9. Sex and the Prostate

The Prostate and Sexual Function

We've seen how proper nutrition and sensible exercise are good for your prostate. You'll be happy to know that sex can be good for your prostate too. But there's a proviso: Indulging in promiscuity and unsafe sexual practices can have a counterproductive effect on prostate health. A man can't have sex with multiple partners, fail to use proper protection, or engage in unsafe anal sex and expect his prostate to remain healthy.

How much sexual activity is the "right" amount? That depends very much on the individual. For some men, once or twice a week may be right; for others, sex once or more a day better suits their needs. Follow your inclination and continue to engage in safe sexual practices.

The Prostate's Role as a Sex Gland

The prostate gland plays a positive, life-affirming role. It is an important accessory sex gland—a fundamental part of a man's sexual mechanism—adding vital nutrients and fluid to sperm. The prostate contains muscular tissue, and, like any muscle, it needs to be kept active and disease-free in order to be maximally efficient.

Not only is moderate, monogamous, safe sex good for your prostate, there is some speculation that it may even help reduce the incidence and retard the development of prostate cancer. A physi-

IS THE PROSTATE GLAND THE MALE G-SPOT?

The prostate is located immediately in front of the rectal wall about three centimeters inside the anus. It can easily be felt by placing one finger inside the anus and probing around the interior wall for a rounded, slightly elevated area.

The prostate is very sensitive and is considered an erogenous zone by some men, who enjoy stimulation of their prostate during sex. Stimulation of the prostate has been touted to increase semen volume and create more powerful ejaculations.

Is the prostate gland a man's ultimate pleasure spot? Whatever some men may say, the prostate is not a hidden "pleasure dome" that opens untold sexual vistas for all men. While a few men claim to achieve orgasm strictly from prostate massage, to other men prostate massage is uncomfortable, giving them the sensation of wanting to urinate.

cian at the Royal Manchester Infirmary in England conducted a research study in which he found a correlation between estimated number of ejaculations and incidence of prostate cancer. A group of 423 men, sixty to eighty years old, was divided into two groups: 274 who had prostate cancer and 149 who were cancer-free. All of the men estimated their ejaculatory frequency during the years in which they had been most sexually active. Men who contracted prostate cancer had, on average, ejaculated much less frequently than men who did not have the disease. Thirty-one percent of the cancer-free men estimated that they had ejaculated five to seven times per week. Only 13 percent of the prostate cancer patients said they had ejaculated that often.

There are obvious scientific problems with this survey. Numerous controllable and uncontrollable risk factors must be taken into account as also having had an influence on the survey group's incidence of prostate cancer. However, the study does provide interesting food for thought on the role of sex in the health of the prostate.

A National Cancer Institute Study of 111 men suggested another health-related link between sex and the prostate: subjects with a history of infection with HPV—the virus that can cause genital warts—had nearly three times the prostate cancer risk of HPV-free men. If a man is diagnosed with genital warts, the Institute for Cancer Prevention recommends that he consider this a potential risk factor and have an early prostate cancer screening.

SEX WITH SOMEONE YOU LOVE

That's what Woody Allen called masturbation—and now the ultimate in safe sex may also protect you from prostate cancer. An Australian study published in the British *Journal of Urology* found that frequent masturbation may indeed protect men against prostate cancer.

It seems that men who ejaculated more than five times a week—especially men in their twenties, thirties, and forties—were a third less likely to develop prostate cancer than those who ejaculated the least frequently. Interestingly, the researchers at the Cancer Council of Victoria in Melbourne did not find similar protection from frequent sexual intercourse.

It's possible that the downside of frequent intercourse negates the benefits of frequent ejaculation. Or, the researchers speculate, it may be analogous to the way a first full-term pregnancy forces breast cells to "fully differentiate and become mature cells. Maybe intense sexual ejaculation at the time when the prostate has finished growing to maturity might actually help it bed down and become a fully developed gland, rather than having too many cells lying around in it."

Coincidentally (or not), the prostate matures during puberty, around the same time many teenage boys discover masturbation. Not only do you not go blind, it's good for you!

DOES EJACULATION AFFECT PSA LEVEL?

We know that having sex or masturbating approximately twenty-four hours before a PSA test will raise PSA blood levels, possibly leading to a false positive or "red flag" test result. Studies have shown that total and free PSA levels increase immediately after ejaculation, with differing rates of return to actual levels. The Institute for Cancer Prevention advises men to abstain from ejaculating for forty-eight hours before a PSA blood test in order to help ensure accurate results.

As men age, their prostate gland is likelier to leak PSA into the bloodstream during orgasm. In fact, men between the ages of fifty and eighty can exhibit a 40 percent increase in the amount of PSA in their blood within an hour after ejaculation. This increase can last for up to forty-eight hours.

IMPOTENCE (ERECTILE DYSFUNCTION)

Erectile dysfunction (ED)—more commonly known as impotence—is the inability to achieve or sustain an erection. Impotence is a very common problem affecting 20 million (one out of five) American men. Half of all men aged forty to seventy experience some degree of erectile dysfunction.

Is impotence simply an inevitable consequence of aging? As most men age, erections do become less frequent and harder to sustain, but erections do not normally disappear altogether because of aging. Most research points to physical causes that are only somewhat age-related.

There are three basic physiological causes of impotence: dysfunction or disturbance of the nerve mechanism; blockage of arterial blood flow into the penis; and increased blood outflow from the penis.

Causes of erectile dysfunction not related to the prostate include diabetes and other hormonal disorders; high blood pressure; heart disease; high cholesterol level and peripheral vascular disease; and any condition that severely impacts the nervous system, such as spinal cord injury, or other severe stress and trauma. Various medications can also help cause or contribute to impotence. But by far the most common cause of impotence is inadequate blood flow to the penis. The major reason for inadequate blood flow is atherosclerosis, the blockage of arteries supplying the penis.

Statistics show that prostate abnormalities are a minor contributor to the overall number of impotence cases. Except for aggressive curative therapy for early prostate cancer or hormone therapy for advanced disease, most disorders of the prostate gland and their treatment will not substantially impair a man's ability to achieve an erection sufficient to have intercourse.

However, impotence and infertility are two of several potential consequences of radical prostatectomy (prostate removal), due to injury of the nerves surrounding the prostate. Radiation therapy and cryosurgery (where the prostate is subjected to extreme cold) can also damage these nerves.

Ability to achieve erection after a prostatectomy will depend somewhat on the age of the patient and his ability to achieve erections *before* the surgery. It will also depend on whether or not nerve-sparing surgery was performed (more on that later). The nerves that are vital to erection run very close to the prostate. If the cancer invades the nerve bundles on both sides of the prostate, the surgeon has no choice but to remove the nerves along with the cancer.

Temporary loss of ability to have an erection firm enough for intercourse is very common following radical surgery and can occur in 60 to 80 percent of cases. The patient will very likely not be able to have a natural, spontaneous erection during the first three months to a year after surgery. However, erectile function can gradually improve for as long as three years after surgery. The good news is that early, daily treatment with either Viagra or alprostadil (a hormone that can be injected into the penis or taken via a small pellet inserted into the urethra) significantly speeds the return of erectile function.

Erectile dysfunction can also result after radiation therapy for prostate cancer. An estimated 30 to 60 percent of patients are affected, depending on the technique employed. The lowest rate of erectile dysfunction is reportedly for brachytherapy—internal radiation using seeds or wires placed directly into or near the tumor.

Transurethral resection of the prostate (TURP), the most common surgery to relieve the symptoms of enlarged prostate, can cause temporary impotence and loss of bladder control. Long-term or even permanent impotence can occur as a result of TURP, but the incidence is generally low, no more than 5 to 8 percent. The rate of long-term incontinence resulting from TURP is less than 1 percent.

There are many good treatments for impotence. Treatment options are divided into four basic categories: pharmacological, mechanical, surgical, and psychological.

Certain medications (such as the much-publicized Viagra) taken prior to intercourse can dramatically improve the ability to achieve erection. Viagra (sildenafil) works by keeping the blood vessels of the penis relaxed, allowing easy blood flow into the penis. Viagra will work only if a man is aroused to begin with. It is reportedly effective in 60 to 70 percent of cases of ED due to physical causes and in 90 percent of cases caused by psychological problems. Men who are not fit enough to have sex because of an existing heart condition should not use Viagra. Consult with your physician before you consider taking this or any other medication related to sexual dysfunction. Other medications and hormonal therapies include yohimbine (oral), testosterone (injection, patch, or oral), prostaglandin E1 (penile in-

OTHER ERECTION AIDS

Other erection aids include a small suppository of alprostadil called Muse inserted into the urethra. It releases a prostaglandin hormone that results in an erection about fifteen minutes later. Unlike Viagra, in men in whom Muse works, the erection happens whether the man is aroused or not.

Other techniques include injection of one or a combination of two or three drugs (papaverine, phentolamine, and alprostadil) directly into the penis. Even though this is done through a very fine needle, not surprisingly, most men are a bit reluctant to try this approach.

The point is, there is help for erectile dysfunction now and there are new drugs currently in clinical testing—but you have to seek help in order to get better.

jection or intraurethral pellet of alprostadil), and phentolamine (oral).

According to the results of a survey reported in the journal *Cancer*, nearly half the men who experience erectile dysfunction after prostate cancer therapy choose not to seek treatment. Embarrassment would appear to be the major reason. Of the men who do seek treatment for their problem, only 38 percent find a therapy that provides at least some degree of help. The majority of men try drugs such as Viagra or the recently approved Levitra and Cialis, but medication helped only 16 percent of the men surveyed.

Some sexual disorders, such as weak erections, premature ejaculation, and impotence, can benefit from prostatic massage or Kegel exercises (as detailed in our healthy prostate fitness regimen in chapter eight).

Treatment for erectile dysfunction is rapidly changing and becoming more sophisticated as our understanding of erectile physiology expands. Men are increasingly aware of the many solutions and remedies available and are becoming more active in seeking help— although they still have a long way to go in terms of "coming out of the closet" on this issue.

NERVE-SPARING OPERATIONS AND THE LATEST NERVE-GRAFTING PROCEDURES

Many men fear they will become impotent as a result of a prostatectomy. Fortunately, this was true more in the past than it is today.

Thanks to refinements in surgical technique, many men who undergo prostate removal will not experience erectile dysfunction.

Dr. Patrick Walsh of Johns Hopkins University developed the nerve-sparing prostate operation. Walsh discovered in the 1980s that the nerves responsible for an erection are on the outside of the prostate, and that severing them could be avoided while still completely removing the prostate and the tumor.

In a Johns Hopkins survey of 503 potent men, thirty-four to seventy-two years old, 68 percent remained potent after radical prostatectomy. As noted, the age of the patient, the stage of the cancer, and surgical factors—the surgeon's skill, and whether one or both neurovascular bundles were preserved during the operation—can all affect potency. Potency was preserved in 91 percent of men younger than fifty; 75 percent of men aged fifty to sixty; 58 percent of men aged sixty to seventy; and 25 percent of men over seventy. In men younger than fifty, the potency rate is similar (about 90 percent in men who kept both neurovascular bundles intact and in men who had only one nerve bundle removed). In men over fifty, however, the sexual potency rate was higher in men who had both neurovascular bundles preserved than in men who lost one bundle to surgery.

When the likelihood of impotence after surgery is adjusted for age, the risk is twice as high if the cancer has penetrated the prostate wall, if it has invaded the seminal vesicles, or if one neurovascular bundle has been removed.

Nerve grafting has long been a standard tool in plastic surgery procedures. A new nerve grafting procedure, discussed in a recent issue of the journal *Urology*, has shown promising results for men undergoing radical prostatectomy. The technique allowed four out of twelve patients to achieve spontaneous, unassisted erections within a year to twenty-eight months after the graft surgery. Another three of the twelve were able to have erections with the aid of Viagra.

Sural nerve grafting—which must take place at the same time the prostatectomy is performed—offsets the removal of the cavernous nerves, responsible for erections, located on either side of the prostate. The surgeon obtains a section of the sural nerve through an incision in the back of the lower right leg. The surgeon then sutures a length of sural nerve onto the stump or stumps of the cavernous (erection) nerves, depending on whether one or both had to be removed with the prostate. The other end of the sural nerve graft is sutured to the far end of the cavernous nerve(s) beyond where they had to be excised, bridging the gap left by the prostate removal. The only significant side effect is numbness in the area on the outside of the ankle of the right foot—a small price to pay to avoid impotence. Four to six weeks after surgery, the patient will begin therapy to restore erectile function. Results will vary.

Sural nerve grafts are currently performed at the University of Tennessee Medical Center, Memorial Sloan-Kettering Cancer Center in New York, the University of Texas M. D. Anderson Cancer Center, and other select hospitals nationwide.

SURGICAL REMOVAL OF THE TESTICLES AND CHEMICAL CASTRATION

Treatment of a prostate tumor may involve surgical removal of the testicles (orchiectomy), which halts about 95 percent of testosterone production. The surgeon makes a small incision in the scrotum, cutting the vas deferens and the blood vessels that supply each testicle. The surgeon then removes the testicles themselves.

Some surgeons perform what is called a subcapsular orchiectomy, which is essentially a cosmetic-effect orchiectomy. The surgeon opens the lining to the testicles and removes the contents of each testicle. The lining is closed again and the surgeon places the emptied shell back inside the scrotum. From all outward appearances, it looks as though nothing has been removed. Even though the basic difference between this and a standard orchiectomy is purely cosmetic, for some men it makes castration easier to accept. There is a chance that some testosterone-producing cells may be left behind in this procedure.

After surgery, patients can usually go home from the hospital the same day or the following day. Bleeding is the only major complication associated with castration. This shouldn't be a problem if the surgeon makes sure that all bleeding has stopped before the scrotum is closed. A compression dressing will be left in place to control bleeding from smaller, harder-to-see blood vessels. A hematoma can still occur, however.

The prostate tumor begins to shrink almost immediately after castration. Any obstructions, symptoms of the disease, or pain related to the disease begin to abate almost immediately.

Castration is irreversible, and for many men, it is simply too radical a treatment to consider under most circumstances. Impotence derived from castration refers not only to the inability to have an erection but to the loss of sex drive as well.

When testosterone production is gone, some of the characteristics associated with being male disappear along with it. Side effects of castration can include tenderness, pain, or swelling (gynecomastia) of the breasts. Another side effect is hot flashes, much like the hot flashes experienced by a woman during menopause, characterized by a sudden rush of warmth in the face, neck, upper chest, and back. Weight gain, loss of muscle mass, and differences in skin tone and hair growth are also common. Long-term effects may include osteoporosis.

There are prescription drugs that inhibit production of testosterone, as well as drugs called antiandrogens. Antiandrogens block the effects of hormones at the actual site of the prostate.

PROSTATITIS AND SEXUAL FUNCTION

Prostatitis is a bacterial infection of the prostate gland. The way in which the prostate becomes infected is not clearly understood. However, engaging in anal intercourse, having multiple sex partners without using a condom, and contracting other bacterial infections, such as urethritis and gonorrhea, are considered risk factors for prostatitis.

Conditions associated with an infected prostate can include impotence and loss of sex drive. Painful erections and ejaculations—pain is felt along the shaft of the penis, in the testes, and in the testicles or scrotum—are among the most dreaded symptoms of prostatitis. Pain may also be evident in the area behind the scrotum and in front of the rectum.

IMPOTENCE WITH A PSYCHOLOGICAL BASIS

If a man can have an erection while asleep or while masturbating but fails to have one in the presence of his sexual partner, his problem is psychological, not physical. At one time impotence was largely thought to be the result of psychological factors. Scientists now know that 85 to 90 percent of cases of impotence are physiological in nature.

Although erection is caused by a reflex mechanism, the brain can sometimes override it. Embarrassment, fear, or insecurity can make a man lose his erection or prevent him from having one in the first

ANATOMY OF THE PENIS AND PENILE IMPLANTS

The penis is not a muscle. It more resembles a highly sensitive blood vessel containing two inflatable cylinders filled with spongy erectile tissue, which fills with blood during moments of sexual stimulation, causing an erection. A third cylinder in the penis contains the urethra, the tube through which urine and semen exit the penis. The head of the penis, called the glans penis, fits neatly over the end of the three cylinders. The three cylinders are enclosed in a tough fibrous sheath, or tunic, important for achieving and sustaining an erection.

When a man is aroused, a signal travels from his brain to his spinal cord, and then along the pelvic nerves to his penis. An erection begins when the small arteries within the penis and the vascular area of the spongy erectile tissue relax. As the vessels widen (dilate), they allow an increase in blood flow as much as six times the normal rate. The erect penis ranges from five to nine inches long. The final phase of rigidity is reached when the muscles over the root of the penis contract, squeezing the exiting blood vessels and trapping the blood in the penis. The erection starts to fade as the arterial network begins to constrict, decreasing the blood flow into the penis, and the other vessels are no longer constricted, thus draining the blood from the penis.

During orgasm, muscles squeeze prostate fluid into the urethra. The milky fluid that carries the sperm out of the penis is partially produced by the prostate.

Once the man is no longer sexually aroused and the excess blood has drained out, the penis returns to its unaroused (flaccid) state.

When something physically interferes with or prevents the penis from filling with blood, or if the blood empties out of the penis too quickly, erectile dysfunction is the result. The complex, sophisticated arousal system of the penis can also be severely impacted when sensitive nerve bundles are damaged as a result of prostate surgery, radiation, or other treatment.

Penile implants are the most invasive and most drastic form of treatment for erectile dysfunction. Whether or not to have an implant is not a decision to be taken lightly. This procedure is reserved for men who have permanent organic impotence. Implant surgery should only be performed by a highly skilled urological surgeon. There are semirigid implants (which cause the penis always to remain in a semirigid state) and inflatable implants. In most cases, sensation should be normal.

Other procedures to restore penile function include arterial revascularization and penile vein ligation.

place. Anxiety may even lead to the release of adrenal hormones that constrict the arterial system, inhibiting an erection.

Some men develop an adjunct psychological problem due to the stress and anxiety of physically based erectile dysfunction. Psychological problems—performance anxiety, guilt, or low self-esteem—can worsen an existing organic condition.

Impotence with a psychological basis or component can often be treated successfully by an experienced sex therapist, by a hospital-based sexual rehabilitation program, or by a sexual dysfunction clinic. There is also an increasing acceptance and use of erection aid devices for both physical and psychological impotence.

INCONTINENCE

Men worry about developing urinary incontinence (involuntary urination) following treatment for prostate cancer. For many men with prostate cancer, bladder control returns within several weeks to several months after radical prostatectomy. In others, longer-range incontinence problems can range from slight to severe. In a major study of men aged fifty-five to seventy-four two years after radical prostatectomy, 10 percent had no bladder control or experienced frequent urine leakage; 14 percent leaked more than twice daily; and 28 percent were wearing pads to keep dry.

Severe incontinence is experienced by an estimated 7 percent of external beam radiation therapy patients. Bladder problems persist in about one third of patients undergoing this therapy, the most common problem being frequent urination. Long-term use of absorbent pads is necessary for an estimated 2 to 5 percent of patients. While severe incontinence is not a frequent side effect (estimated at 7 percent), frequent urination is experienced by one third of patients undergoing brachytherapy (radiation therapy with radioactive material sealed in seeds or wires).

TREATING INCONTINENCE

Talk to your physician about the best methods for dealing with incontinence. While the condition may never be corrected completely, in virtually every case it can be helped to a good degree. Treatment of incontinence depends upon the type, cause and severity of the condition.

The Institute for Cancer Prevention recommends dietary modification (including avoidance of caffeine, alcohol, and chocolate), bladder retraining, and pelvic floor muscle exercises as a natural defense against incontinence.

Other treatment options include antispasmodic drugs and surgery (the latter should almost always be the option of last resort). Men who suffer incontinence as the result of an enlarged prostate can be treated by prescription medications (including Proscar, Flomax, Hytrin, Uroxatral, and Cardura). Widespread use of these medications has substantially reduced the number of men who opt for surgery. Procedures utilizing microwave and laser therapies have also contributed to the decreased popularity of surgery as an option.

A SIMPLE BUT EFFECTIVE BLADDER-TRAINING METHOD TO COMBAT INCONTINENCE

If you're suffering from incontinence, there's a simple, effective way to help alleviate the condition: when you feel the urge to urinate, try holding it in for five minutes. If you feel that this is impossible, give in to the urge and relieve yourself. Many times, however, you'll find that you are actually able to hold the urine in for that extra five minutes. After you gain facility with the five-minute delay, gradually work your way up to ten-minute or even fifteen-minute

---

THE THREE TYPES OF INCONTINENCE

- **Stress incontinence:** Caused by dysfunction of the bladder sphincter (the muscular valve that keeps urine in the bladder). There is urine leakage when a man coughs, sneezes, laughs, works out, or is distracted. This is the form of incontinence most associated with prostate surgery, which may damage the muscles or nerves of the sphincter valve.
- **Overflow incontinence:** Caused by blockage or narrowing of the bladder outlet by cancer, enlarged prostate, or scar tissue resulting from surgery. It takes a man longer than normal to initiate his urine stream, or sometimes the urine dribbles out in a weak stream.
- **Urge incontinence:** An urgent need to urinate immediately. This can be a symptom of enlarged prostate, prostate cancer, or any number of urinary tract conditions.

intervals. This can be a natural way to strengthen your bladder, very much like Kegel exercises. Kegel exercises are wonderful for strengthening the bladder muscles—and you can do them virtually anywhere.

There are other simple things you can do to make incontinence less of a problem. Empty your bladder before bedtime or before strenuous or vigorous activity. Avoid drinking excessive amounts of fluid. Because fat in the abdomen can push on the bladder, losing weight can help improve bladder control.

OTHER AIDS FOR INCONTINENCE

Collagen and other material can be surgically injected to tighten the bladder sphincter. An artificial sphincter can even be implanted surgically if the incontinence is really severe.

There are incontinence products such as pads that can be worn under clothing and bed pads that can protect linens and mattresses. The most efficient incontinence products should provide absorbency and comfort and not be too bulky, too expensive (see if these products are covered by your insurance), or too difficult to find in local stores.

There are sheaths called condom catheters, as well as compression devices, that are placed on the penis to control incontinence. Self-catheterization may be an option for certain types of incontinence. The incontinence sufferer inserts a thin tube in his urethra to drain and empty the bladder. It is easy to learn this safe and generally painless technique.

You'll discover that winning the battle against incontinence—no matter how severe the condition—is neither as daunting nor as complicated as you might have imagined.

INFERTILITY

A small percentage of men have infertility problems related to the prostate. However, the vast majority of fertility problems are not due to prostate conditions.

We covered the potential consequences of radical prostatectomy and castration when we discussed impotence. There are other circumstances related to the genitourinary system and the prostate that can lead to infertility.

GENITAL TRACT OBSTRUCTIONS AND INFERTILITY

A condition called azoospermia (lack of sperm in the ejaculate) can result from an acquired reproductive tract obstruction due to vasectomy, failed vasectomy reversal (some men who have chosen to have a vasectomy later decide they want the procedure reversed in order to restore fertility), or scar tissue due to infection and inflammation.

There are two primary surgical procedures with jawbreaking names (vasovasostomy, vasoepididymostomy) that remove or bypass obstructions in the genital tract. These procedures are generally performed to restore fertility and sometimes to relieve pain.

Advances in techniques, instruments, and diagnostic procedures have made surgery for genital tract obstruction more effective and less invasive.

SEX, INFERTILITY, AND THE ENLARGED PROSTATE

Will surgery for benign prostatic hyperplasia (BPH) interfere with your ability to have sex or to reproduce? It is estimated that enlarged-prostate surgery can affect sexual function in up to 30 percent of cases. The good news is that most men will eventually return to normal sexual function. But it may take as much as a year, although sexual function generally returns from within a few weeks to a matter of months after surgery. Recovery time depends largely on the type of surgical procedure, how long the condition was present, and how chronic the symptoms were before the surgery was performed.

TURP AND RETROGRADE EJACULATION

A prevalent side effect of transurethral resection of the prostate (TURP)—the most common surgery to relieve the symptoms of enlarged prostate—is retrograde ejaculation, or "dry climax." Semen is forced backward into the bladder during orgasm instead of out through the penis, leading to infertility.

During normal sexual activity, sperm from the testes enters the urethra near the opening of the bladder. Since a sphincter normally closes off the bladder entrance during ejaculation, semen exits through the penis. Enlarged prostate surgery impairs this sphincter muscle as it widens the neck of the bladder. Following surgery, the semen sometimes takes the path of least resistance and enters the wider opening in the bladder rather than going out through the penis. This semen is later expelled from the bladder along with urine. With this condition, there can be a difference in orgasmic sensation.

IS IT ALL IN THE SEX HORMONES?

There are two major theories of the possible cause and effect between sex hormone levels and risk or incidence of enlarged prostate. As a man ages, his testosterone level decreases relative to his amount of circulating estrogen. Estrogen is the female sex hormone, which is also present in much lower levels in the male. A higher male estrogen to testosterone ratio may bolster the effect of the testosterone derivative DHT. DHT promotes cell growth and glandular enlargement in the prostate as it interacts with estrogen.

The second hormonally based theory of the origin of prostate enlargement centers around prostate gland development requiring the conversion of testosterone into DHT in the presence of an enzyme called 5alpha-reductase. As a man ages, the amount of DHT in the prostate gland remains high, even as circulating testosterone level drops. A higher ratio of DHT to testosterone in the prostate may promote cell growth and lead to greater enlargement. Tellingly, scientists have noted that men who do not produce DHT do not develop an enlarged prostate.

VASECTOMY AS A PROSTATE CANCER RISK FACTOR

About one in six American men has had a vasectomy. A handful of studies have indicated that a vasectomy may be a moderate risk factor for prostate cancer. However, a more recent, large-scale study found that men who undergo vasectomies are no more likely to develop prostate cancer than men who do not. The study, conducted under the auspices of the U.S. National Institute of Child Health and Human Development, surveyed more than 2,000 men in New Zealand. New Zealand has the highest rate of vasectomies of all nations, as well as mandatory reporting of all new cancer cases. The sampling was certainly large enough to detect a risk factor for prostate cancer associated with vasectomy, but no such linkage was found.

10. Prostatitis: A Little Tenderness Goes a Long Way

An Insufficiently Understood Disease

Prostatitis is, simply stated, an inflammation of the prostate gland. This disease of the prostate is surprisingly widespread in American men but not well understood. Inflammation of the prostate is extremely rare in preadolescent boys but common in mature men. It is estimated that doctors diagnose about 2 million cases of prostatitis each year. Despite its prevalence, prostatitis is poorly studied, difficult to diagnose, and hard to treat.

The Three Faces of Prostatitis

Prostatitis is actually a blanket term for three separate conditions. Two types are bacterial (caused by bacteria), and one is not. Because prostatitis exists in these three forms, diagnosis and treatment of the disease can be especially difficult. Each type of prostatitis has a different cause and requires a specific treatment strategy.

Acute Bacterial Prostatitis (ABP)

This is the most serious form of the disease, but, fortunately, the least common and easiest to treat. The onset of symptoms is usually sudden and severe. This form of prostatitis is caused by a bacterial infection, usually by the bacterium *Escherichia coli*, more commonly known as *E. coli*. *E. coli* are commonly found in the urinary tract and the large intestines. This kind of prostatitis is thought to be caused by *E. coli* or other bacteria migrating to the prostate from the bowel or via the urethra.

Ignoring these symptoms (below) will surely lead to the development of more serious conditions. The inability to urinate can lead to urinary tract infection and infection in the bloodstream (bacteremia). You could also develop a prostatic abscess, an accumulation of infected pus inside the prostate. The abscess might have to be drained using a needle passed into the prostate from the rectum or perineum, or it may have to be removed using a type of surgery called TURP (transurethral resection of the prostate), a procedure frequently used to treat enlarged prostate or BPH (see Chapter 11). ABP can be fatal if left untreated for too long.

CHRONIC BACTERIAL PROSTATITIS (CBP)

This type of prostatitis is also caused by bacterial infection by *E. coli* or other kinds of bacteria. Unlike acute bacterial prostatitis, however, the symptoms are not as severe and develop more slowly. Chronic bacterial prostatitis usually targets men over the age of

---

SYMPTOMS OF ACUTE BACTERIAL PROSTATITIS

Symptoms often start suddenly, and medical help should be sought immediately. Sometimes hospitalization may be necessary for a few days in order to bring the disease under control. Symptoms include:

- Fever
- Chills
- A general flu-like feeling
- Pain in the lower back
- Pain in the perineum (the area between the scrotum and the anus)
- Pain or a burning sensation during urination
- Inability to urinate or decreased urine flow
- Inability to empty the bladder during urination
- Frequent and urgent need to urinate
- Blood or pus in the urine
- Painful ejaculation

forty. It can be caused by infections in the urinary tract, the bladder, or the blood. Sometimes the infection is the result of a trauma to the urinary tract or the insertion of a catheter during medical procedures. In addition, calcified stones that form in the prostate called prostatic calculi can become infected. Another cause is related to a structural defect in the prostate that allows bacteria to collect inside the gland. CBP may also be linked to fungal and viral organisms such as chlamydia, ureaplasma, mycoplasma, herpes simplex, cytomegalovirus, and adenovirus, but they are not thought to directly cause this type of prostatitis. Sexually active younger men who have contracted a sexually transmitted disease such as gonorrhea are more likely to develop CBP, although STDs are not a direct cause of the condition.

Unlike acute bacterial prostatitis, which responds well to treatment and is quickly cured, CBP keeps coming back again and again. You can sometimes get chronic bacterial prostatitis after having been successfully treated for a case of acute bacterial prostatitis. This occurs because antibiotics used to fight the infection are unable to penetrate deeply enough into the tissue of the prostate to destroy the bacteria. Colonies of the bacteria survive deep inside the pros-

SYMPTOMS OF CHRONIC BACTERIAL PROSTATITIS (CBP)

Symptoms of chronic bacterial prostatitis build up slowly over time and can vary from patient to patient. Symptoms include:

- Frequent urination
- Pain or burning sensation while urinating
- Difficulty starting or continuing urination
- Frequent nighttime urination
- Diminished flow of urine
- Sudden or compelling urge to urinate
- Painful ejaculation
- Occasional blood in semen
- Pain in the lower back
- Pain along the shaft of the penis or in the scrotum
- Pain in the perineum (the area between the scrotum and the anus)
- Recurring bladder infections

tate and cause reinfection. Bacteria can also persist on the inside of prostate stones.

CPB is not as serious an illness as acute bacterial prostatitis and is usually not life-threatening, but the symptoms of the disease are severe enough to make you want to seek medical treatment without delay. Infection of the prostate frequently leads to infection of the urinary tract and other unpleasant conditions that have a negative impact on your quality of life.

CHRONIC NONBACTERIAL PROSTATITIS (CNP)

This is the most common type of prostatitis, but it is also the most difficult to diagnose and treat. Unlike the other varieties of the disease, chronic nonbacterial prostatitis apparently is not an infectious disease caused by bacteria. There is no bacteria in the patient's urine or prostatic fluid, but his urine specimens contain white blood cells, indicating inflammation. The exact cause of CNP is unknown, and it does not respond to treatment with antibiotics.

A number of factors may be linked to CNP. Some medical researchers suspect that a still undetectable bacterial or viral organism causes the disease. Anxiety and stress may cause tightening of the urinary sphincter muscles that causes fluids to back up in the urethra and irritate the prostate. Heavy lifting on or off the job may con-

---

SYMPTOMS OF CHRONIC NONBACTERIAL PROSTATITIS (CNP)

CNP has many of the same symptoms as chronic bacterial prostatitis, although there are some variations.

- Frequent urination
- Pain or burning sensation while urinating
- Sudden or compelling urge to urinate
- Painful ejaculation
- Pain in the lower back
- Pain in the perineum (the area between the scrotum and the anus)
- Pain in the rectum
- Pain along the inner thighs
- Pain in muscles or joints
- Decreased libido or impotence

tribute to CNP, as may occupations that involve exposing the prostate to a lot of vibrations, such as truck driving or operating heavy machinery. Certain recreational activities such as jogging or bicycling may also irritate the prostate.

Some forms of chronic nonbacterial prostatitis are related to sexual activity. This can be due to a lack of sexual activity, which causes unejaculated semen to build up and inflame the prostate. This condition is called congestive prostatitis. Conversely, too much sexual activity can strain and irritate the prostate, leading to exhaustive or overuse prostatitis.

To further confound diagnosis, the symptoms of chronic nonbacterial prostatitis are practically indistinguishable from a related condition called prostatodynia, or chronic pelvic pain syndrome (CPPS). Diagnostic testing can distinguish between the two conditions. Prostatodynia is covered more fully in Chapter 12.

WHICH KIND DO I HAVE?

A urologist once called prostatitis the most imprecise diagnosis in medicine. Proper diagnosis may prove elusive, and doctors must be especially careful to distinguish among chronic bacterial prostatitis, chronic nonbacterial prostatitis, and prostatodynia, all of which have very similar symptoms.

To ensure a proper diagnosis, your doctor will begin by asking questions. He or she will want to know about your medical history, your family's medical history and your occupation. You will be asked in detail about the nature of your symptoms, any recent changes in your lifestyle, and your sexual habits.

Next, your doctor will conduct a thorough physical exam. He or she will check your abdomen and pelvic area for any unusual tenderness. Then a digital rectal exam (DRE) will be performed in order to check the condition of the prostate. In the DRE procedure the doctor inserts a gloved and lubricated finger into the rectum and examines the prostate for anything unusual. Acute bacterial prostatitis can easily be detected by the DRE because the prostate will often feel enlarged and tender to the touch, but other forms of prostatitis may not be as easily detectable because they do not cause this kind of swelling and tenderness. In addition to the DRE, other tests may have to be performed in order to make an accurate diagnosis.

THE STAMEY-MEARES FOUR-GLASS TEST

The Stamey-Meares four-glass test is a special urinalysis procedure that is considered the "gold standard" used to diagnose the various types of prostatitis. It was devised by Meares and Stamey in 1968 and has been in use as a diagnostic tool ever since. The test seems complicated, but it can be performed in the doctor's office in about half an hour. It involves taking three separate samples of urine and a sample of fluid from the prostate.

You will be asked to retract the foreskin of your penis (if there is one) and cleanse the penis. Then you must begin urinating and collect a sample of the first ounce of your urine in a sterile cup, wait a bit, then collect a second urine sample in midstream in a second cup. After this, the bladder is voided until it is almost, but not quite, empty.

The next phase involves obtaining a sample of your prostate fluid. To do this, the doctor will insert his or her gloved and lubricated finger into the rectum and vigorously massage and press the prostate until a sample of the fluid is discharged from the penis. The fluid is collected and placed on laboratory slides for analysis. This part of the procedure is not done if you have acute bacterial prostatitis because this condition causes the prostate to become swollen and irritated, and prostate massage would be too painful and could possibly release harmful bacteria into the bloodstream.

Finally, a third urine sample will be collected as you empty your bladder completely. This sample will also contain some fluid from the prostate mixed in with the urine. The end result will be two samples of urine, a sample of prostatic fluid and a sample containing prostatic fluid and urine. These four samples represent the "four glasses" of the Stamey-Meares test.

The first urine sample also contains fluid from the urethra, while the second urine sample, having flushed the urethra, primarily contains urine from the bladder. The third and forth samples contain fluids from the prostate. All four samples are sent to the lab to look for the presence of bacteria and white blood cells. They will allow your doctor to determine if the infection is located in the urethra, the bladder or the prostate.

If bacteria are found in any of the samples, a diagnosis of acute bacterial prostatitis or chronic bacterial prostatitis will be made. The location of the infection will be pinpointed, and the bacteria will be identified so that an appropriate antibiotic can be prescribed to counter it.

If no bacteria are found in any of the samples, but white blood cells are found in the sample of prostatic fluid, then the diagnosis will be chronic nonbacterial prostatitis. The presence of white blood cells indicates a noninfectious inflammation of the prostate. No antibiotic treatment will be required because there is no infection present.

If no bacteria or white blood cells are found in any of the samples, you probably don't have prostatitis at all but a related condition called prostatodynia, which is discussed in Chapter 12. These and other tests can also determine if you have other medical conditions that should be treated, such as benign enlargement of the prostate (BPH), inflammation of the urethra (urethritis), or urinary tract infection.

An alternative to the Stamey-Meares procedure, called the pre- and post-massage test (PPMT), has recently come into use. It is basically a simplified version of the four-glass test that involves first taking a midstream urine sample, then performing a DRE to rectally massage the prostate, and then taking a second urine sample after the massage. The PPMT is somewhat less expensive than the Stamey-Meares test because there are only two, rather than four, samples sent to be analyzed in the lab. It is also easier on the patient because the process of obtaining fluid from the prostate for analysis involves vigorous massage and manipulation that can be painful or uncomfortable, and there is less of this with PPMT. The accuracy of the PPMT in comparison to the four-glass test as a diagnostic tool is still being evaluated.

TREATMENT STRATEGIES FOR BACTERIAL PROSTATITIS

Acute bacterial prostatitis is the easiest type to diagnose and treat. You may have to spend a few days in the hospital while your fever is brought down and your condition stabilized. You may need to rest in bed for a while and drink plenty of fluids to keep your body hydrated. You may also have to take stool softeners to take the strain away from bowel movements and mild painkillers to relieve discomfort. In cases where urinary retention occurs, or if you are unable to urinate at all, a catheter may have to be inserted to drain the bladder. You may also have to abstain from sexual activity for a short time.

ANTIBIOTICS

Antibiotics are used as the first line of treatment in combating the infection. The Stamey-Meares test will determine exactly which type of bacteria is causing the problem. It may be *E. coli*, a variety of staphylococcus (staph), streptococcus (strep), or one of a number of other bacteria. Antibiotics commonly used to treat ABP include ciprofloxacin (Cipro), doxycycline (Vibramycin), norfloxacin (Noroxin), ofloxacin (Floxin), and trimethoprim-sulfamethoxazole (Bactrim, Septra).

It is usually difficult to treat the prostate with antibiotics because these drugs cannot penetrate deep enough inside the gland to be completely effective. This is because of the blood-prostate barrier, maintained by a membrane called the prostatic epithelium. This membrane is designed to keep harmful substances out of the prostate, but keeps out antibiotics as well. During acute bacterial prostatitis, however, the blood-prostate barrier breaks down to some extent, allowing the antibiotics to penetrate deep inside the gland. For this reason, many doctors prescribe antibiotics for a period of six weeks to allow the medicine to penetrate into the interior of the prostate tissue and kill off the infection completely. If the antibiotics are taken for only a few days, the infection can recur in the future as episodes of chronic bacterial prostatitis.

In cases of chronic bacterial prostatitis the same kinds of antibiotics are prescribed, but they must be used for a longer period of time. At this point, however, the bacteria may have been able to gain a foothold inside the prostate and the infection will be much harder to eradicate. For cases that do not immediately respond to treatment, your doctor may recommend a regimen of long-term, low-dose antibiotic therapy. Your doctor may also perform prostate massage while you are taking antibiotics, a procedure that makes it possible for the drugs to penetrate more deeply into infected prostatic tissue.

Sometimes surgical removal of infected sections of the prostate may be required, and in extreme cases an open prostatectomy may be required to remove the entire prostate.

Further complications can arise if you have prostate stones (calculi). Bacteria can persist inside these stones unaffected by antibiotics, causing prostatitis infections to recur again and again. The long-term solution is to remove the stones surgically by using a procedure commonly used to treat BPH (enlarged prostate) called transurethral resection of the prostate, or TURP.

CHRONIC NONBACTERIAL PROSTATITIS

This variety of prostatitis is the most difficult to treat. Because there is no apparent bacterial infection, antibiotics are probably not effective to treat the condition. Nevertheless, most doctors prescribe antibiotics early in the therapy for a couple of weeks as a precaution. Treatment strategies for nonbacterial prostatitis are aimed at relieving symptoms rather than curing the disease because the cause of the condition is unknown.

TREATMENT OPTIONS FOR CHRONIC NONBACTERIAL PROSTATITIS (CNP)

ALPHA-BLOCKERS

These are medications that help relax the muscles of the prostate and the bladder neck. They are prescribed for men who are having difficulty urinating, and are frequently used to treat enlarged prostate (BPH). Alpha-blockers can be effective in removing urinary obstructions so that you don't have to urinate as frequently. The most frequently prescribed alpha-blockers for prostatitis are doxazosin (Cardura), tamsulosin (Flomax), and terazosin (Hytrin). In some cases an anticholinergic drug such as oxybutynin (Ditropan) or 5alpha-reductase inhibitors may be prescribed.

PAIN RELIEVERS

Analgesic medicines not only relieve pain and discomfort but also help reduce inflammation of the prostate tissue as well. An over-the-counter pain medication such as aspirin, acetaminophen (Tylenol), or ibuprofen (Advil) can be used, or your doctor may prescribe other nonsteroidal anti-inflammatory drugs (NSAIDs) such as celecoxib (Celebrex), indomethacin (Indocin), naproxen (Naprosyn), or rofe-coxib (Vioxx).

EXERCISE

Exercises that stretch and relax the lower pelvic muscles can help relieve symptoms. A physical therapist can recommend the appropriate exercises for this purpose. After working with the therapist, you can continue to perform the exercises at home.

SITZ BATHS

Some patients find that sitz baths improve their symptoms. Taken from the German word *sitzen,* meaning "to sit," this therapy involves sitting in a warm bath for about fifteen to thirty minutes two or three times a day. For chronic nonbacterial prostatitis, temperatures of up to 115 degrees are optimal. Sitz baths are also used to treat bacterial prostatitis, but at slightly cooler temperatures (around 95 degrees F).

RELAXATION THERAPY

Although the cause is not clearly understood, the relaxation of tight or irritated muscles can help relieve the symptoms of prostatitis. Therapists sometimes recommend biofeedback therapy to help loosen overtightened muscles. Biofeedback is a method used to teach people how to control their body responses. During a biofeed-

---

MICROWAVES

A technology used to shrink enlarged prostates may also be useful for treating chronic prostatitis. It's microwave therapy.

Although bacteria can't always be found in chronic prostatitis, there are some who believe that there are still germs lurking in the prostate that are causing the ongoing problems. Since microwave therapy is believed to be lethal to many organisms (microwaves are used to sterilize urinary catheters and surgical scalpels), several investigators are trying microwave therapy, applied through tiny antennae inserted into the urethra, in an attempt to kill bacteria in the prostate. It's called transurethral microwave therapy (TUMT).

Patients with nonbacterial prostatitis who don't respond to traditional therapy may benefit from this approach. Early results are promising, with a 25 percent rate of complete and sustained improvement in a group of forty-five patients using TUMT.

back session, a therapist attaches electrodes and other sensors to your skin on various parts of the body. These superficial electrodes are connected to a monitoring device that gives you feedback on your bodily functions, including tension in your muscles. Once the electrodes are hooked up, the therapist will use techniques designed to relax your muscles. The monitor will indicate when your muscles are completely relaxed, and the therapist will teach you how to maintain this level of relaxation by watching the monitor. Once you have learned how to achieve this state of relaxation, you will be able to maintain it without having to be hooked up to the feedback machine.

PSYCHOTHERAPY

Some doctors recommend that you undergo psychiatric counseling or stress management courses that can enable you to cope with stress more effectively. Relaxing the mind can help relax muscles in the prostate and lower pelvic area. Doctors may prescribe a tranquilizer, such as diazepam (Valium) or amitriptyline (Elavil), or an antidepressant medication, such as fluoxetine (Prozac), to obtain a similar relaxation effect.

PROSTATE MASSAGE

Prostate massage can help relieve the symptoms of CNP by relieving congested ducts inside the gland. If you are taking antibiotics during the early phase of CNP treatment, massage will allow the drugs to pass deeper into the prostatic tissue. Massage therapy may have to be performed as frequently as three times a week to be effective.

The massage procedure is similar to that performed during a digital rectal exam (DRE) or during the Stamey-Meares or pre- and post-massage test (PPMT). To massage the prostate, the doctor inserts a gloved, lubricated finger into your rectum in order to access the gland. He or she will gently massage the prostate from top to bottom and from side to side. The massage is much less vigorous than the technique used during the PPMT and four-glass tests, which are aimed at extracting prostatic fluid, and are not as uncomfortable to the patient.

DIET AND LIFESTYLE CHANGES

In addition to medical treatment, many men find that certain changes in their diet and lifestyle can help minimize or control their symptoms. See Chapter 4 for the Institute for Cancer Prevention's Prostate Health Pyramid; Chapter 5 for a detailed discussion of nutrition and the prostate; and Chapter 6 for details of the prostate Transition Diet.

• **Drink plenty of water.** In addition to your usual six-to-eight-glass intake, try to drink another four glasses of water or clear liquids each day. This helps dilute acids, salts, and other irritants in your urine.

• **Go to the bathroom at frequent intervals.** Increased water intake will help flush out the urinary tract.

• **Limit your alcohol intake.** Alcohol can irritate the prostate.

• **Avoid long periods of sitting.** This may include driving and bicycle riding. If you have a desk job, you may be obliged to take standing or walking breaks at regular intervals.

• **Avoid trauma to the lower pelvic region.** Operating heavy machinery that produces intense vibration in the pelvic area can impact the prostate. So can some common exercises such as jogging or other relatively high-impact exercises.

• **Change your sexual habits.** "Congestive" prostatitis, thought to be caused by a buildup of semen in the testicles that may irritate the prostate, can be relieved by an increase in the number of your ejaculations. In the absence of other options, masturbation can be used to achieve this goal. Conversely, "exhaustive" or "overuse" prostatitis, caused by excessive ejaculation, can be alleviated by decreasing your level of sexual activity.

• **Change your diet.** Some patients report that avoiding certain foods and beverages helps relieve their symptoms. These include acidic foods and drinks such as coffee, cranberry juice, colas, citrus fruits and juices, and tomatoes. Highly spiced foods should also be avoided.

GAY MEN AND PROSTATITIS

Gay men's health issues have traditionally received short shrift. Certain health issues of concern to gay men continue to receive inadequate attention. One such problem is prostatitis.

Unprotected anal sex is considered a risk factor for prostatitis. Gay men may also risk getting prostatitis if:

- They insert unsterile sex toys or other objects into their urethra or rectum.
- They neglect a urethritis condition (a sexually transmitted urethral infection).
- They have contracted other bacterial infections, such as gonorrhea.
- They have sex with multiple partners, especially unprotected sex.

Buildup of prostate fluids that become a component of ejaculate can create an environment for bacterial growth. Like their straight counterparts, gay men should pursue a vigorous, active—but safe—sex life. Safe sex means wearing a condom and not participating in sex with multiple partners. If you're without a partner—or choose to be without one for a period of time—masturbation at least every couple of days is a good idea for prostate health (see the sidebar on page 168).

IF IT'S NOT PROSTATITIS, WHAT ELSE MIGHT IT BE?

There are some sexually transmitted diseases (STDs) that may make gay men think they have prostatitis. These include:

- **Epididymitis.** The epididymis is a small organ attached to the testicle. An *E. coli* infection can be transmitted to gay men who are the insertive partner during anal intercourse. It is usually accompanied by urethritis (see below). Symptoms include testicular pain and tenderness. Non–sexually transmitted epididymitis can result from urinary tract infection, and is often found in men over thirty-five who have recently undergone urinary tract surgery.
- **Urethritis.** This is an inflammation of the urethra caused by chlamydial infection. Symptoms may include discharge from the tip

of the penis and discomfort during urination. Having urethritis can make it easier to catch and pass along other STDs. Sexual penetration with an infected partner has a 20 percent transmission rate for males with a single encounter.

• **Chlamydia.** This is a bacterial infection of the male sexual organs that can spread to the prostate gland or the epididymis. The anus and the rectum may be infected through anal intercourse. Chlamydia will show no symptoms unless the urethra is infected. It is estimated that at least 20 percent of men infected with chlamydia or gonorrhea are also infected with HIV.

TIPS FOR GAY MEN
• Avoid anonymous sex.
• Always use a condom during anal intercourse.
• Familiarize yourself with the symptoms of STDs.
• Don't have sex if you show any symptoms.
• Contact your physician immediately if symptoms appear.

LIVING WITH PROSTATITIS

Prostatitis can be a frustrating condition for doctors to treat and for patients to endure. Bacterial prostatitis infections can keep recurring, requiring long-term treatment with antibiotics that may not be effective. Causes of chronic nonbacterial prostatitis are not clearly understood and current treatments for the condition are designed only to treat symptoms. Patients who see the quality of their lives diminished by the illness sometimes despair and wonder if their condition will ever improve. Many men just have to learn to "live with it." Here are a couple of additional points to consider:

• **Prostatitis does not lead to prostate cancer.** There's no evidence that having any form of prostatitis puts you at greater risk for developing prostate cancer or any other prostate disease. Prostatitis can, however, elevate PSA blood levels, which can confuse diagnosis on tests used to screen for prostate cancer. The test may have to be redone after you've been treated with antibiotics. If your prostatitis is chronic, you may have to have a percent free PSA test.

• **You can't pass prostatitis to your partner during sexual inter-**

course. Although bacterial forms of prostatitis are infectious diseases, the condition is not contagious and can't be passed along to
your partner when you have sex. Not understanding this, many men
with prostatitis stop having sex entirely for fear of transmitting the
disease to their partner. If you have prostatitis, there's no reason why
you can't enjoy a normal sex life. Certain forms of the disease, however, can interfere with the development of semen and lower your
fertility.

• **Prostatitis is a treatable condition.** Even if it cannot be cured,
you can usually get relief from its symptoms by following your
doctor's recommended treatment. It does not, in and of itself, lead to
more serious conditions of the prostate. As prostatitis is studied in
more depth, advances in medical science may discover a cure or a
comprehensive treatment for this mysterious, bothersome ailment.

11. When Size Matters: Benign Prostatic Hyperplasia (BPH)

What is BPH?

Although prostate cancer is the most life-threatening condition of the prostate, the most common prostate disease is called benign prostatic hyperplasia, commonly referred to by the acronym BPH. This condition has been known to medical science for quite some time. Founding fathers Benjamin Franklin and Thomas Jefferson may have suffered from this ailment. BPH occurs in about 50 percent of men in their sixties and nearly 80 percent of men in their eighties. More than 350,000 operations to alleviate this illness are performed in the United States each year, making it the most common surgery for men over the age of fifty-five.

The term "benign prostatic hyperplasia" refers to a nonmalignant enlargement of the prostate gland. It must be stressed that this type of enlargement is not cancerous and that growth is confined to the prostate and does not spread to surrounding tissues. There is no statistical evidence that BPH increases the risk of getting prostate cancer. The two conditions are entirely separate and distinct, although you can have cancer and BPH at the same time.

An enlarged prostate is not necessarily a problem in itself. Many men with severely enlarged prostates are unaware of the condition and have no recognizable symptoms. Problems only emerge when the enlargement begins to impede the flow of urine through the urethra, the slender tube that carries urine from the bladder, passes it through the prostate and into the penis during the process of urination. Swelling of the prostatic tissues causes the constriction of the urethra and produces difficulties with the normal flow of urine.

How BPH Develops

During early childhood, a boy's prostate is very small, about the size of a pea. With the onset of puberty, the male hormone testosterone is released into the body in large quantities. This causes the prostate to grow until, at age twenty, it is about the size of a walnut. Designed to produce some of the fluid that makes up semen, the gland is situated just below the bladder and surrounds the urethra. Although the prostate is technically not part of the urinary system, it surrounds the urethra somewhat like a straw passing through the central hole of a doughnut.

From about age twenty to age forty, the rate of prostate growth slows to practically nil. After forty, however, it begins to expand once more. Researchers are not sure why this happens, but it is thought that it is caused by a complex interaction of hormones within the prostate. Testosterone has been fingered as one of the culprits. Although the body produces significantly less testosterone in men after age forty, researchers theorize that in older men testosterone is converted into another male hormone called dihydrotestosterone, or DHT. It is thought that DHT, possibly in connection with the hormone estrogen, a female hormone that is also present in males, stimulates the enlargement of the prostate. Another substance thought to be responsible is an enzyme called 5alpha-reductase, which is instrumental in converting testosterone to DHT. Also implicated are substances called growth factors that govern cell growth and cell death within various human tissues. Somehow, between the action of DHT, estrogen, and growth factors, cells in the prostate are inhibited from dying in the normal fashion, while new cells continue to be produced, causing the gland to enlarge.

Into the Transition Zone

Simple enlargement of the prostate might not cause symptoms of BPH. The prostate can swell to the size of a small grapefruit in some men without producing any noticeable symptoms. In others, even a little enlargement produces a lot of symptoms. It is the specific location of the growth that produces the symptoms of BPH.

BPH occurs with growth in an area of the prostate called the transition zone. This is the inner portion of the gland that surrounds the urethra like a ring. In young men, the transition zone makes up roughly 5 percent of a normal prostate. With the onset of middle age, tissues in the transition zone begin to expand, forming glandular nodules along the prostate cells that line the urethra. As BPH progresses, the nodules cluster into lobes that constrict the passage of urine through the urethra. Due to the location of the transition zone in the center of the prostate, abnormal growth in this area may not be detected by a doctor during the digital rectal exam used to diagnose BPH because only the outside portion of the gland is felt during the procedure.

WHO GETS BPH?

Aging seems to be the primary factor in the development of BPH. Simply put, the longer men live, the more likely they are to get BPH. The condition rarely occurs in men under the age of forty. An exception to this rule arises in men who seem to have a genetic predisposition to the disease. Studies indicate that about 7 percent of men need treatment for BPH because they have inherited a gene that facilitates prostate enlargement. Male relatives of these men were found to be four times as likely as other men to require prostate surgery, while the brothers of the men were six times as likely. For this reason, providing a detailed family history to your doctor is essential in diagnosing BPH.

Environmental factors may also play a part. For instance, Japanese men have historically had a much lower incidence of BPH (as well as prostate cancer) than Caucasian men. This disparity vanishes, however, when Japanese men emigrate from Japan to Western countries. Some researchers attribute this to a change in diet and theorize that there is a link between BPH and an increase in the consumption of foods containing large amounts of animal fat, which is missing from most Asian diets. Consumption of soy products by Japanese men may also be a factor that prevents BPH.

Symptoms of BPH

Complaints due to BPH develop gradually. At first, many men experience few symptoms because the powerful muscle of the bladder pushes urine through the constricted urethra more forcefully in order to compensate for the restricted flow. Over time, however, the bladder muscle becomes strained and less efficient at forcing urine out of the body, leading to a marked decrease in urine flow. This, in addition, causes the bladder wall to become less elastic and less able to retain urine. Symptoms of BPH emerge in response to these conditions. Urination becomes more frequent and more urgent. Some of the more annoying and embarrassing symptoms commonly experienced by men with BPH are the frequent need to urinate at night (nocturia) and the inability to postpone urination. This, in turn, results in episodes of involuntary urination, or "urge incontinence." As BPH progresses, men sometimes lose the capacity to empty the bladder completely during urination, a condition that can lead to much more serious symptoms, including chronic urinary tract infections, kidney damage, and inability to urinate at all (urinary retention).

Prominent symptoms of BPH include:

- A weak urine stream
- Difficulty starting urination
- Stopping and starting again during urination (interrupted stream)
- Dribbling at the end of urination
- Frequent and/or urgent need to urinate and wetting (urge incontinence)
- Increased urination at night
- A sense of not being able to empty the bladder completely

When to See a Doctor

Many men, aware of changes in their urination patterns, suspect that they have BPH but do not consider their symptoms severe enough to seek medical attention. But BPH can progress to a stage where it becomes more than a mere annoyance. If it is left untreated, serious complications can develop.

Acute urinary retention is a condition in which the urethra is constricted so much that the patient is completely unable to urinate. When this happens, urine can back up into the kidneys and even cause kidney damage and/or failure. Prostate cancer and prostatitis can also cause this condition. Treatment involves the insertion of a catheter to drain the bladder, which can be painful because of the constricted urethra; also, the catheter may then have to be worn for an extended period of time. Surgery may also be necessary. In addition, should the patient suffer a blow to the stomach while his bladder is overfilled, his bladder could rupture and the contents spill into the abdominal cavity, causing serious infection and even death.

Urine retention can also lead to the formation of bladder stones. These are produced when crystals of uric acid or calcium precipitate in the urine and form hard, rocklike deposits. Bladder stones can be

THE AMERICAN UROLOGICAL ASSOCIATION SYMPTOM QUESTIONNAIRE

The American Urological Association has formulated a short questionnaire that will assist your doctor in diagnosing BPH and in assessing the severity of your condition. The test is not complicated and should take only a few minutes for you to complete. Again, you should be completely honest when you fill out this form so that your doctor can accurately assess your condition. Take it along the next time you get a general checkup.

SCALE

0: Not at all
1: Less than one time in five
2: Less than half the time
3: About half the time
4: More than half the time
5: Almost always

Over the past month, how often have you had a sensation of not emptying your bladder completely after you finished urinating?
  0   1   2   3   4   5

Over the past month, how often have you had to urinate again less than two hours after you had finished urinating?
  0   1   2   3   4   5

Over the past month, how often have you found you stopped and started again several times when you urinated?

   0   1   2   3   4   5

Over the past month, how often have you found it is difficult to postpone urination?

   0   1   2   3   4   5

Over the past month, how often have you had a weak urinary stream?

   0   1   2   3   4   5

Over the past month, how often have you had to push or strain to begin urination?

   0   1   2   3   4   5

Over the past month, how many times did you most typically get up to urinate from the time you went to bed at night until you got up in the morning?

   0   1   2   3   4   5

TOTAL SCORE _____

SCORING KEY

Mild symptoms: 0 to 7 total points
Moderate symptoms: 8 to 19 total points
Severe symptoms: 20 to 35 total points

dissolved or broken up using endoscopic means, avoiding the need for open surgery. Other conditions that may appear include recurrent urinary tract infections and the passing of blood during urination. Overflow incontinence, the involuntary discharge of urine, may also develop. These conditions potentially are extremely serious, and if they are present the patient needs medical help immediately.

At some point the symptoms of BPH will probably become severe enough to prompt a visit to the doctor. In order to diagnose BPH properly, the patient must be honest with the physician. Although some men might feel embarrassed discussing their frequency of urination, this information is important in diagnosis and treatment. You may even want to keep a symptom log or diary that records how often you urinate, how long your urination lasts, how weak the stream is, and so forth. It is vital for your doctor to diagnose BPH correctly, so as to eliminate the possibility of more serious conditions that can mimic the symptoms of BPH, including bladder stones, bladder infection (cystitis), bladder tumor, heart failure, diabetes, a neurological problem, prostatitis, or prostate cancer.

During the initial visit the doctor will want to discuss your urinary symptoms in depth but will also want to know about any other health problems or medical conditions, what medications you are currently taking, and your family's medical history, especially the incidence of prostate problems in your close male relatives. In addition, your doctor will probably give you a general physical examination, a blood test to check your kidney function, a urine test to determine whether an infection is present, and a PSA test to check for prostate cancer.

THE DIGITAL RECTAL EXAM (DRE)

Your doctor will also want to perform a digital rectal examination (DRE) to find out if your prostate is enlarged and to check for the possibility of prostate cancer or prostatitis. In this procedure, the doctor's gloved, lubricated index finger is gently guided into the patient's rectum. The finger is then positioned so that the doctor can feel the back of the prostate. Bear in mind that the DRE is a somewhat limited tool in diagnosing the severity of BPH. Although the doctor may detect that the prostate is enlarged, remember that the prostate growth that most seriously impacts the patient's urinary symptoms occurs in the transition zone, in the central core of the prostate. The patient's prostate may appear to be normal-sized when examined by the doctor's finger yet have significant growth in the transition zone, causing obstruction of the urethra. The DRE also allows the doctor to check the tone of the anal sphincter, which may indicate medical conditions unrelated to the prostate, such as neurological disorders like multiple sclerosis and Parkinson's disease.

If the results of these tests indicate that you have BPH, your doctor may wish to perform additional tests to confirm the diagnosis and to ascertain the severity of the condition.

URINARY FLOW TEST

As the name suggests, this procedure measures the strength and volume of your urine flow. The test involves having the patient urinate into an electronic machine specially designed for this purpose.

Five or six ounces of urine must be expelled by the patient to ensure an accurate reading. The test is used to identify men whose urine flow rate is not seriously diminished and who would not benefit from treatment. A flow rate of 15 milliliters per second (ml/sec) is considered normal; a rate of 10–15 ml/sec indicates moderate symptoms; and anything less than 10 ml/sec usually signifies severe BPH. This test enables your physician to monitor your urine flow rate patterns over time. Consult with your physician to determine if he has access to this machine or if he can recommend a specialist who does.

POSTVOID RESIDUAL VOLUME TEST

This test is used to determine whether or not you are able to empty your bladder completely and, if not, how much urine remains in the bladder. There are two forms of this test. One procedure involves the insertion of a small catheter through the urethra and into the bladder, where the volume of residual urine is measured. The other involves the use of ultrasound imaging of the lower abdomen to accomplish the same result. Ultrasound is more widely used but is considered less accurate than direct measurement using a catheter. If significant amounts of residual urine are detected, BPH is severe and will require intensive treatment.

ULTRASOUND IMAGING

This imaging technique uses high-frequency sound waves to produce an image of the prostate. These "sound pictures" can be taken either externally, through the abdomen, or more often, transrectally, by using a wandlike device inserted into the rectum. Ultrasound can measure the overall size of the prostate and can also detect other conditions, such as obstruction of the kidney, kidney or prostate stones, and hidden tumors in the upper urinary tract.

URODYNAMIC STUDIES

Your doctor may suspect that your symptoms are not due to BPH but may instead be related to bladder dysfunction. In this case he or she may want to perform a series of urodynamic tests that measure bladder pressure and function. Cystometry is a procedure that uses a small catheter inserted through the urethra and into the bladder to measure pressure changes. Water is injected directly into the bladder in order to monitor changes in pressure. Pressure-flow studies use a small catheter placed in the bladder to measure bladder pressure as you urinate. This is done in order to find out if the patient's urinary symptoms are due to the urethra's being obstructed by BPH or to other bladder problems.

CYSTOSCOPY

In this procedure the penis is anesthetized and a thin, lighted tube called a cystoscope is inserted through the urethra and threaded into the bladder area. The cystoscope, which functions something like the periscope in a submarine, allows the physician to directly observe conditions inside the urinary tract. Using the cystoscope, the doctor can examine the prostate for enlargement, stones, or other abnormalities, check the urethra to determine the degree of obstruction, and inspect the bladder for stones, tumors, or other problems.

INTRAVENOUS PYELOGRAM

The intravenous pyelogram technique involves injecting a special dye into the patient's vein and taking an X ray of the urinary tract. The dye makes urine visible, revealing its passage from the kidneys through the ureters, bladder, and urethra and any points of blockage in the system. Because some men have a severe allergic reaction to the iodine in the dye, this procedure is more often used with men who have blood in their urine.

TREATMENT OPTIONS

Once the diagnosis of BPH has been confirmed by your doctor, you must decide whether to live with the symptoms of BPH or to seek treatment. In cases of severe BPH, in which urine is retained in the bladder, the need for medical or surgical treatment becomes urgent, but men who have less severe symptoms may also opt to improve their quality of life by seeking treatment for BPH. Treatment options fall into five basic categories: "watchful waiting," medication, surgery, nonsurgical procedures, and diet and alternative treatments.

WATCHFUL WAITING

This option is most appropriate for men with the least severe symptoms of BPH. Your doctor will schedule frequent checkups in order to monitor your symptoms closely and make sure that you're not developing any complications. The symptoms of BPH may improve over time, or they may worsen, at which point your doctor may advocate more intensive treatment.

During this period of watchful waiting there are some simple lifestyle changes that you can adopt that may help control the symptoms of BPH and prevent your condition from getting any worse.

MEDICATIONS

Until recently, surgery was the only option for men suffering from BPH. Drugs used to treat the condition have been in existence only since the mid-1980s. As a result, there are no long-term studies of how well they work and what their long-term side effects might be. For the most part, medications are used to treat men with mild to moderate symptoms of BPH, while surgery is preferred to treat more severe cases. In general, surgery is considered the most effective treatment for BPH, especially for those with severe symptoms, but for many men with moderate symptoms, who are unable or unwilling to undergo surgery, medication is their preferred option.

Unlike surgery, which happens once, medication must be taken on a daily basis and its effectiveness ends as you stop taking the drug. This means that you must take the medication for the rest of your life. Also, some medication can take weeks or months to have the desired effect.

LIFESTYLE CHANGES THAT CAN IMPACT THE SYMPTOMS OF BPH
- **Limit your consumption of beverages.** Avoid drinking water and other beverages after 7 P.M. to reduce the frequency of your trips to the bathroom at night.
- **Empty your bladder as fully as possible every time you urinate.**
- **Limit your alcohol consumption.** Alcohol increases urine production and may cause congestion in the prostate.
- **Be careful with nonprescription cold medicines.** The ones that contain decongestants can exacerbate the symptoms of an enlarged prostate. Always read the warning labels on these types of medications carefully.
- **Be active.** A sedentary lifestyle causes urine to be retained in the body. Studies show that even moderate exercise can relieve some of the urinary problems caused by BPH.

The drugs used to treat BPH employ two basic strategies. One is to shrink the prostate by interfering with hormones that cause the gland to enlarge. The other is aimed at preventing the prostate muscle tissue from constricting the urethra.

Finasteride (Proscar)

Finasteride was the first drug designed specifically to treat symptoms of BPH. It was developed by Merck & Co. in the mid-1980s and approved for treatment by the FDA in 1992.

The discovery of the drug came from a study of a small group of men living in the Dominican Republic. These men were born lacking the ability to produce the enzyme 5alpha-reductase, the substance that converts testosterone into its more potent form, dihydrotestosterone. As a result, the men were born with male sex organs that were so markedly underdeveloped they were actually thought to be girls. Some of them were even raised as girls, until, to everyone's surprise, they reached puberty and their genitals grew to the extent that they were then recognized as males.

Studies of these men revealed an intriguing fact: none of them ever developed BPH. This led chemists to speculate that they could develop a pill that would mimic the genetic condition of these men and prevent prostate growth.

How Finasteride Works

Finasteride works by blocking the action of 5alpha-reductase, the enzyme that converts testosterone into dihydrotestosterone (DHT), the hormone responsible for prostate growth. Once DHT is suppressed, the size of the prostate shrinks and pressure on the urethra is reduced, providing relief from the symptoms of BPH. The drug does more than simply relieve symptoms; it actually halts the progression of the disease. Because testosterone levels in the blood are not affected by the drug, most men who take finasteride do not experience impotence, although it is a possible side effect.

In some studies, finasteride has been shown to be an effective treatment for men with BPH. About 50 percent of men taking the drug report at least a 50 percent improvement in their symptoms, and more than 70 percent show some relief. Finasteride causes the prostrate to shrink approximately 20 percent after one year and 30 percent after three years.

However, other studies have found that while finasteride may indeed shrink the prostate, that does not correlate very well with symptom relief unless the prostate was very large to begin with. That's why finasteride is now used primarily in men who have a significantly enlarged prostate.

The Pluses and Minuses of Finasteride

Finasteride is most effective in men with a moderately or markedly enlarged prostate, while men with less enlargement may not notice any change in their condition. There are few side effects, but about 4 to 5 percent of men report impotence and around 5 percent experi-

---

PROSCAR/PROPECIA AND BIRTH DEFECTS

When a drug is labeled with a warning about possible birth defects, people tend to panic. It's probably a reaction to the thalidomide scare of the early 1960s, when several thousand babies were born with serious limb defects due to in utero exposure to the drug.

Finasteride (Propecia, Proscar) works by inhibiting an enzyme that converts testosterone into DHT, the form of testosterone needed for the normal development of masculine features in a male fetus. So if a male fetus is exposed to finasteride while it is in the womb, it may not develop normal male sex organs.

While it is true that finasteride is found in the seminal fluid of men taking the drug, male monkeys given massive doses of finasteride did not produce deformed male offspring. It does not produce any detrimental effect at conception.

For finasteride to have a teratogenic effect (cause birth defects), again, the fetus has to be exposed to the drug in the womb. That's why pregnant women are advised not to handle finasteride tablets, because theoretically they could absorb the drug through the skin, and if they were pregnant (remember, they may not realize it early on), it could harm the fetus. I use the word "theoretically" because this has been shown only in animal studies and most experts think that a woman would be unlikely to absorb finasteride through unbroken skin. Still, it's much better to be safe than sorry, especially when it comes to the health of one's baby.

There is also a theoretical, though highly unlikely, risk that a woman may absorb finasteride from a male sexual partner's semen. However, the amount of the drug found in the semen is very small and is not thought to be enough to pose a risk to a fetus, even if the drug were absorbed. Recently, similar drugs that inhibit 5alpha reductase are being marketed, although the experience with these drugs is very limited.

ence a decrease in libido. These sexual side effects soon disappear if the patient discontinues using the drug. Other side effects that are occasionally reported are swollen lips, skin rash, and tenderness of the breasts. There is another interesting (and unintended) side effect. Some bald men who took finasteride in a 5 mg dose to treat BPH reported renewed hair growth. The same DHT that stimulates prostate growth is toxic to hair follicles; the enzyme that produces DHT from testosterone is present in those follicles and is also inhibited by finasteride. In a 1 mg dosage, finasteride is sold as the drug Propecia, a medication the FDA approved to regrow hair.

The drug does not provide immediate relief from BPH symptoms. It takes about six months of daily use for finasteride to have any effect on the prostate. The medication is taken in pill form once a day in a dosage of 5 mg, and if its use is discontinued, the symptoms of BPH will return. The medication is moderately expensive and must be taken for the rest of the patient's life.

Alpha-Blockers

The FDA has approved four other drugs for the treatment of BPH: terazosin (Hytrin), doxazosin (Cardura), tamsulosin (Flomax), and alfuzosin (Uroxatral). All of these prescription medications belong to a group of drugs called alpha-blockers. These drugs work by relaxing the smooth muscle cells within the walls of arteries and similar muscle cells in the capsule of the prostate. Terazosin and doxazosin are called nonselective alpha-blockers, which means that they affect both the artery and the prostate smooth muscle and so may be more likely to cause a drop in blood pressure. Tamulosin and alfuzosin are called selective alpha-blockers, which means they should only affect the smooth muscle of the prostate and thus are less likely to cause low blood pressure and drug interactions. Alpha-blockers interfere with the action of neurotransmitter substances called alpha-1 adrenoceptors in the prostate, causing the smooth muscles of the gland to relax their hold on the urethra and allowing urine to flow through it more freely.

Unlike finasteride, which must be taken for months before the patient notices any benefit, alpha-blockers work almost immediately, often within one or two days after the medication is first taken. About 75 percent of patients report an increase in urinary flow and a decrease in how often they have to urinate. Alpha-blockers provide relief by treating the symptoms of BPH, but, unlike finasteride, they do not physically shrink the size of the prostate.

Although doctors are still uncertain about the long-term effects of this relatively new class of drugs, alpha-blockers appear to be safe. They may not be appropriate for patients with low blood pressure or heart problems, but a physician should make this decision. Side effects can include headaches, dizziness, fatigue and nasal congestion. Some users of tamsulosin may experience dry ejaculations.

A Dynamic Duo

Recent clinical trials have found that combining finasteride with the alpha-blocker doxazosin can be more effective in treating BPH than either taken alone. This may work because the two drugs work on different aspects of BPH simultaneously. The two-drug "cocktail" reduced BPH progression by 67 percent in the study, compared with 39 percent for doxazosin alone and 34 percent for finasteride alone.

SURGERY

If your symptoms are too extreme or do not respond to lifestyle changes or medication, your doctor may recommend surgery. At one time in the not-too-distant past, surgery was the only treatment for BPH.

Advances in modern medicine have led to surgical procedures that are minimally invasive and do not require general anesthesia. These procedures are called transurethral because they are performed by accessing the prostate through the urethra rather than through an open incision of the abdomen. Today, the overwhelming majority of prostate surgeries are performed using transurethral techniques.

Before performing any prostate surgery, your doctor will want to review your medical history and current condition thoroughly. Make sure that you are completely open and honest with your doctor during these interviews. He or she will want to know if you've had any problems with unusual bleeding in the past, even during dental work. If you are taking aspirin on a daily basis, you should discontinue taking it at least ten days before surgery, as aspirin can cause excessive bleeding. Your doctor may also want to examine your urinary tract prior to surgery using ultrasound or cystoscopy to check the condition of your kidneys, bladder, and prostate.

Surgery is not for everyone. A patient's age and overall health may rule it out. Men with certain serious health conditions, such as uncontrolled diabetes, cirrhosis of the liver, a major psychiatric disorder, or severe lung, kidney, heart, or blood pressure problems are not good candidates for surgery.

Transurethral Resection of the Prostate (TURP)

This is the most common form of prostate surgery. It is successful in improving symptoms in about 80 percent of cases. TURP is most appropriate for men with moderate to severe BPH, but not for those with grossly enlarged prostates.

The patient is usually given spinal anesthesia to numb the lower body. Then an instrument called a resectoscope is inserted into the urethra and threaded into the prostate. The resectoscope, which is about half an inch in diameter and twelve inches long, contains a fiber-optic light and a lens that enables the surgeon to see inside the patient's body. There is also a tiny valve that controls the flow of irrigating fluid. At the tip of the instrument is an electrical loop used to cut tissue and seal off blood vessels.

During the operation, the surgeon uses the loop to slice away sections of the obstructing prostate tissue one piece at a time. These tissue fragments are sent to a pathologist and examined for prostate cancer. A newer TURP technique uses a special "roller ball" at the tip of the resectoscope to vaporize the prostate tissue electrically instead of slicing it. The procedure takes about ninety minutes.

After the operation a Foley catheter is inserted into the urethra and the bladder is irrigated with a saline solution for twenty-four hours in order to prevent blood clots from forming. In addition, a urinary catheter may have to stay in for a few days. The patient can expect to stay in the hospital for one to three days following surgery. Before leaving the hospital the patient should be able to urinate on his own, although some pain, discomfort, or a burning sensation may be experienced during urination. This usually disappears within a few days. The patient may notice blood passed in the urine, which is normal and will gradually diminish over a period of days to weeks.

Complications of TURP

Moderate to severe bleeding may occur during surgery or during the recovery period. Sometimes a blood transfusion may be required. Bleeding seems to be related to the size of the prostate; larger glands tend to bleed more profusely than smaller ones. Another   2 complication is sometimes termed "TURP syndrome," a rare condition experienced by about 2 percent of patients that is caused when the body absorbs too much of the irrigating fluid used during the TURP procedure, which dilutes the blood and, more important, lowers the sodium level in the blood. The symptoms are nausea, confusion, vomiting, high blood pressure, falling heart rate, and vision problems. Diuretics or a saline solution are used to restore the body's normal fluid and electrolyte balance.

Some patients experience an inability to urinate after TURP sur-   3 gery. This may be due to the trauma of surgery causing the bladder to become slack. A temporary catheter may be used to give the bladder a few days' rest until the bladder tone recovers. Other patients may experience urinary incontinence for a variety of reasons. Drugs   4 may be used to stop involuntary contractions of the bladder, and Kegel exercises can help strengthen the pelvic muscles to relieve the condition. Urinary tract infections and urethral stricture may occur   5 in rare cases.

Two of the most common (and distressing) complications are related to sexual activity. Impotence, the inability to maintain an erec-   6 . tion, is reported by about 5 to 8 percent of patients, especially older ones. For many men normal sexual function will return within a few weeks or months, but for some impotence can be a permanent condition.

A more frequent side effect of TURP is called retrograde ejacula-   7 tion, also known as dry orgasm, a condition experienced by 75 to 80 percent of patients after this procedure. As the term suggests, this refers to an absence of liquid semen during orgasm. This is caused by the semen being pushed backward into the bladder during orgasm instead of being normally expelled through the penis. Many men find this upsetting, but retrograde ejaculation presents no hazard to the patient's health and has no adverse effect on sexual performance and relatively little impact on pleasure. Due to the absence of semen, however, the patient essentially loses his ability to father children. But since sperm can sometimes "make it out" during orgasm, some form of contraception should still be used to be sure of avoiding pregnancy.

Symptoms of BPH improved markedly in 80 percent of patients

after TURP. Because the procedure is minimally invasive, there are relatively few major risks associated with the operation itself. Another benefit of TURP is that the pieces of sliced-off prostate produced during the surgery can be collected and used to screen the patient for prostate cancer.

On the downside, TURP treats only the symptoms of BPH and does nothing to regulate prostate growth. In fact, the prostate may continue to grow after the surgery, so that 10 percent (1 in 10 men who had the operation) need another operation within ten years. Because of this, some physicians feel that TURP is not as effective in the long term as other surgical procedures, such as open prostatectomy. However, the vast majority of these patients who require surgical intervention can be managed by this operation or other minimally invasive procedures.

Transurethral Incision of the Prostate (TUIP)

Like TURP, transurethral incision of the prostate (TUIP) involves spinal anesthesia and the use of the resectoscope inserted through the urethra and into the prostate. But unlike TURP, in the TUIP procedure the surgeon does not shave slices from the prostate but instead makes one or two longitudinal cuts in the gland. The cuts help

---

BLOCKING THE PAIN: SPINAL AND EPIDURAL ANESTHESIA

During TURP, TUIP, and other transurethral procedures, general anesthesia, in which the patient is rendered completely unconscious, is not usually required. Instead, spinal or epidural anesthesia, in which the patient remains conscious and aware, is preferred.

In spinal anesthesia, a shot of local anesthetic is injected into the small of the back through the dura, the membrane that lines the spinal cord, and into the spinal fluid. Within minutes, the entire lower body feels numb and heavy, and the feeling lasts for the duration of the operation. After surgery, the patient should take care to lie flat in bed until the numbness wears off completely; otherwise he may experience severe headaches.

Epidural anesthesia involves inserting a small tube between the vertebrae of the spine near the small of the patient's back. A local anesthetic is administered through this tube and over the spinal membranes, causing numbness of the lower body. While spinal anesthesia is given in a single injection, in epidural anesthesia the anesthetic drips into the patient's body continuously, so that the degree of numbness or pain relief can be adjusted.

enlarge the opening of the urethra and permit an increased flow of urine.

TUIP is more effective for treating younger men with mild to moderate prostate enlargement. This is because, unlike the TURP procedure, TUIP surgery is less likely to result in the retrograde or dry ejaculation that drastically reduces fertility. In general, TUIP causes less in the way of complications than TURP, and sometimes only an overnight hospital stay is required.

TUIP is not as effective as TURP in relieving the symptoms of BPH. Patients report that the overall increase in urine flow is marginal compared to their condition before surgery. Like TURP, TUIP relieves only the symptoms of BPH. The prostate may continue to grow and to obstruct urine flow. The TUIP procedure may have to be repeated more often than TURP. Also, because TUIP surgery does not involve cutting sections from the prostate, unlike TURP it does not produce tissue samples that can be analyzed in a prostate biopsy.

Open Prostatectomy

Once this was the only treatment of any kind for BPH, but today its use has been eclipsed by less invasive transurethral surgeries such as TURP and TUIP, which cause fewer complications. Open prostatectomy is indicated in cases where the prostate is extremely enlarged or if there are other exacerbating factors, such as bladder stones. The term "open" means that, unlike in a transurethral procedure, an incision is made in the patient's abdomen through which portions of the prostate are removed. General, rather than local, anesthesia is usually used, which renders the patient unconscious.

This type of surgery is more commonly used to treat prostate cancer, in which case the entire prostate is removed by the surgeon. This is referred to as radical prostatectomy. To treat BPH, however, a partial prostatectomy procedure is used in which only the inner portion of the gland that obstructs urinary flow is removed and the outer portion is left intact.

During a partial prostatectomy, the surgeon makes an incision in the lower abdomen, exposing the bladder. Then the bladder is cut open, allowing access to the prostate. The surgeon inserts instruments through the bladder incision to excise the prostate tissue surrounding the urethra from the center out. Bladder stones may also

RECOVERING AFTER SURGERY

After you have had a TURP, a TUIP, open prostatectomy, or another procedure, it may take a couple of weeks to a few months for you to make a full recovery. You should take it easy for a few weeks after you get home from the hospital and consult your doctor about when it is safe to resume your normal routine. Some people suffer setbacks because they try to do too much after surgery. During this period, following a few simple rules will help your body heal itself.

• Drink at least eight glasses of water a day to flush the bladder.
• Avoid straining when moving your bowel.
• Eat lots of fruits, vegetables, grains, and high-fiber foods to avoid constipation. If constipation persists, ask your doctor if you can take a laxative.
• Don't do any heavy lifting or perform any action jarring to the pelvic area.
• Don't drive, ride a bicycle, or operate heavy machinery.
• Ask your doctor when it will be safe to resume sexual activity.

be removed at this time. There are variations of this procedure in which the surgeon bypasses the bladder and accesses the prostate more directly.

Excess bleeding during open surgery is always a concern, and a blood transfusion may have to be given at some point. After surgery, the patient may experience bladder spasms and stress incontinence, in which urine leaks out of the penis during moderate physical activity, coughing, or sneezing. Scar tissue may form in the bladder neck (bladder neck contracture) or in the urethra (urethral stricture).

Like the TURP procedure, open prostatectomy can result in dry ejaculation or impotence. After surgery, the prostate can regrow and begin to cause urinary problems again, but open prostatectomy is considered more effective in providing long-term relief from the symptoms of BPH than either TURP or TUIP.

Heat and Laser Therapies
Advances in medical technology have provided a number of new treatments for BPH that utilize microwaves, radio frequencies, and/or lasers to shrink or destroy enlarged prostate tissues. These new therapies are more effective than medication, yet less invasive than surgery, but because they are so new their long-term effect on

BPH has yet to be evaluated. Some of these procedures can be performed on an outpatient basis.

Lasers vaporize prostate tissue and shrink the gland. In comparison with other types of surgery, laser techniques cause less bleeding. They can be useful in treating men who take anticoagulant medications or who have significant heart disease. Some therapies, however, may require the wearing of a catheter for extended periods.

Photoselective Vaporization of the Prostate (PVP)

What distinguishes this technique from other laser technologies is the high energy at which the laser operates and the wavelength it emits. The energy is absorbed only by hemoglobin in the blood vessels of the gland itself and the light penetrates only a millimeter or two into the tissue, minimizing collateral damage to tissues the urologist doesn't want to remove.

The high energy allows for true vaporization of the prostatic tissue and simultaneous coagulation, making PVP virtually bloodless. The procedure is done under local anesthesia and takes twenty to fifty minutes, depending on the size of the gland. It has had very few complications.

Some have reported results with PVP that were as good as or better than using TURP, quoting an improvement of the American Urological Association (AUA) symptom score of 92 percent; quality of life improvement of 90 percent; peak urinary flow rate improvement of 196 percent; and posturination residual volume improvement of 93 percent. Additionally, in these studies all patients went home within twenty-three hours, many on the day of the procedure; and more than 30 percent were sent home without a catheter. Of those who did receive a catheter, the mean catherization time was just fourteen hours. A Mayo Clinic study has found the results to be stable for at least five years postoperatively. Also, the range of patients that can be treated using PVP is greater than with any other known technology. In a study done at New York Weill Cornell Medical Center on men with very large prostates (who are not treatable by TURP) and patients on anticoagulants, PVP was a safe and effective treatment. For some of these men, PVP may be their only safe alternative. Note that many alternative techniques initially have "fantastic results" but do not stand up as well later on.

Interstitial Laser Therapy

Interstitial laser therapy focuses laser energy on the inside of the enlarged prostate in order to heat the tissue and clear the urethra. It is effective in treating men with large prostates, reducing prostate volume and increasing urine flow. As with other laser treatments, bleeding is minimal, making it a good treatment for men who have heart disease or who are taking anticoagulants. On the downside, this procedure causes inflammation of the prostate tissue that may cause the patient to have to wear a catheter for about a week. Urinary tract infections are also commonly reported.

Transurethral Microwave Therapy (TUMT)

In this procedure the patient is given local anesthesia and a special catheter is inserted into the urethra. This catheter contains a tiny microwave antenna and a cooling system that circulates water to protect the urethra from the heat during the treatment. A device that emits microwave energy, called a Prostatron, is inserted into the rectum. The Prostatron is hooked up to a computer that monitors microwave levels and controls the flow of energy to the antenna in the catheter. The computer-regulated microwaves then heat the prostate tissues, destroying the inner portion of the gland. The patient may feel some heat in the prostate area, have a strong desire to urinate, or experience bladder spasms during the procedure.

The TUMT procedure takes about a hour and can be performed on an outpatient basis. The patient can go home as soon as he is urinating normally, but about 30 percent of men have to wear a urinary catheter for a few days. Frequent urination and blood in the urine are common during recovery. Unlike TURP, TUMT was not reported to cause impotence or dry ejaculation, but patients may notice a change in the amount of semen they ejaculate during orgasm. Because the heated prostate tissue swells before it shrinks, the patient may not experience any relief from his urinary symptoms for several weeks. In fact, things may get worse before they get better. The long-term risks and benefits of this technique are still being evaluated. The TUMT procedure is not recommended for men who have a pacemaker.

Transurethral Needle Ablation (TUNA)

This outpatient technique is very similar to TUMT. It uses low-level radio-frequency energy transmitted through two needles inserted into the prostate that heat and destroy parts of the gland's enlarged tissue. The needles are deployed at the end of a catheter and then used to heat the areas of the prostate adjacent to the urethra that are causing urinary problems. During the TUNA procedure, as with TUMT, the urethra is protected from the heat.

TUNA may not be as effective as other surgical procedures in treating BPH, but on the plus side there are fewer side effects than with TURP surgery, and the patient can still have a TURP later, if needed. No incontinence or impotence has been observed. Side effects may include urinary retention, blood in the urine and painful urination, but less than with TURP. A very small number of men also experience dry ejaculation after surgery. As with other recent procedures, its long-term effectiveness is unknown. TUNA is not recommended for men with very large prostates.

Transurethral Electrovaporization of the Prostate (TVP)

This is basically a variation on the TURP procedure, but instead of using an electrified loop to section the prostate, TVP employs a special metal instrument inserted through a catheter that uses a high-frequency electrical current to vaporize areas of the prostate while sealing off tissues to prevent bleeding. While TVP may prove to be as effective as TURP, the TVP procedure is simpler and has fewer complications. Because it causes little bleeding, it is recommended for some higher-risk patients, such as men taking blood-thinning medication. As with other recently invented procedures, the long-term risks and benefits of TVP are still being evaluated.

Transurethral Ultrasound Aspiration of the Prostate (TUAP)

With TUAP, a periscope-like probe called an endoscope is inserted into the urethra to locate enlarged prostate tissues, which are then treated with high energy ultrasound. The ultrasound energy liquefies prostatic glandular tissue, which is high in water content, leaving the capsule of the prostate, which is higher in collagen, untouched. An aspirator device in the endoscope then vacuums up the BPH tissue.

TUAP causes no incontinence or urinary problems, but about 85 percent of men who have had this procedure reported retrograde or dry ejaculation, which makes it unsuitable for men who are concerned about their fertility. Also, ultrasound does not work as well in men whose BPH is located near the bladder neck.

Transurethral Evaporation of the Prostate (TUEP)

Similar to the electrovaporization (TVP) process, TUEP uses laser energy instead of electricity to vaporize prostate tissue. The procedure is considered relatively safe and causes limited bleeding. Improvement in urine flow is usually noted soon after the procedure.

Visual Laser Ablation of the Prostate (VLAP)

In this technique, a laser is used to dry up and destroy enlarged prostate tissue, which is then expelled from the body over a period of weeks or even months. A big disadvantage of this procedure is that as the dead prostate tissue is eliminated, it causes swelling that leads to urine retention. Consequently, the patient must wear a urinary catheter for several days. A burning sensation during urination may be felt for days or weeks after having the procedure.

NONSURGICAL PROCEDURES

There are other options for patients who are unable or unwilling to have surgery or take medication. These procedures involve inserting objects into the body rather than cutting or destroying prostate tissue. They can typically be performed in a doctor's office in about fifteen minutes.

Balloon Urethoplasty (Balloon Dilation)

In this procedure a catheter with a deflated balloon on the end is inserted into the area of the urethra adjacent to the prostate. The balloon is then inflated, stretching the urethra and compressing prostate tissue to enable increased urine flow. The procedure can be performed in a urologist's office and takes about fifteen minutes. Relief from BPH symptoms usually lasts only a short time, however, which has led to a decline in the popularity of this procedure. The effect is similar to placebo.

Prostatic Stent

This is a thin mesh tube, usually made of nickel-titanium alloys, that is inserted into the urethra to widen it and keep it open. It is designed so that once the device is in place, the epithelial tissue of the urethra will grow over the stent to keep it in place. A prostatic stent can be an option for older men for whom surgery is problematic. It can be inserted in ten or fifteen minutes on an outpatient basis. There is little or no bleeding, and the procedure does not require a catheter.

A BIG PROSTATE DOESN'T ALWAYS EQUAL BIG TROUBLE!

When Proscar (finasteride) was first approved for the treatment of BPH, it was a big deal. Finally, here was a drug that shrank enlarged prostates. And shrink them it did—but still not all men got relief from their symptoms.

That's when further studies showed a somewhat puzzling finding: a big prostate doesn't necessarily mean terrible symptoms. When ultrasound was used to determine the size of test subjects' prostates, it turned out that size did not correlate very well with the severity of symptoms, based on the American Urological Association symptom questionnaire. Some men with pretty big prostates had relatively few symptoms, and some with only slightly enlarged prostates suffered a lot. That's why shrinking the prostate with Proscar did not always produce a happy camper, although for men with very large prostates who had a lot of symptoms, shrinking the gland with medication did seem to help.

Complications can arise if the stent is not positioned properly; the patient may need to have a second procedure to remove or realign it. Urethral tissue can also overgrow the stent and render it useless. Some men reported no relief from their symptoms and others experienced irritation while urinating or developed frequent urinary tract infections.

Diet and Alternative Treatments

In addition to the orthodox medical treatments, several herbal treatments and dietary supplements have been used to treat BPH. Researchers have also looked at the role of diet in preventing or treating it.

Herbal Remedies

Traditional cultures throughout the world have used a number of herbal remedies to treat BPH for many years. While there is anecdotal evidence that these substances may provide some benefit, there are few controlled clinical studies to confirm this. These herbal remedies include saw palmetto, cernilton, radix urticae, African plum, stinging nettle, pygeum bark, and pumpkin seed oil.

Nutritional Supplements

Zinc was shown to reduce prostate enlargement in a recent study. Patients given zinc supplements reported an improvement in their symptoms, and 75 percent showed a decrease in prostate size. Dietary sources of zinc include whole grains, some seafood, nuts, beans, and fortified breakfast cereals.

Magnesium is another mineral that may play a role in suppressing the symptoms of BPH. Good natural sources of magnesium are soybeans, tofu, peanuts, broccoli, Swiss chard, spinach, and tomato paste.

Amino acids such as alanine, glutamic acid, and glycine have been shown to shrink prostate size and relieve the symptoms of BPH in recent clinical trials. In one study, men with BPH who took amino acid supplements reported less urgency to urinate and less frequent urination at night, and 92 percent showed some reduction in prostate size. Foods rich in these amino acids include soybeans, lentils, and fish.

All of these nutrients can be taken in supplement form if they cannot be obtained through food sources alone.

Other Dietary Factors

Although the connection between diet and BPH is much less clear cut than between diet and prostate cancer, diet may play a significant role in enlargement of the prostate. For the best foods recommended for good prostate health, consult the Prostate Health Pyramid in Chapter 4 and "The Nutrition Connection" in Chapter 5.

Soy products contain phytochemical substances called isoflavones that are known to affect hormone levels in the prostate. Isoflavones are believed to prevent the development of prostate cancer and may also play a role in suppressing BPH by regulating testosterone levels. Eating and drinking soy products such as soy milk, tofu, and soy nuts can help protect you against both of these serious prostate conditions.

Many men report that their BPH symptoms improve when they avoid certain types of food and drink, including coffee, alcohol, and spicy foods. Eliminating or lessening your intake of these items may help your condition. Overuse of the dietary supplement DHEA can also aggravate BPH.

While the onset of BPH seems inevitable as men's life spans grow longer, preventive measures, new kinds of sophisticated surgery, revolutionary nonsurgical procedures, and innovative medications are helping to make the burden bearable.

Medical science may soon discover ways to use diet and nutrition to prevent or even eliminate BPH entirely.

Putting It All Together

With so many treatment options to choose from, deciding on the best treatment can be difficult. Some factors to consider are:

How Severe Are Your Symptoms?

If you can live with frequent trips to the bathroom and other minor inconveniences caused by mild to moderate BPH, watchful waiting or minimally invasive treatments may be best. If your symptoms are severe enough to cause organ damage, frequent urinary tract infections, urinary bleeding, or bladder stones, you may have to consider surgery on a more urgent basis. Many men opt for treatment due to sleep deprivation from multiple trips to the bathroom during the night.

How Large Is Your Prostate?

The size of your prostate is a factor that will influence your choice of treatment. Some medications or procedures are more effective for men with large prostates, while others may work better on small to midsized enlargements. Treatments that are best suited for more enlarged prostates include finasteride (Proscar), transurethral resection of the prostate (TURP), open prostatectomy, transurethral microwave therapy (TUMT), and laser therapy.

Treatments that work better on small to moderately sized prostates include alpha-blockers, transurethral incision of the prostate (TUIP), transurethral needle ablation (TUNA), transurethral electrovaporization of the prostate (TVP), and laser therapy.

How Old Are You?

Younger men may want to pursue a different treatment strategy than older men. Older patients may prefer treatments that provide more immediate relief and may be less concerned about long-term effects, impotence, or infertility. They also recover from surgery and other invasive procedures more slowly. Younger men will be more likely to consider treatment options with fewer long-term consequences, including the possibility of having to repeat the surgical procedure. They are also likely to be more concerned with the possible sexual side effects of treatment.

How's Your Health?

Men with certain health conditions are not good candidates for surgery and do not recover as quickly. In general, surgery is not recommended for men with uncontrolled diabetes, cirrhosis of the liver, serious lung, kidney, or heart disease, or major psychiatric disorders. Men who are taking certain types of medication or who are allergic to specific drugs are not good candidates.

Do You Want to Be a Father?

If you are concerned with your fertility, you will want to avoid procedures that may compromise your ability to father children. These include TURP, TUIP, open prostatectomy, and certain laser therapies, all of which can cause retrograde (dry) ejaculation. Unlike impotence, which can sometimes be reversed, this condition is usually permanent. In certain rare cases, TUNA, interstitial laser therapy, and alpha-blocking medication also can cause retrograde ejaculation, although it's reversible if you stop taking the alpha-blockers.

How's Your Sex Life?

Impotence is an unfortunate side effect of some prostate treatments. TURP treatment in particular can cause impotence in approximately 5 to 10 percent of men who have the surgery, but this condition can reverse itself over time. In addition, various types of surgery can damage nerves or blood vessels next to the prostate, which can also cause impotence.

Your Body, Your Choice

Ultimately you must decide, in consultation with your doctor, which BPH treatment is most appropriate for you. You will have to take a careful look at the risks, benefits, and costs of the treatments, which may impact your life in profound ways. Talk to other men with BPH who have had these treatments to get some firsthand input. Keep in mind that if one treatment doesn't work, you can always switch to another one that may be more effective for you. While at one time the only treatment option for men with BPH was surgery, today there are many approaches and options for treating the condition.

12. Prostatodynia (Chronic Pelvic Pain Syndrome)

Of all the noncancerous conditions of the prostate, prostatodynia is the most mysterious and least understood. Although its symptoms closely resemble those of chronic nonbacterial prostatitis, prostatodynia may not be a condition of the prostate, or even of the urinary tract, at all. Efforts to define exactly what prostatodynia is are leading to a redefinition of the categories of prostatitis-related disorders. Under this new classification system, prostatodynia is referred to as chronic pelvic pain syndrome (CPPS), although we'll still refer to it as prostatodynia for convenience. Other terms for the condition that are seldom used today are prostatalgia and prostatosis.

Symptoms of Prostatodynia

The term prostatodynia means, simply, "painful prostate," and the defining symptom of the condition is pain in the lower pelvic area in the general vicinity of the prostate. Whether the pain actually has anything to do with the prostate or is due to other factors is debatable. There is no related urinary tract infection, and urine samples show no traces of bacteria. Similarly, there is no evidence of inflammation of prostate tissue that would be signaled by the presence of white blood cells in urine or prostatic fluid samples. Unlike some other disorders of the prostate, prostatodynia affects young to middle-aged men. Symptoms include:

- Frequent urination
- Pain or burning sensation while urinating
- Sudden or compelling urge to urinate
- A feeling of not being able to empty the bladder
- Pain in the lower back
- Pain in the perineum (the area between the scrotum and the anus)
- Pain in the rectum
- Pain in the penis or scrotum
- Pain in the general pelvic area
- Painful ejaculation
- Pain in joints
- Impotence (erectile dysfunction)

Some physicians consider prostatodynia a kind of catchall diagnosis that encompasses a variety of real and/or psychosomatic symptoms. The symptoms of prostatodynia are so similar to those of chronic bacterial and nonbacterial prostatitis (CNP) that some doctors consider them to be slightly differing aspects of the same illness. Sophisticated testing is needed to differentiate between prostatodynia and CNP.

DIAGNOSIS OF PROSTATODYNIA

A standard technique often used to diagnose prostatodynia is the Stamey-Meares four-glass test, which is also used to diagnose various types of bacterial and nonbacterial prostatitis. The test involves taking three samples of your urine and one sample of your prostatic fluid.

First, one sample of your urine is taken when you start to urinate, then another is taken in midstream. At this point the doctor will rectally massage the prostate until prostatic fluid is expelled and collected for analysis. Next, a fourth sample of urine mixed with prostate fluid is taken. Most urologists no longer do all these steps, however.

If bacteria are found, the diagnosis will be bacterial prostatitis. If white blood cells, indicating inflammation of the prostate, are found in the prostatic fluid or fluid and urine samples, chronic nonbacterial prostatitis will likely be diagnosed. A diagnosis of prostatodynia will result if no traces of bacteria are found in any of the urine samples and no white blood cells are found in the samples containing fluid from the prostate. But you should realize that prostatodynia is a diagnosis of "exclusion," meaning that it's what doctors are left with when all other causes of the symptoms have been eliminated.

WHAT CAUSES PROSTATODYNIA?

The absence of physical evidence in connection with prostatodynia gives medical science very little to go on in figuring out what causes this disease. Given the catch-all nature of the diagnosis, prostatodynia may just be a blanket term that applies to a number of separate and distinct conditions that are all lumped together for the sake of convenience. Current research efforts to solve the mystery of prostatodynia are following several very different paths.

PROSTATODYNIA AND INTERSTITIAL CYSTITIS

Interstitial cystitis (IC) is a disease that might be considered a female version of prostatodynia. It shares many of the same symptoms, including frequent and urgent urination and pain in the pelvic area, but 90 percent of IC patients are women, none of whom, of course, has a prostate gland. As with prostatodynia, the causes of interstitial cystitis are unknown. IC is linked to the absence of a protective layer of protein called glycosaminoglycan (GAG) that lines the inner surface of the bladder. The function of the layer of GAG is to prevent urine from seeping into the bladder wall, but in interstitial cystitis, much of this GAG layer is lost and urine is able to seep into the bladder muscles. This seepage causes inflammation and pain in the bladder area. Similarities between the symptoms of IC and those of prostatodynia have led some researchers to believe that the two conditions may be related and that prostatodynia is simply a type of IC that occurs in men.

PROSTATODYNIA AS A TENSION DISORDER

Another theory is that prostatodynia is caused by chronic tension or spasm in the pelvic floor muscles. It has long been noted that patients suffering from prostatodynia are type A personalities, individuals who tend to be hard-driven, tense, and continually stressed. These men are frequently found to have trigger points or knots of contracted muscle fiber in the pelvic area. These trigger points are painful when pressed, and muscle spasms can be very painful all by themselves. Some researchers think that tension in the pelvic muscles causes the constriction of the urethral sphincter—one of the muscles that controls urination—and the bladder neck. There is also some evidence to suggest that prostatodynia may be related to strain or dysfunction of the iliopsoas muscle, a large muscle that runs from the lower back down to the pelvis.

A DISORDER OF THE IMMUNE SYSTEM?

Some researchers believe that the symptoms of prostatodynia are the result of a dysfunctional or overfunctioning immune system. This would make prostatodynia similar to illnesses such as diabetes, rheumatoid arthritis, asthma, allergies, and lupus. Some researchers think there may be a link between prostatodynia and Reiter syndrome, a form of chronic inflammatory arthritis that can cause inflammation of the genital area. Also, retention of semen in the body during periods of sexual abstinence might possibly provoke a response by the immune system.

AN INFECTIOUS CONDITION?

Some researchers think that prostatodynia is the result of a hidden infection of the prostate by unknown bacterial, fungal, or viral microorganisms that remain undetected during diagnosis.

URETHRAL STRICTURE

This is a condition in which the urethra, the tube that carries urine from the bladder to the penis, becomes narrowed and constricted by a buildup of fibrous scar tissue. This leads to problems with expelling urine and urine retention in the bladder that can cause irritation and inflammation of the prostate. It is a common disorder among men and usually results from an infection or trauma of the urethra.

OTHER POSSIBLE CAUSES

Because diagnosis is so elusive, some doctors believe that the condition is merely psychosomatic and that the symptoms are all in the patient's mind. Other possible causes of prostatodynia include a rare type of tumor, a food allergy, or a yeast infection, and there are a

MEDICAL CONDITIONS THAT MIMIC PROSTATODYNIA

Some medical conditions can mimic the symptoms of prostatodynia. These include depression, fibromyalgia, interstitial cystitis, hernia, urethral stricture, drug/food reactions, stress, bladder cancer, prostatic cyst/abscess, ejaculatory duct cyst, urethritis, allergic reaction, spinal stenosis, urethral stone, seminal vesicle cyst/vesiculitis, benign prostatic hyperplasia (BPH), radiation cystitis, sexually transmitted diseases, myofascial pain syndrome, and pelvic joint pain.

number of other medical conditions that have symptoms that are similar to those of prostatodynia.

DRAWING A NEW DIAGNOSTIC MAP OF PROSTATITIS-TYPE DISORDERS

In an attempt to clarify the interrelationships of the various prostate disorders related to prostatitis, the U.S. National Institutes of Health (NIH) recently proposed a new classification system for these disorders that is designed to aid doctors in the diagnosis of prostatitis and prostatodynia.

ASYMPTOMATIC PROSTATITIS

The NIH proposal included a new category of prostate disease called asymptomatic prostatitis. Diagnostically, it can be looked at as the opposite of prostatodynia. Whereas with prostatodynia the patient has symptoms but there is no evidence of inflammation, with asymptomatic prostatitis there is evidence of inflammation withou' the patient experiencing any symptoms.

Asymptomatic prostatitis is usually detected through a pr biopsy performed to investigate another problem, usually r cancer. The biopsy is usually performed because high prostate-specific antigen are found in the patient during which may be an indication of prostatic cancer. The ' that the patient does not have cancer but instead d ence of inflammation in the prostate that causes P evated.

With asymptomatic prostatitis, the patie

symptoms or experience the discomfort associated with other types of prostatitis. The condition usually clears up after taking antibiotics for two weeks, after which the PSA levels return to normal.

TREATMENT OPTIONS FOR PROSTATODYNIA

Because so little is known about the nature of prostatodynia, treatment is aimed at relieving symptoms rather than curing the disease. A variety of medications, as well as physical and psychiatric therapies, are used to treat the condition.

MEDICATIONS
Alpha-Blockers

This class of drugs was developed to treat high blood pressure, and they have more recently been used to treat benign enlargement of the prostate (BPH) and chronic nonbacterial prostatitis (CBP). Alpha-blockers work by relaxing the muscle cells of the bladder and urethra, allowing urine to flow more freely to relieve urinary symptoms. The alpha-blockers most commonly used to treat prostatodynia are doxazosin (Cardura), tamulosin (Flomax), and terazosin (Hytrin). You may have to keep taking this medication indefinitely because your symptoms can return as soon as you stop taking it.

Analgesics and Anti-Inflammatory Medications

Analgesic medicines not only relieve pain and discomfort but also help reduce inflammation in muscle tissue. Over-the-counter pain medications such as aspirin or acetaminophen (Tylenol) can be used, or your doctor may prescribe a nonsteroidal anti-inflammatory drug (NSAID) such as rofecoxib (Vioxx), ibuprofen (Advil), or celecoxib (Celebrex).

Antibiotics

Although prostatodynia, by definition, is not an infectious disease, many doctors prescribe at least one blind trial of antibiotics early in the therapy, sometimes only for the sake of completeness. A dissenting medical opinion holds that antibiotics can pose an additional level of risk for the patient and are not an appropriate treatment option for prostatodynia.

Muscle Relaxants and Tranquilizers

These medications are prescribed to relieve tension in the pelvic floor muscles. They also alter mood and relieve the symptoms of mental stress. Diazepam (Valium) is the most commonly prescribed drug in this class used to treat prostatodynia.

Interstitial Cystitis Medications

Medicines used specifically to treat interstitial cystitis, which is thought to be a related condition, have also been used to treat prostatodynia. These include pentosan polysulfate (Elmiron) and dimethyl sulfoxide (DMSO). Some clinical trials have shown these drugs to be effective, but more research is needed to determine if they are a viable treatment option.

Physical Therapy

Because prostatodynia is thought to be a condition related to spasms in the pelvic floor muscles, one approach is to treat it primarily as a muscular condition. A physical therapist can teach you exercises designed to relax these muscles and provide relief from your symptoms.

Psychiatric Counseling

Another avenue of treatment involves recommending that the patient undergo psychiatric counseling or attend a stress management course that can enable him to cope with stress more effectively. As prostatodynia seems to afflict stressed-out men with type A personalities, psychotherapy can be an effective treatment.

Sitz Baths

Some men find that sitz baths improve their symptoms. From the German word *sitzen*, meaning "to sit," sitz baths simply involve immersing your lower body in warm to hot water two or three times a day for fifteen to thirty minutes. For the treatment of prostatodynia, a bath taken in water as hot as can be comfortably tolerated seems to provide the most relief from symptoms, possibly by relaxing the pelvic floor muscles.

Increased Water Intake

This may help to dilute the concentration of irritants in the urine that exacerbate the irritative symptoms of prostatodynia.

Changes in Diet and Lifestyle

Anecdotal evidence suggests that avoiding acidic and spicy foods and drinks can provide some relief. The patient should try to abstain from highly spiced, peppery foods and beverages with a high acid content, such as citrus juices, colas, and coffee. Overindulgence in alcohol should also be avoided. The Institute for Cancer Prevention recommends following the dietary recommendations of the Prostate Health Pyramid, emphasizing fiber and antioxidant-rich foods in the diet, as well as foods high in lycopene, magnesium, zinc, lecithin, and amino acids.

The patient might have to cut back on sports or exercise activities that can irritate or inflame the lower pelvic area, such as weight lifting, jogging, or bicycle riding. Sitting for long periods of time, especially while driving, should be avoided. If the patient has a desk job, frequent breaks of standing or walking around can help relieve stress in the lower pelvic muscles.

SOLVING THE ENIGMA OF PROSTATODYNIA

Prostatodynia is a riddle wrapped in a mystery. The causes and disease process of the condition are still unknown. Diagnosis and treatment are still question marks. It is possible that prostatodynia is a complex condition with multiple causes that may require multiple treatment strategies. The prostate may not even be involved at all.

But don't despair. There are a variety of treatment options, and it may take time to figure out which one works best for you. Be patient. Since medical science does not yet know what actually causes prostatodynia, a cure will be possible once the mystery of its cause has been solved.

IV.

PROSTATE CANCER

13. Guarding Against Prostate Cancer

THE INSTITUTE FOR CANCER PREVENTION ON PROSTATE CANCER

The Institute for Cancer Prevention was founded in 1969 as the American Health Foundation to reduce the incidence, morbidity, and mortality of all kinds of cancer through prevention, research, and education. In the past thirty-five years, it has focused a good part of its energy on prostate cancer. Much of what the institute has discovered is in the pages of this book.

WHAT IS PROSTATE CANCER?

Prostate cancer (prostatic carcinoma) is the malignant growth of the glandular cells of the prostate. Prostate cancer typically develops and grows slowly over a number of years, but it can sometimes grow rapidly and spread outside the prostate gland. It may spread locally to the bladder and seminal vesicles, which carry sperm from the testicles, and then migrate to the lymph nodes of the pelvis and to bones of the spine, pelvis, and elsewhere.

Men substantially increase their risk of developing the disease as they age into their middle years and beyond. But many younger men also have some latent cancer cells in their prostate.

Researchers examined the prostates of younger men who died in accidents or from other premature causes and found that among men aged thirty to forty, 30 percent had some cancer cells in their prostate. In the vast majority of cases these were latent cancer cells, not yet at the stage where they would grow, multiply, and spread. In some of these men, the latent cancer cells would probably never have multiplied or spread, but it's impossible to tell whose cancer would have spread. Even when cancer goes beyond the latent stage, it is very difficult to determine what course it will take.

Metastasis is the spread of cancer to distant sites in the body. Cancer cells can invade neighboring tissues or take root in other parts of the body. If prostate cancer cells didn't spread at all, the mortality rate from the disease would be very low.

What makes prostate cancer spread? Not all the reasons are known. The male hormone testosterone stimulates hormone-dependent prostate cancer. As long as the body produces testosterone, prostate cancer may continue to spread.

Not surprisingly, the reported incidence of prostate cancer among men increased between 1992 and 1998 with the advent and popularization of the PSA blood-screening test.

WHO GETS PROSTATE CANCER?

Fifteen percent of American men will eventually be diagnosed with prostate cancer, 75 percent of them after the age of sixty-five. Because prostate cancer does tend to grow slowly, many men over the age of sixty-five diagnosed with prostate cancer will actually die of other causes.

Prostate cancer can run in the family: a man whose father had prostate cancer has twice the normal risk of getting the disease. Race also plays a role: African Americans are at higher risk than Caucasians and Asians (the lowest-risk group).

ENCOURAGING STATISTICS ON PROSTATE CANCER
- Fewer than 10 percent of men diagnosed with prostate cancer die within five years of diagnosis. Nearly 80 percent survive at least ten years, and upward of 60 percent survive at least fifteen years.
- More than seventy percent of prostate cancers are diagnosed while they are still localized.
- Of the approximately 6 percent of men whose prostate cancer is already advanced and has spread to noncontiguous parts of the body at the time of diagnosis, almost 35 percent will survive at least five years.

A Note on Symptoms

Prostate cancer often goes undetected for many years without producing overt symptoms. It grows unobtrusively, most commonly in the outer section of the gland, where it is less likely to affect urine flow. Because it usually grows in the outer section of the prostate, it can often be felt during a digital rectal exam.

Fortunately, prostate cancer is clinically not as common as benign prostate disease, but the majority of elderly men have it. In its intermediate or advanced stage, prostate cancer can exhibit symptoms similar to benign enlargement (frequent nocturnal urination, weak or interrupted urine stream). Benign enlargement can coexist with prostate cancer, although one does *not* cause the other. There are a number of urinary tract infections that can cause the same or similar symptoms. Most often early prostate cancer does not produce any symptoms; when it coexists with benign enlargement, patients may experience the usual symptoms of BPH.

Symptoms of intermediate or advanced prostate cancer include:

- Blood in the urine or semen
- A painful or burning sensation when passing urine
- Pronounced loss of appetite and weight
- Impotence
- Severe incontinence
- Pain in the pelvic bone, hips, buttocks, spine, ribs, lower back, or upper thighs, or along one side of the penis
- Painful ejaculation
- A discharge emanating from the urethra

The Institute for Cancer Prevention's Prostate Cancer Prevention Program

Prostate cancer is highly curable if detected early. If you haven't been diagnosed with the disease, anything you can do to help ensure against developing prostate cancer is, by definition, preventive in nature. That's why prevention is the best cure.

The truth is that death from prostate cancer may be prevented. The goal of prevention is to block carcinogenesis, the step-by-step transformation of normal prostate cells into cancerous ones.

Prostate cancer is the perfect candidate for a prevention program because there is a prolonged interval—usually many years—before latent cancer cells become active or between the time a prostate cancer tumor is small and nonaggressive and when it becomes large and aggressive (if it ever becomes so).

Men who may derive the most benefit from preventive therapy are those who are at increased risk for developing prostate cancer in the first place. This includes African Americans; men with a family history of the disease; men with prostatic intraepithelial neoplasia (PIN)—cells that aren't cancerous but are not quite "regular" either; men with extremely early stage cancers—which may or may not grow and spread—who want to impede tumor growth; and men with previously treated cancers who want to avoid a recurrence.

While there is as yet no quick-fix preventive for prostate cancer, all men can take serious preventive strides against the disease by following the six-step Institute for Cancer Prevention program:

1. **Have regular prostate cancer screenings,** especially when you reach your middle years. Because of the high incidence of prostate cancer in aging men, it is recommended that all men aged fifty-plus have regular screenings.

Although the Institute for Cancer Prevention advocates routine annual screening for prostate cancer, some prominent scientific and medical organizations do not.

However, there is one thing virtually all medical experts agree on: Every man needs balanced information on the pluses and minuses of prostate cancer screening techniques in order to make an informed decision.

2. **Eat the foods recommended in the Prostate Health Pyramid,** including plenty of antioxidant foods, while avoiding red meat and fatty foods. **Follow the Transition Diet** to help ensure a smooth transition to a prostate-healthy diet until the foods recommended in the pyramid become a comfortable part of your daily nutritional routine.

3. **Follow the Prostate Health Exercise Regimen.** Increasing evidence indicates that exercise may actually help prevent prostate cancer.

4. **Carefully assess your individual risk factors.** Make specific adjustments in your lifestyle if you fall into one or more of the high-risk

groups. For example, if you're an African American, you should start screening for prostate cancer at an earlier age than other men. If you are obese, you should lose your excess weight through a consistent combination of exercise and diet. If you live in a part of the country where the incidence of prostate cancer is higher than normal, you should familiarize yourself with all the available environmental risk factor research. You might also attend local seminars on environmental issues, where you'll have the opportunity to ask questions. Prostate cancer cluster zones—areas where there is an unusually high incidence of prostate cancer—might exist because of selenium-poor soil, a paucity of sunlight compared to other regions of the country, environmental toxins, or any number of other environmentally linked factors.

5. **Relax!** Stress certainly plays a role in weakening the immune system, leaving the door open to carcinogenic cell formation. Researchers theorize that stress can produce tension in the lower pelvic muscles, affecting the normal functioning of the prostate gland and possibly causing prostatitis. Meditation, yoga, and biofeedback are alternative treatments to reduce stress.

We do know that there is a rapidly growing awareness of the health benefits that can be achieved by reducing stress. Scientists are discovering that distinct regions of the brain perceive the presence of stressors and are able to communicate with the cells of the immune system. We are learning much more about the stressor-induced risks of disease development, the biochemical effect stress has on the immune system, and techniques that can reduce the harmful effects of stress on the immune system by interacting with stress-responsive areas of the brain.

In a recent study, forty-eight medical students were inoculated with a series of three hepatitis B vaccine injections. Specific hepatitis B antibody and T-cell responses were measured (T-cells play a major role in a variety of cell-mediated immune reactions). Students who were characterized as being in the lower-stressed/lower-anxiety group exhibited antibodies after the first injection. Their immune system was working quite efficiently. These same students had higher overall antibody levels and a more vigorous T-cell response at the end of the third inoculation. The student group that was characterized as having higher stress and anxiety levels did not exhibit nearly as efficient an immune system response to the hepatitis B vaccines. The study concluded that stress could influence risk for infectious diseases.

6. **Have a healthy, active sex life.** This does not give you license to engage in sex with multiple partners or to practice unsafe sex. Only a monogamous or sexually selective lifestyle (avoiding prostitutes and getting a sense of the sexual history of your partners) can be a key element in good prostate health.

LET THE SUNSHINE IN

According to cancer cluster studies and clinical tests, ultraviolet radiation and vitamin D may protect against prostate cancer. Most of the vitamin D we need to sustain life is manufactured by the body, with the assistance of the sun's ultraviolet radiation.

Statistics are clear about this: Caucasian men living in the southern half of the country—where the sun, on average, shines brighter

---

VITAMIN E AND SELENIUM: PRIME PREVENTIVES IN THE WAR AGAINST PROSTATE CANCER

In 2001, the National Cancer Institute launched a seven-to-twelve-year trial study of 32,000 men in an attempt to determine how effectively selenium and vitamin E supplements can reduce the incidence of prostate cancer.

Selenium supplementation was first studied in the 1980s as a potential skin cancer preventive for residents of the Southeast, where the soil is selenium-poor. Although selenium supplements were found to have no effect on the incidence of skin cancer, cancers of the prostate, lung, and colon all decreased in the study group. The original study used high-selenium yeast; the current NCI study is using a selenium-rich supplement of selenomethionine, the most abundant form of selenium found in the yeast.

Vitamin E's potential as a prostate cancer preventive also became apparent in a clinical trial designed to test its efficacy against a different type of cancer (in this case, lung cancer). 29,000 male Finnish smokers took a daily vitamin E supplement. The supplement had no clinical impact on lung cancer, but the subjects did exhibit a substantial one-third reduction in the incidence of prostate cancer and a 41 percent reduction in prostate cancer mortality rate.

In another study, researchers at the Johns Hopkins School of Hygiene and Public Health found that men with high blood levels of gamma-tocopherol (a form of vitamin E) had only a quarter of the risk of prostate cancer of men with lower blood levels of the vitamin.

and longer than in the northern half—tend to have lower prostate cancer rates. People living in major cities have higher rates of prostate cancer than rural areas.

This may also help explain why African-American men and older men have a relatively high incidence of prostate cancer. The melanin in dark skin can block the sun from reaching a specific pro-hormone in the skin. Without it, the production of vitamin D is inhibited. Older men and urban dwellers usually spend more time indoors, tending to get less direct sunlight than younger men.

PREVENTION: IS IT IN THE GENES?

Cells multiply continuously. Key genes that help regulate cell growth have been identified as p53 and bcl-2. If bcl-2 dominates, cells will be prone to develop cancer; if p53 dominates, cell growth will be controlled and cancer will not develop. Finding agents that will activate gene p53 and deactivate gene bcl-2 may be the key to preventing cancer or even curing existing cancer.

CONTROLLING HORMONES TO PREVENT CANCER

Hormonal therapy—the standard treatment for more advanced cases of prostate cancer—is known to produce significant side effects and is therefore not considered practical for prostate cancer–preventive therapy. But the potential preventive properties of certain hormones should be discussed, if only in a "what if" context.

High levels of androgens (male hormones such as testosterone) may contribute to risk of prostate cancer. But if this were strictly true, younger males would develop prostate cancer at a substantial rate, since they have the highest testosterone levels. Some clinical data indicates that prostate cancer actually depends not on testosterone but on dihydrotestosterone (DHT) for growth.

Some research has indicated that the hormone progesterone may have the ability to prevent or even reverse prostate and other cancers by inhibiting the body from converting testosterone to DHT. Males naturally produce about half the amount of progesterone that females do.

Researchers have noted that men with high levels of the hormone insulin-like growth factor–I (IGF-I) are more likely to develop prostate cancer. As its name implies, IGF-I hormone is somewhat similar to insulin, but it differs in that it controls cell growth, not sugar metabolism. However, not all clinical studies have found a linkage between elevated IGF-I levels and incidence of prostate cancer.

PREVENTIVE DRUGS: THE JURY IS STILL OUT

The factor that ultimately determines whether a drug is used for specific medical treatment is its toxicity level and its major side effects, balanced against its effectiveness against a certain disease. When a man is suffering from advanced prostate cancer, adverse reactions are acceptable, considering that the alternative to drug therapy may be death. But when a drug is given to a healthy man for preventive purposes, its side effects should always be minor or nonexistent. Prevention is not really prevention when it causes as many or more problems than it solves.

There are several drugs with genuine preventive potential that have few side effects or no side effects to speak of. Finasteride (Proscar) is the drug showing the most clinical promise in actually preventing prostate cancer. Its side effects are either rare or minor.

Finasteride is already being used extensively to treat enlarged prostate. Finasteride blocks the chemical 5alpha-reductase, which converts testosterone into its more powerful form, DHT. Testosterone and DHT are androgens that stimulate the growth of normal as well as cancerous prostate cells. Males born without 5alpha-reductase don't get prostate cancer.

Finasteride inhibits 5alpha-reductase and depresses blood DHT concentrations dramatically, to near castration levels. Sexual side effects from finasteride are uncommon. Most men can enjoy the benefits of the drug while retaining potency and sex drive.

However, every coin has a reverse side. Some scientists have suggested that finasteride may have a counterproductive effect, increasing rather than decreasing the concentration of testosterone in the prostate, thus providing fuel for cancer cells to multiply. These same scientists also question whether a decrease in blood DHT necessarily means a decrease in DHT within the prostate itself. Nevertheless, a large clinical trial showed that finasteride can indeed help prevent prostate cancer (see page 264).

Other preventive agents with the potential to instead make matters worse include synthetic retinoid drugs, specifically the experimental drug 4-HPR. Retinoids have shown clinical promise in inhibiting cancer cell growth but may actually enhance cancer growth in certain men. Retinoids also have too many pronounced side effects to be widely prescribed as a preventive medication.

DFMO is a drug which reportedly binds to and blocks catalysts that stimulate cancerous as well as noncancerous cell production. We will learn more about its potential to prevent or arrest prostate cancer subsequent to further clinical tests.

A high-fat, low-fiber diet irritates the lining of the colon. Did you know that this inflammation is promoted by a class of compounds called eicosanoids? Some scientists also suspect that eicosanoids promote the spread of cancer cells. They are studying a potent anti-inflammatory protein called uteroglobin—found in the uterus, respiratory tract, and prostate—that may be effective in blocking potentially cancer-promoting inflammation.

Other promising cancer-preventing drugs are currently being tested. It will be years before their preventive value, if any, is determined.

THE PSA TEST: CUTTING THROUGH THE CONTROVERSY

The basics of the prostate-specific antigen (PSA) biomarker screening test for prostate cancer were discussed in Chapter 3. Now let's talk about the pros and cons of the test.

Since its inception, PSA testing to screen for prostate cancer has been the subject of controversy. Some physicians believe that the PSA test is too flawed a screening tool. Here are some of the reasons why:

TRINOVIN: A DIETARY SUPPLEMENT THAT HELPS PREVENT CANCER?

Trinovin is a dietary supplement that has recently been the focus of research for its possible chemopreventive properties. Trinovin, derived from a legume of the red clover plant, is a combination of four phytoestrogens purported to mimic the effect of the hormone estrogen, delaying or preventing the growth of prostate cancer cells.

Although a few small-scale trials have shown promising results, no large-scale, randomized trials have been conducted to date. Trinovin has no reported significant side effects.

- **Many factors can affect PSA levels.** This includes certain medical procedures, such as a digital rectal exam prior to a PSA test; an enlarged prostate or other urinary tract condition; a prostate infection; or ejaculation within forty-eight hours prior to the test. All these factors and more can lead to false-positive test results.

- **Many false-positive results occur.** As noted, a high PSA level does not necessarily indicate the presence of cancer. False-positive results occur when the PSA level is elevated but no cancer is actually present. A man whose PSA level tests significantly higher than the norm may experience anxiety until comprehensive biopsy results are obtained, whether or not he turns out to have prostate cancer. Of men aged fifty or older, 15 of every 100 will exhibit elevated PSA levels; of these 15, 12 will be false-positives and only three will turn out to indicate cancer. The PSA test may also reveal a cancer that is not clinically significant or a very slowly growing tumor that is unlikely to be life-threatening. Many men have latent prostate cancers that, even though they are detectable, don't spread or cause significant health problems.

FALSE-POSITIVE ANXIETY

A lot has been written, in both the scientific and lay press, about the anxiety caused by false-positive results from relatively nonspecific cancer-screening tests.

In twenty-three years of interviewing cancer patients and people who have been screened, I have heard many stories about "cancer anxiety." While stress caused by a test result that turns out to be incorrect is undeniable, the great majority of people who find themselves in this situation have told me that they would rather go through whatever testing is necessary to find out whether or not they have cancer. If they have to go through some anxiety while it's all being worked out, that's a price they're willing to pay.

In any case, when it comes to PSA results, physicians should explain clearly that an elevated PSA does not necessarily mean cancer. Furthermore, any stress can be minimized by expeditious scheduling and quick reading of biopsies, as well as quick communication of results to the patient.

Yes, the PSA test is imperfect, and many men will undergo needless anxiety over a false-positive result; but it's all we have for now, and it could save your life—so go get tested.

• **Unnecessary biopsies may be performed, and aggressive therapy may be used, even when such treatment may not be necessary.** If the PSA test shows an abnormally high result, a biopsy will be recommended. Even if the cancer has not spread outside the prostate gland, the patient is faced with the decision to undergo treatment, such as surgery or radiation therapy, or to engage in "watchful waiting" (careful monitoring of the progress of the cancer). Surgery and radiation can both have significant side effects and complications. It is estimated that about 30 to 50 percent of men have some microscopic evidence of prostate cancer cells by age fifty, and as high as 70 to 90 percent in men over eighty. The vast majority of men who live long enough will have microscopic evidence of prostate cancer. Critics of the PSA test—and critics of widespread screening for prostate cancer in general—allege that large numbers of men suffer the side effects of unnecessary treatment because of too much emphasis on flawed screening procedures.

• **False-negative results.** A man may test in the normal range, indicating he does not have prostate cancer, when in fact he does.

• **Early detection does not necessarily mean a reduction in mortality rate.** Finding even a small tumor or early-stage prostate cancer does not guarantee that the patient's life will be saved. Since the use of early detection tests for prostate cancer became common, the prostate cancer mortality rate has, in fact, dropped. It has not yet been proven, however, that this is a direct or indirect result of PSA screening.

• **Detection of late-stage prostate cancer may be a case of too little, too late.** A PSA test result may simply be too late to do much good for a man with a fast-growing, aggressive cancer that has already spread to other parts of his body. Of course, if men get a PSA test regularly, as recommended, prostate cancer would usually be detected at a very early stage and there would be far fewer cases of "too little, too late."

GRADING PROSTATE CANCER

Many pathologists grade prostate cancers according to the Gleason system. This system assigns a Gleason grade, using numbers from 1

PSA SCREENING AND CANCER MORTALITY RATES:
THE BOTTOM LINE

What effect, if any, have the introduction and popularization of PSA testing had on the prostate cancer mortality rate? We do know that, beginning in 1989, the rapid popularization of PSA testing led to a substantial increase in new diagnoses of preclinical prostate cancer. That should come as no surprise. Estimates are that, on average, PSA screening detects prostate cancer five years earlier than it would otherwise be detected.

Survival of cancer is generally defined as staying alive for five years after initial diagnosis. For example, if a prostate cancer was initially detected in the year 2000 by PSA testing, it won't be until 2005 that the patient is considered to have "survived" his cancer. But that is the point at which, on average, the cancer would have been detected without the PSA. Thus that "increased" survival may not actually translate into a longer total life span.

However, it makes sense that early prostate cancer detection can lead to earlier and more effective treatment, which in turn would show dividends of true lower mortality rates.

This we do know: in the last six years, the United States experienced an unexplained decrease in prostate cancer mortality for the first time in thirty years (an estimated 6.7 percent reduction in mortality rate). This argues strongly in the PSA test's favor.

The Institute for Cancer Prevention concedes that the PSA test isn't perfect. It is, however, a prime weapon in the war against prostate cancer. **The institute supports PSA testing, as well as current clinical research that seeks to devise accurate tests involving other biomarkers for the detection of prostate cancer.**

to 5, based on how much—or how little—the arrangement of cells in cancerous tissue resembles normal prostate tissue. If the cancerous tissue looks close to normal, it is assigned a grade of 1. If the cancerous tissue cells spread throughout the prostate and show a wide variety of malignant characteristics, it is classified as a grade 5 tumor. Grades 2 through 4 exhibit an increasing degree of intermediate features, signifying a more malignant level of cancer as the numbers rise.

If the cells don't look cancerous but don't quite look normal either, they are reported as "suspicious." This is usually categorized in two ways: either as "atypical" or as prostatic intraepithelial neoplasia (PIN).

PIN is generally characterized as either low-grade or high-grade.

Many men begin to develop low-grade PIN at an early age but do not necessarily develop prostate cancer. With atypical findings or high-grade PIN, cancer may already be present somewhere in the prostate gland. With high-grade PIN, for example, there is a 30 to 50 percent chance of finding prostate cancer in a subsequent biopsy. Repeat biopsies are often recommended in such cases.

THE PSA TEST UNDER FIRE

The PSA test has always been an imperfect screening test for prostate cancer. But the reluctance of many men to have a digital rectal exam, combined with the ease of a simple PSA blood test, has led many men and their doctors to adopt the PSA test as the screening tool of choice.

Its sensitivity was originally thought to be fairly high, but its specificity wasn't great since we've already read that anything from an infection to ejaculation can drive up your numbers, leading to anxiety, repeat testing, and perhaps even unnecessary biopsy. Now a spate of recent studies has muddied the waters even more.

First came a report in *The Journal of the American Medical Association* by Memorial Sloan-Kettering researchers showing that a man's PSA levels commonly show a fair amount of normal fluctuation over time. They studied nearly a thousand men who had five consecutive PSA tests over a four-year period. While a fifth of the men had an elevated PSA level at some time during the study, the level of nearly half of them spontaneously returned to normal on subsequent tests.

The message here is that because there are natural variations in PSA levels, an elevated reading should be confirmed several weeks later before moving on to a biopsy. The authors note that a delay in diagnosis of a few weeks or months is unlikely to alter treatment efficacy since prostate cancer is almost always very slow-growing.

Then came a Wake Forest University study in *The Journal of the National Cancer Institute* that showed that genetics cause some men to test higher on the PSA test, even when they don't have prostate cancer or any other elevating factor. Using DNA sequencing, researchers identified three variations in a part of the gene that controls PSA levels. The researchers found that up to 20 percent of men may have genetic variants that cause levels of PSA that are about 30 percent higher than other men's, which could lead to needless biopsies.

Testing for the genetic variants, which is quick and inexpensive, may one day be a routine part of screening for prostate cancer and could lead to higher cutoff numbers before a biopsy is recommended. Confused? Wait, there's more!

(continued on next page)

Finally, a study in *The New England Journal of Medicine* argued for the converse—that the PSA level at which a prostate biopsy is recommended should be *lowered,* particularly for younger men. Worse yet, the study seemed to show that the PSA test may actually miss up to *82 percent* of tumors in men older than sixty. At least that's how the results were widely reported.

But a closer reading of the study is needed to put it into perspective. Since not all men who have a PSA test done will undergo a biopsy to check for cancer, the authors say this makes the PSA test look better than it really is. So they performed a sophisticated statistical data analysis using a mathematical model to "correct" for this apparent statistical bias. That's how they arrived at the 82 percent missed cancer estimate, not by actually finding those "missed" cancers.

Finally, they recommended lowering the PSA level at which a biopsy would be done, saying this would increase the sensitivity of the test. It would also submit millions of additional men to a prostate biopsy, with all the potential costs, complications, and anxiety that would come with that.

So what should men do? First of all, the message here is *not* "Well, the PSA test misses most prostate cancers anyway, so why should I bother?" **Do not stop having PSA tests, but realize that its numbers are not enough all by themselves.** A DRE is an important part of prostate cancer screening, as is the rest of your clinical picture, including your family history, the rate at which your PSA levels have been increasing (PSA velocity), your age, genetic testing when it becomes available, and so on.

The entire PSA story is still evolving, as is our understanding of prostate cancer, for that matter. The PSA and digital rectal exam (DRE) are imperfect, but clearly we are finding more and more prostate cancers at earlier stages, when they are treatable, modifiable through diet and lifestyle changes—and, yes, curable.

Because prostate cancers often have areas with different grades, a grade is assigned to each of the two areas that make up most of the cancer. These two grades are added together to yield the Gleason score (also called the Gleason sum), which is between 2 and 10. The higher your Gleason score, the more likely it is that your cancer will grow and spread rapidly. Scores of 2 through 4 are often grouped together as low; 5 and 6 are considered intermediate; and scores of 7 to 10 are considered high.

The pathologist will send your doctor a report that stages the cancer. Three capital letters are used frequently in this report: T, N, and M.

T, for "tumor," signifies the extent of the cancer in, and adjacent

THE STAGES OF PROSTATE CANCER

Prostate cancer staging is a complex process. Accurate staging is critical to establish optimal treatment. Physicians may describe the clinical stage of the cancer by using either Roman numerals or capital letters.

STAGE	CHARACTERISTICS
STAGE I/STAGE A	The cancer cannot be felt during a rectal exam. It may be found by accident when surgery is performed for other reasons, such as enlarged prostate. There is no evidence the cancer has spread outside the prostate.
II/B	The tumor involves more tissue within the prostate; it can be felt during a rectal exam; or it is found when a biopsy is performed as a result of a high PSA level. There is no evidence that the cancer has spread outside the prostate.
III/C	The cancer has spread outside the prostate to nearby tissues.

to, the prostate gland. N stands for "nodes," signifying if the cancer has spread to nearby lymph nodes. M stands for "metastasis," signifying whether the cancer has spread to other organs or tissues, such as the lungs or bones. These letters are followed by a number indicating the extent of the condition, and perhaps by a lowercase letter to indicate the location of the cancer.

TUMOR STATUS

T1a: Nonpalpable tumor is found incidentally after prostatectomy or TURP done for BPH in less than 5 percent of tissue sample.

T1b: Nonpalpable tumor is found incidentally after prostatectomy of TURP done for BPH in more than 5 percent of tissue sample.

T1c: Nonpalpable tumor is identified by needle biopsy due to elevated PSA.

T2a: Tumor involves one lobe of the prostate and can be felt by a DRE.

T2b: Tumor involves both lobes of the prostate and can be felt by a DRE.

T3a: Tumor extends through the prostate capsule.

T3b: Tumor is found in the seminal vesicles.

T4: Tumor has spread to surrounding structures, such as the bladder neck or external sphincter.

LYMPH NODE STATUS
NX: Regional lymph nodes cannot be assessed.
N0: There is no regional lymph node metastasis.
N1: There is metastasis in regional lymph node or nodes.

STATUS OF DISTANT METASTASES
MX: Distant metastasis cannot be assessed.
M0: There is no distant metastasis.
M1: There is distant metastasis.
M1a: Tumor is found in lymph nodes beyond the pelvic region.
M1b: Tumor is found in bone.
M1c: Tumor has spread to other distant sites.

THE WHITMORE-JEWETT STAGING SYSTEM
Here's another common prostate cancer staging system:

Stage A: Cancer may incidentally be found during surgery for enlarged prostate.
A1: Cancer is small and low-grade.
A2: Cancer is high-grade or found throughout the tissue specimen.

Stage B: Cancer is detected by a digital exam and is limited to the prostate.
B1: Cancer is limited to one side of the prostate.
B2: There is cancer on both sides of the prostate.

Stage C: Cancer has spread to tissues directly surrounding the prostate.

Stage D: Cancer has metastasized to the lymph nodes or to bone.
D1: Cancer has spread only to the pelvic lymph nodes.
D2: Cancer has spread to the bones.

Prostate Cancer Q&A: Things You Need to Know

What's the most typical outcome for a man diagnosed with prostate cancer?

His chances are very good indeed. Early-stage prostate cancer is a highly treatable disease with a high cure rate. Early screening and detection help make the outcome even more encouraging.

Does an elevated PSA mean I should have a bone scan as well as a biopsy?

No. Bone scans should generally be restricted to patients with a PSA level higher than 10, but your physician will decide.

I've heard of men having a PSA test after their prostate was removed. Why?

Assuming that the prostate has been completely removed, there may still be prostate cancer cells in other parts of the body, and these cells may still be secreting PSA. In this case, the PSA test will show a reading. If that reading is sufficiently high enough, it may indicate the need for further treatment. A high PSA level—or a rising PSA level over a series of follow-up tests—may indicate continuing cancer growth.

PSA levels vary greatly from one man to the next, and possibly even from one test to the next. With cancer patients, doctors are less interested in the exact PSA level than they are in changes over time. If the prostate has been surgically removed and there has been no spread of cancer cells elsewhere in the body, the PSA should fall to very low levels within three weeks after the operation. Radiation treatments cause a slower drop.

Can a urinary tract infection elevate my PSA level?

Yes. As noted, many things unrelated to prostate cancer can raise your PSA level, and a urinary tract infection is one of them. The prostate gland can react negatively to a urinary tract infection, leading to possible prostatitis (inflammation of the prostate gland), and an elevated PSA level.

Are there any medications that lower PSA level, leading to a false-negative reading?

Medications such as saw palmetto (an herbal medicine used for prostatitis) and finasteride (Proscar, Propecia; used to treat BPH and balding, respectively) can give a false lower reading. Inform your physician that you are taking these medications or any other medications that may possibly affect your PSA level.

Is there any validity to the notion that some men are having their PSA serum blood level checked too often?
The Institute for Cancer Prevention feels that any school of thought that discourages regular prostate health screening is counterproductive. But according to data from the Prostate, Lung, Colorectal and Ovarian (PLCO) Cancer Screening Trial, sponsored by the National Cancer Institute, some men may not need to repeat the test as often as previously thought. Based on results from nearly 30,000 men enrolled in the PLCO trial who had annual PSA tests as part of the study, men whose last PSA test was less than 1 ng/ml may want to consider screening less often than annually. But all men *should* continue to be screened.

We keep hearing so many mixed messages from the media. Are prostate cancer rates rising or declining?
Mortality rates are declining, but the incidence of new cases appears to be on the rise. However, the reasons for this are not cause to panic or proof that prostate cancer is "spreading." The larger the population of men over sixty-five—and that population is rapidly rising—the more men who will be diagnosed with prostate cancer.

The increasing popularity of the PSA test over the last fifteen years means that more men are being diagnosed with prostate cancer. Some of these men have only the slight presence of a slowly growing cancer and would not have been diagnosed for years, if ever, if not for the high sensitivity of the PSA test.

Can blood protein patterns help distinguish the presence of prostate cancer?
A recently devised test may be useful in determining when to perform a biopsy in men with elevated PSA levels. The test proved useful not only in men with normal-to-high PSA levels but also in men whose PSA levels were only marginally elevated.

Complex patterns of proteins found in patients' blood serum may help distinguish between prostate cancer and benign conditions. Reportedly, researchers were able to differentiate between samples taken from patients diagnosed with cancer and patients diagnosed with enlarged prostate.

Researchers analyzed serum proteins with mass spectroscopy, a technique used to sort proteins and other molecules based on their weight and electrical charge. Researchers were able to correctly identify 36 of 38 (95 percent) cases of prostate cancer and 177 of 228 cases (78 percent) of benign disease. Though this test is not yet available, it could be evaluated by the Food and Drug Administration (FDA) as early as 2004.

What is a complete androgen blockade?
Some of the body's androgens (male hormones) are produced in the adrenal glands, but most are produced in the testes. To completely block all androgen production in the body of prostate cancer patients, an antiandrogen—typically flutamide, bicalutamide, or nilutamide—is used to block androgen receptors.

If a man is already diagnosed with prostate cancer and he begins to feel pain in other areas, such as his back or legs, is this an indication that the cancer is spreading?
Not necessarily; the pain may stem from another source, especially if he has experienced pain in those regions before. It is certainly prudent to have a bone scan in this case (or a follow-up bone scan), since, unfortunately, the cancer may indeed be spreading. Pain in the lower body or groin is one of the symptoms of advanced prostate cancer.

How common are bowel disorders as a result of radiation treatment for prostate cancer?
Moderately common. As many as 20 percent of men who receive external beam radiation therapy for prostate cancer experience gastrointestinal problems that can include constipation, blood in the stool, diarrhea, cramps, or urgency to have a bowel movement. State-of-the-art equipment may lower that figure.

What are the most common forms of medical malpractice lawsuits in the diagnosis and treatment of prostate cancer?
- Misinterpreting PSA blood test or biopsy results
- Failing to diagnose the presence of cancer in a biopsy procedure

- Failing to provide or recommend a biopsy when a patient exhibits a sufficiently elevated PSA level
- Failing to recommend appropriate treatment options for a prostate disease or condition or utilizing inappropriate treatment options in relation to the degree and stage of the cancer

Is radiotherapy for prostate cancer patients who have already been treated with surgery or hormone therapy of any benefit?
There is at least one major long-term clinical test now under way, involving 650 patients worldwide, to help determine if additional radiation treatment is of benefit. Subjects will be divided into two treatment groups. Group 1 will be treated with hormone therapy. Group 2 will have radiotherapy in addition to the hormone therapy. The two groups will be compared to determine if there is any statistically significant difference between treatment success rates.

What are my chances of getting prostate cancer and another form of cancer at the same time?
Though not a common occurrence, this certainly does happen. A mutation of the p53 gene can lead to a variety of cancers, including prostate cancer and lymphoma.

If I undergo hormone therapy, will I eventually become resistant to the drugs?
Hormone therapy is a common treatment for men with advanced prostate cancer. Different men react to hormone therapy in different ways. It may work successfully for one man longer than for another. However, most men undergoing hormone treatment will eventually develop hormone resistance, and the treatment will become less effective—or quite ineffective—in controlling the cancer. It takes some men much longer to develop hormone resistance (for some a matter of months, for others a matter of years).

With intermittent hormone therapy, drugs are administered for six months; then there is a six-month layoff, after which therapy resumes.

IN THE WAKE OF PROSTATE CANCER: COPING AND GETTING ON WITH YOUR LIFE

Prostate cancer is almost never a death sentence. It is one of the least virulent and most treatable and curable of cancers. Psychological adjustment to the disease is a relatively smooth process for some men.

But we're not going to soft-pedal the truth and tell you that it is an *easy* process. It never is, even for the strongest of us; even for those of us blessed with a wonderful support system of family and friends.

You'll overcome your negative emotions even more quickly by realizing that many of the ways to prevent prostate cancer discussed earlier in this chapter are equally as beneficial for slowing down the progress of the disease and maintaining maximal health after you have been diagnosed and while you're being treated.

- **Eat a prostate-healthy diet.**
- **Get plenty of exercise.**
- **Enjoy your sex life.** If you're experiencing sexual problems as a result of surgery or radiation treatment, be aware that there are lots of effective therapies to treat your condition.
- **Practice relaxation and stress-reducing techniques** such as meditation and deep breathing.
- **Reach out to others.** Besides those in your immediate circle, there are support groups. You can talk to other men who are experiencing the physical and emotional trauma of prostate cancer. Sharing the experience not only lets you know that your tribulations and fears are by no means unique but can provide information and comfort.

14. TREATING PROSTATE CANCER

A TREATMENT DILEMMA

According to American Cancer Society (ACS) statistics, prostate cancer affected an estimated 220,900 American men in 2003, with nearly 29,000 deaths from the disease.

According to the ACS, an American male has a 16 percent chance of developing prostate cancer in his lifetime. Those odds are still unacceptably and unnecessarily high. But if you do become one of the 16 percent, let's consider what course should be followed.

DETERMINING THE RIGHT TREATMENT FOR EACH PATIENT

There are a number of increasingly sophisticated treatment options available for prostate cancer patients. Surgery, for all its long history in the United States, is just one of them and should never be considered without attention to other options.

Before making an important treatment decision, get a second opinion. Let another physician review your diagnosis and discuss treatment options with you. Some health insurance companies require a second opinion; many others will cover a second opinion if the patient requests it.

There is no single prescribed routine for the treatment of prostate cancer. In addition to the stage and grade of the cancer, the choice of therapy depends on the age of the patient, health considerations that may be unrelated to the cancer, and a number of other individual factors, including lifestyle.

When the cancer is localized (when there is no evidence that it has spread to the lymph nodes or elsewhere), treatment options include:

- **"Watchful waiting,"** or **surveillance** (careful observation before deciding on treatment, or deciding against aggressive treatment altogether)
- **External beam radiation therapy**
- **Brachytherapy** (the implanting of radioactive seeds into the prostate)
- **Surgery,** such as radical prostatectomy (removal of the prostate gland)

EXPECTANT THERAPY

WATCHFUL WAITING

When it comes to prostate cancer, sometimes the best thing to do is to keep a very close watch on the cancer and continue to follow appropriate dietary and lifestyle measures. The Prostate Health Pyramid and the Healthy Prostate Fitness Regimen have been developed specifically by the Institute for Cancer Prevention as adjuvant treatment modalities as well as preventive tools. "Watchful waiting"—also known as surveillance or deferred treatment—may be recommended by a physician when the tumor is small (in an early stage) and is not growing quickly (is a low-grade tumor); when there is only scant microscopic evidence of cancer cells; or when the disadvantages of treatment outweigh the benefits. It is especially suitable for older men with limited life expectancy. Many older men have other medical conditions that make surgery risky. In addition, they are unlikely to die of the cancer during their limited life.

As we know, prostate cancer most often occurs in older men and usually tends to be slow-growing. For men over seventy, other conditions and diseases may be far more of a threat to life and health than low-grade prostate cancer. These health conditions may need to be addressed more directly than the prostate cancer.

DON'T CONFUSE WATCHFUL WAITING WITH DOING NOTHING

While the numbers for prostate cancer in this country seem alarming, they are actually much higher than even the latest statistics indicate. In fact, most men will die *with* prostate cancer.

Let me explain that last statement: most men will die *with* prostate cancer but not *of* prostate cancer. We know that because autopsy studies that have looked at the prostates of men who died of other causes found that many had undetected cancer in their prostate that was not their cause of death. Furthermore, the percentage of men with prostate cancer increased with age until it was nearly as high as their age (70 percent of seventy-year-olds may have prostate cancer, 80 percent of eighty-year-olds, and so on.).

What that translates into is that many, many men have a form of prostate cancer that is often referred to as *somnolent* (literally "sleepy"), that is, very slow growing and may never become life-threatening. Most men with prostate cancer will die of any number of other things long before their cancer becomes an issue.

That's where watchful waiting becomes a reasonable approach to managing prostate cancer. Rather than doing nothing, you and your doctor keep a close eye on your tumor through regular screening, so that intervention can be planned at the first sign that the cancer may be becoming more aggressive or is beginning to spread or enlarge significantly. Plus, you will be following the diet and lifestyle recommendations carefully laid out in this book, so that your cancer is that much less likely to ever become life-threatening.

Watchful waiting is a far more common approach to managing prostate cancer in many European countries than it is in America. Some people would say that it has to do with their systems of socialized medicine, which favor less aggressive and less costly treatments. Perhaps—but I would argue that there are cultural reasons as well.

For some reason, we in America have developed a "get it all out" and "kill it all" attitude toward cancer. Many are the women who still choose mastectomy over lumpectomy (complete breast removal versus breast-conserving surgery) because they do not want to live with even the slight possibility that some cancer was left behind.

That mentality also permeates the medical profession and the general public in this country. So when a PSA level and subsequent biopsy indicate prostate cancer, *few are the men or doctors who will be able to psychologically handle the thought of "just watching" their cancer.*

But as we argue in this chapter, that may just be the best approach. We can learn something from our brothers "across the pond."

Surveillance may prove a viable, prudent option even for some young men. As with older patients, watchful waiting would depend on the cancer's stage and grade; how rapidly the cancer is likely to grow (which often can't be determined accurately); the patient's overall health level; a close analysis of the patient's biopsy results; and the patient's personal choice, based on his informed inclination and heavily influenced by a frank consultation with his physician.

Of those initially managed by watchful waiting, about 40 percent ultimately go on to active treatment. Predictors of shifting to active treatment include younger age, higher level of formal education, baseline higher PSA, PSA rate of change, and higher Gleason grades.

Long-term studies are currently under way to compare the success rate of various treatment modalities with the efficacy of watchful waiting. The mainstream medical community may be surprised at the results—perhaps discovering that when it comes to treatment, less can be more.

RADIATION THERAPY

EXTERNAL BEAM RADIATION (XBRT, EBR), RADIOTHERAPY

External beam radiation therapy is often recommended for older men with additional health issues or for men with more advanced prostate cancer. Its initial impact is less traumatic than that of surgery. Like surgery, radiation is localized therapy.

External beam radiotherapy is done over several days. A typical course of treatment might be five times a week for six or seven weeks. The patient doesn't feel anything during radiation therapy, which usually takes place at a radiotherapy unit attached to or affiliated with a hospital. The specialist who provides the treatment may make ink marks on your skin to use as a guide for the X-ray beam. This beam delivers the high-energy radiation necessary to kill underlying prostate cancer cells. While the X-rays are ideally targeted at the prostate only, they may cause some damage to the tissues around the gland. However, modern conformal radiotherapy (see p. 258) minimizes this complication.

While you will not feel the therapy itself, you will feel its side effects. Impotence does not usually occur immediately after radiation therapy. It tends to gradually develop over the course of one or more years. Upward of 60 percent of men become impotent within two years of external beam radiation therapy. With surgery, impotence, if it is going to happen, occurs immediately but may improve over time.

Many patients experience extreme fatigue, especially in the latter weeks of treatment. Some men suffer from diarrhea and bleeding due to damage to the rectum and small bowel or experience frequent, uncomfortable urination due to bladder injury. Bladder problems persist in about one third of patients. Longer-term complications include a narrowing of the urethra that makes urination difficult. It is typical for the skin in the treated area to become red, dry, and tender. Radiation also commonly causes hair loss in the treated area. This loss may be temporary or permanent.

Sometimes radiation treatment can damage the intestines and cause lactose intolerance, a condition in which the body can't digest or absorb milk sugar (lactose). Symptoms of lactose intolerance include diarrhea, gas, and cramping.

CONFORMAL RADIATION THERAPY

This is external beam radiation therapy with higher radiation doses and more accurate targeting of diseased tissue, with a reduced rate of the radiation dose to normal surrounding tissue and reportedly fewer side effects. Conformal radiation therapy takes several forms: three-dimensional (3D) conformal radiation; intensity-modulated radiation therapy; and proton beam radiation.

Proton beam radiation bombards diseased tissue with protons—the parts of atoms that carry a positive electric charge—instead of with X-rays. As of 2004, there are only a few medical centers in the United States that have the technology for proton beam therapy available. To date, no clinical comparison has been made on the effectiveness of proton beam therapy versus 3D X-ray therapy.

BRACHYTHERAPY

Brachytherapy goes by many names: internal radiation therapy, seeding, seed implants, interstitial radiation therapy (IRT), and implant radiation. Radioactive material (radioisotopes) sealed in needles, seeds, or wires is placed directly into or near a prostate cancer tumor.

In an earlier era, seed implants were performed using an "open" implantation method, involving surgery to expose the prostate gland. Manual placement of seeds, which was imprecise, meant that there were areas where the seeds were too far apart to be effective against certain cancer cells. In the 1970s, ultrasound template guidance was introduced; this allows seeds to be distributed uniformly throughout the prostate and eliminates the need for surgical incisions and guesswork.

That's the good news; now for the bad news. Brachytherapy can cause impotence, urinary incontinence (severe incontinence is not a typical side effect, but frequent urination may persist in one third of patients who have brachytherapy), as well as bowel problems (significant long-term bowel problems reportedly occur in less than 5 percent of patients). Impotence was reportedly less likely to develop after brachytherapy (about 20 to 40 percent estimated incidence) than after radical prostatectomy or external beam radiation. However, results from more recent, longer-term studies indicate a much higher rate of impotence with longer years of follow-up after treatment.

After initial implantation, seed radiation is present in the prostate for two to six months. Two commonly used types of radiation seeds are palladium seeds and iodine seeds. Iodine seeds are used for prostate cancers of Gleason grade 6 or less (less advanced cancers); palladium seeds are used for grade 7 or greater (more advanced cancers). Implantation takes about an hour. Even after the radiation effects fade, the seeds remain in the prostate permanently, without any known complications or side effects.

If the patient has an enlarged prostate in addition to prostate cancer, the extent of the enlargement will be evaluated with a transrectal ultrasound probe, and further evaluated with a CAT scan of the pubic arch, to gauge possible interference with seed implantation. If the prostate gland is simply too large to effectively allow for seed implantation, the size of the prostate will be reduced by a monthly injection of a drug such as Lupron and with further supplementation of a drug such as Casodex for a period of three months.

Brachytherapy is more expensive than other treatment options, but it is covered by most medical insurance. Seed implantation patients typically require less hospitalization time and can return to work more quickly than patients who have had a prostatectomy or undergone EBR.

Is It Safe for Me to Be Around Other People?

There are no restrictions on the patient's contact with other adults, although some caution should be shown with small children and pregnant women, maintaining a distance of six feet or more following seed implantation. Ask your physician how long you should take such precautions. Isotopes emit low-level radiation, most of it confined to the prostate. Very small amounts of radiation might reach others if a seed is expelled in the urine or a minute amount travels through the air.

Occasionally the patient will require an additional short treatment with external radiation after seed implantation only if his Gleason score is higher than 6 or if his PSA reading is over 10.

HORMONE THERAPY

Hormone therapy, or hormonal therapy, involves the use of drugs that prevent the release of testosterone; drugs that counter the effects of testosterone; or a surgical procedure called orchiectomy, surgical removal of the testicles.

ORCHIECTOMY

Surgically removing the testicles cuts off the source that produces the majority of male hormones and fuels prostate cancer. Although both testicles are removed, the scrotal sac is left in place. An orchiectomy is a relatively brief procedure performed under local or general anesthetic.

About 90 percent of the men who have this operation suffer from impotence, and a severely reduced or complete lack of libido. Some men also experience hot flashes (which usually fade in time and can be reduced by antiandrogens), breast tenderness and growth of breast tissue, osteoporosis, anemia, loss of muscle mass, weight gain, and extreme fatigue. Intense psychological ramifications and decreased mental acuity often accompany the physical side effects.

Given the roll call of major side effects, orchiectomy is a hormone cessation therapy reserved for advanced cases of prostate cancer, where the cancer has metastasized dramatically.

Unlike the use of injections to reduce androgen (male hormone) levels, orchiectomy is not reversible.

ANTIANDROGENS AND ANDROGEN BLOCKADE

An androgen blockade is most often used for men with advanced, metastasized prostate cancer, when it is no longer possible to cure the disease with surgery or radiation. In some instances, medicines that block the action of testosterone can be used to check cancer spread and shrink cancerous growths even when cancer is present throughout the body. Antiandrogens block the body's ability to utilize testosterone. Antiandrogen therapy uses a hormone-blocking drug, often taken in combination with a luteinizing hormone-releasing hormone (LHRH) analog (see next section).

Strictly speaking, an androgen blockade is not considered curative. Some prostate cancer cells are able to grow independently of testosterone. These cells are referred to as androgen-independent, hormone-resistant, or hormone-refractory cells. Typically, men receiving hormone therapy have their cancer go into remission for two to three years, with occasional men experiencing a much longer-term remission.

Men who are treated with a total androgen blockade may experience more side effects than men who are treated with a single method of hormonal therapy. Antiandrogens can cause nausea, vomiting, diarrhea, and breast growth and tenderness. Ketoconazole, if used extensively, may cause liver problems. Aminoglutethimide can cause skin rashes. Any hormone therapy that lowers androgen levels will contribute to osteoporosis in older men.

Antiandrogen side effects in patients already treated by orchiectomy and with LHRH agonists include diarrhea (a common side effect), nausea, liver problems, and tiredness.

LHRH ANALOGS

Luteinizing hormone-releasing hormone (LHRH) analogs are a class of drugs used to shut down testosterone production. The resulting decrease in testosterone level tempers the spread of cancer, and helps relieve pain and other symptoms associated with advanced prostate cancer.

When first taken, an LHRH agonist may actually have a counterproductive effect for a short time. This phenomenon is referred to as "flare." To prevent flare, the doctor may give the patient an antiandrogen along with the LHRH agonist. Gradually, LHRH treatment will cause testosterone levels to fall and symptoms to abate.

Side effects of LHRH analogs are similar to those of orchiectomy. Like other hormone-based treatment options, LHRH analogs may cause impotence. Hot flashes are the most common side effect associated with LHRH analogs.

FDA-approved hormone blockers, often used in combination, include Lupron (leuprolide acetate), Zoladex (goserelin acetate implant), Viadur (leuprolide acetate), Casodex (bicalutamide), Eulexin (flutamide), and Nilandron (nilutamide).

New drugs to block the effects of male hormones and stifle prostate cancer growth are being developed or have been approved recently by the FDA. One such drug, Abarelix, is an analog GnRH (gonadotropin-releasing hormone) and acts to block receptors in the anterior pituitary gland. Abarelix is believed to work in a similar fashion to LHRH agonists, but it appears to lower testosterone levels faster and does not cause a surge of testosterone production before suppressing it.

HORMONE-RESISTANT OR REFRACTORY PROSTATE CANCER

In hormone-resistant prostate cancer, the cancer may progress and PSA levels rise despite reduced testosterone levels. The cancer no longer responds to the hormonal therapy. However, hormone-resistant prostate cancer may respond to a *change* in hormonal therapy—for example, intermittent androgen blockade or antiandrogen withdrawal, both discussed below.

When nothing in hormonal therapy seems to work, other treatments may have to be considered, including chemotherapy, experimental treatment, or purely palliative (treating the symptoms and easing the pain) as opposed to curative therapy.

ANTIANDROGEN WITHDRAWAL

Prostate cancer may start to progress again after patients have been on antiandrogen therapy for a period of time. In this case, the cancer has simply become resistant to the antiandrogen and the antiandrogen therapy may be stopped.

INTERMITTENT ANDROGEN BLOCKADE

This is also known as intermittent (noncontinuous) androgen suppression or intermittent hormonal therapy. An intermittent blockade can include administration of a single hormonal drug (such as an LHRH analog) or a combination of hormonal drugs (such as LHRH and an antiandrogen). Administration of intermittent therapies will depend largely on the patient's ongoing PSA values and the monitoring of prostate cancer symptoms. Once predetermined results are achieved, hormonal therapy is discontinued until there is further evidence of cancer progression.

NEOADJUVANT HORMONAL THERAPY

The aim of neoadjuvant hormonal therapy is to shrink the prostate in order to more effectively perform some other primary treatment. Some surgeons and radiation oncologists use hormonal therapy before employing surgery or radiation therapy. For example, hormonal therapy is sometimes used before surgery to shrink the prostate cancer tumor so it can be removed more effectively. Hormonal therapy may be used before external radiation therapy to shrink the tumor or the prostate itself. It may also be used prior to brachytherapy to shrink the gland for more effective seed placement. Similarly, it may be used prior to cryosurgery (freezing the prostate to cure the cancer) to shrink the gland and make it easier to perform cryosurgery.

Estrogens (hormones that promote female sex characteristics) can also prevent the testicles from producing testosterone. Estrogen therapy is seldom used today in the treatment of prostate cancer because of a host of serious side effects, including effects on potency and sexual characteristics, such as the inducement of "hot flashes." Side effects such as a higher-pitched voice and breast growth are rare.

Other treatments focused on the hormone IGF-I—a biomarker for increased prostate cancer risk—have potential, according to researchers from McGill and Harvard Universities.

FINASTERIDE AND PROSTATE CANCER: THE MAGIC BULLET?

Finasteride is a 5alpha-reductase inhibitor used in hormone therapy to stop the conversion of testosterone to dihydrotestosterone (DHT). It has been effective in the treatment of enlarged prostate. Sold under the brand name Proscar, finasteride is also the active ingredient in Propecia (the well-known hair-growth product).

Finasteride has been found to reduce PSA blood serum levels by about 50 percent within twelve months. Because the PSA blood test

BONE DENSITY AND PROSTATE CANCER TREATMENT

It's not just a female thing: Men also need hormones to maintain bone density. Men who lose androgens are at risk of developing osteoporosis. It is important to prevent the loss of bone during hormone treatment for prostate cancer.

In a small-scale Australian study, researchers observed a dozen men with prostate cancer who were receiving total androgen suppressive treatment. The subjects were also given doses of etidronate, an antiosteoporosis medication used by menopausal women. The men had experienced significant losses in bone mineral density in their spines and hips before receiving the etidronate. After etidronate supplementation, spinal bone density increased in the men by an average of 8 percent, with lesser but still significant increases in the bone density of their hips. Similar results would have to be seen in a much larger scale study to be deemed valid.

In another study, scientists at Massachusetts General Hospital observed forty-seven men with prostate cancer who were treated with the androgen suppressant leuprolide. About half received leuprolide alone; the other half received leuprolide and pamidronate (both etidronate and pamidronate are bisphosphonates, drugs that increase bone density). Subjects receiving leuprolide had a decrease in bone density of 3.3 percent in the spine and 2.1 percent in the hip. Those who also received pamidronate showed no decrease in bone mineral density in either site. According to the study, pamidronate was shown to preserve bone density in men with prostate cancer receiving treatment with leuprolide.

is routinely used as a biomarker to detect prostate cancer, taking finasteride can produce a false negative on the PSA test, and the cancer may go undetected.

Now there may be a much more significant connection between finasteride and prostate cancer. There are rather substantial clinical indications that taking finasteride may actually *prevent* some men from developing prostate cancer.

THE PROSTATE CANCER PREVENTION TRIAL

Because of its exceptionally low level of side effects, finasteride was the first pharmaceutical ever to be tested in a major clinical trial for prevention of prostate cancer. Since prostate cancer is linked to hormonal change, it was posited that finasteride, which lowers DHT levels, might inhibit cancer development.

Starting almost a decade ago, the Prostate Cancer Prevention Trial (PCPT) was organized by the National Cancer Institute. The trial involved 18,000 men who were at least fifty-five years old, and free of any apparent prostate disease. The minimum age limit was fifty-five because older men are much more likely to develop prostate cancer than younger men. Ninety-eight out of every 100 cases of prostate cancer are diagnosed in men fifty-five years of age and over.

Half the subjects were given finasteride and the other half a placebo. Prostate health was closely monitored over the years in order to see if finasteride might have an effect on the development of cancer. None of the men in the trial, or their doctors, knew whether they were taking finasteride or a placebo. This is what is known as a double-blind study.

The two groups of men were compared to see if there was any difference in the rates of prostate cancer development.

In June 2003, the Prostate Cancer Prevention Trial was actually stopped earlier than scheduled (it was originally scheduled to terminate in May 2004) because of a clear finding that finasteride reduced the incidence of prostate cancer. According to results reported in *The New England Journal of Medicine,* subjects who took finasteride reduced their chances of getting prostate cancer by nearly 25 percent compared to men who took a placebo. Finasteride was declared by NCI researchers to be the first drug to reduce the risk of prostate cancer.

There is one very interesting caveat to these findings. Trial participants who did develop prostate cancer experienced a somewhat higher incidence of high-grade tumors. Researchers are continuing to analyze data to find out whether finasteride actually *caused* the higher-grade tumors in these specific subjects. Of concern is that finasteride reduced only the less aggressive hormonally responsive tumors, but not the more aggressive hormonally resistant ones. Of ten men who died from prostate cancer during the study, five were given finasteride and five were given a placebo.

The reduction in prostate cancer risk was seen regardless of age, family history, race/ethnicity, and PSA level at the time of entry into the study.

CHEMOTHERAPY

Chemotherapy is the intravenous injection or oral ingestion of therapeutic drugs to kill cancerous cells. Unfortunately, these same drugs can also damage or kill healthy cells. Chemotherapy has often been reserved for men with advanced prostate cancer who have already tried multiple therapies that have ceased to be effective, such as hormone suppression. It has become a more common treatment with the recent development of oral medications that have fewer side effects than prior chemotherapy regimens.

The side effects depend on the type of drug used, the amount taken, and the length of treatment. Side effects generally associated with chemotherapy include nausea, vomiting, loss of appetite, hair loss, increased susceptibility to infection, mouth sores, fatigue, and tenderness or irritation at the injection site. The patient may have low blood cell counts because chemotherapy can damage the blood-producing cells in bone marrow. This damage can result in an increased chance of infection from a shortage of white blood cells; bleeding or bruising after minor cuts or injuries caused by a shortage of blood platelets; and fatigue resulting from a low red blood cell count.

Most of the side effects disappear once treatment stops, and there are remedies for some side effects. Antiemetic drugs can be used to prevent or reduce nausea and vomiting. Other drugs can be given to boost blood cell counts.

NEW DRUGS IN DEVELOPMENT FOR THE MANAGEMENT OF PROSTATE CANCER

More than a hundred new drugs and vaccines for treating prostate cancer are currently in clinical trial. There are drugs that may choke off the blood supply to prostate tumors, and drugs that may bolster the immune system to attack prostate tumors.

Some of the new drugs on which the most clinical information is currently available include suramin, bicalutamide, and nilutamide. Suramin is in clinical trials for the management of patients with advanced prostate cancer who have failed to respond to standard hormonal therapies. Bicalutamide and nilutamide are antiandrogens believed to have clinical effects similar to those of flutamide. They are already available in some countries. Older pharmaceuticals cur-

CHEMOPREVENTION

We've mentioned Proscar as a drug that blocks the enzyme that converts testosterone into its more toxic form, DHT. That same drug
(generic name finasteride), repackaged in a lower dose and called
Propecia, also fights baldness. The same enzyme that transforms
testosterone in the prostate also resides in the hair follicles of balding men. The DHT that's
formed is toxic to the hair follicles, and that's what leads to male-pattern baldness.

Now finasteride has been found to offer some protection against prostate cancer in a
very large, federally funded study. This makes finasteride only the second drug shown to
reduce the risk for a specific cancer. The other cancer preventive is tamoxifen, which many
high-risk women take to protect themselves against breast cancer and which, despite some
risks, has been approved for that use by the Food and Drug Administration.

However, finasteride may encourage the growth of more aggressive tumors, although
it's possible that the drug only makes cancers look more aggressive than they really are.
Another possibility is that the drug prevents primarily the less aggressive cancers, and so
only the aggressive, more likely to metastasize, tumors are the ones that grow (and those
are the ones that eventually kill patients). Still unanswered is the effect, if any, on cancer
survival.

An editorial in *The New England Journal of Medicine* said it was too soon to recommend men be put on finasteride solely in an attempt to prevent prostate cancer. Still, men
with strong risk factors for prostate cancer may want to discuss it with their doctor.

rently used to treat other conditions are being tested for their potential value in the treatment of prostate cancer. One example is mitox-
antrone. A recent study even indicated that an aspirin a day might
help delay the progression of prostate cancer.

COX-2 inhibitors with brand names such as Vioxx and Celebrex
are drugs given for arthritis relief. The COX-2 enzyme is needed at
several junctures in the cycle for a normal prostate cell to develop
into a cancer cell, and then a cell that metastasizes. A study reports
that COX-2 inhibitors decrease cancer risk in patients with colon
polyps. There are now studies testing COX-2 inhibitors as a possible
cancer preventive method for men with elevated PSA.

Other nonsteroidal anti-inflammatory drugs (NSAIDs) such as aspirin and ibuprofen (Advil, Motrin) also inhibit the COX-2 enzyme.
In fact, the cancer protective effect of these drugs was originally ob-

ARSENIC: A PROSTATE CANCER FIGHTER?

Arsenic as a treatment for prostate cancer? Stranger things have happened.

Researchers at Montefiore Medical Center tested fifteen prostate cancer patients with arsenic trioxide therapy. The men had already failed to respond to hormone treatment, and some of the fifteen had unsuccessfully tried radiation therapy and chemotherapy.

Two patients showed a promising response, and another experienced a significant fall in PSA level following the arsenic treatment. Arsenic treatment also showing promising results in another trial involving patients with recurrent leukemia.

Stay tuned on this one. They may be onto something!

served in people who took a lot of aspirin. The difference in these older NSAIDs is that they also inhibit the COX-1 enzyme, which is protective of the stomach lining. Thus, while COX-1 inhibitors may be just as effective in protecting against cancer as the newer COX-2 inhibitors, they may also be more likely to cause stomach upset and bleeding.

ON THE HORIZON: THE PROSTATE CANCER VACCINE

Prostate cancer vaccines are largely unproven and currently available only in clinical trials. However, there are some very interesting experimental prostate cancer vaccines in development.

Researchers at the University of Illinois at Chicago have tested a vaccine for prostate cancer. This vaccine attempts to activate the immune system in targeted fashion, attacking only prostate cancer cells, in order to recognize and destroy cells that are expressing high PSA levels.

Researchers at Duke University removed immune cells from cancer patients, sensitized these cells to the cancer, then reinjected the cells into the patients' bloodstream. The reinjected cells activated other immune cells to attack only the cancerous cells.

A vaccine designed to stimulate immune response against prostate cancer showed promising results in some patients with advanced instances of the disease, according to a study published in the

Journal of Clinical Oncology. The vaccine was prepared by mixing a genetically engineered protein with the patient's own dendritic cells (cells that play a role in the body's immune response). Thirty-one patients with advanced prostate cancer who were not responsive to hormonal or other treatments developed a strong immune response to prostatic acid phosphatase (PAP), a protein on the surface of prostate cells. Side effects included mild urinary complaints, fever, and fatigue. The study did not encompass long-term consequences of the vaccine, if any.

Prostate-specific membrane antigen, or PSMA, is an antigen found on prostate cancer cells. Injection of dendritic cells combined with PSMA may induce a cellular immune response in prostate cancer patients. Or dendritic cell vaccine therapy may have a synergistic effect when combined with other therapies. Not all subjects in a recent clinical trial responded to the vaccine, but some were observed to have a reduction in localized and distant metastases, and a drop in PSA levels.

Researchers at the Johns Hopkins Oncology Center developed a vaccine using a genetically engineered virus that was reportedly successful in attacking prostate cancer cells. The virus vaccine was given to patients whose cancers had continued to grow even after their prostates had been removed. Scientists took cancer cells from the patients' own tumors and grew them in the lab. Then they used a virus to insert an additional gene (which causes the immune system to attack tumors) into the DNA of the cancer cells. Within a month, the researchers saw signs that anticancer immune cells were circulating in the blood. The study could not confirm that the vaccine could improve prostate cancer survival.

Another virus vaccine was developed by clinical researchers at the University of Iowa Hospitals and Clinics, based on a similar idea, namely that activation of the immune response to prostate-associated antigens will initiate an antitumor response capable of destroying existing prostate cancer cells.

Indiana University Cancer Center investigated a vaccine for treating metastasized prostate cancer. Variant vaccines were tested: One used the vaccinia virus—a relatively harmless virus found in smallpox vaccines—and the second used fowlpox vaccine.

Other prostate cancer vaccines in clinical trial include genetically modified viruses containing prostate-specific antigen (PSA). The pa-

CANCER VACCINES: INSPIRING HOPE FOR THE FUTURE

The reason cancer vaccines are so potentially exciting is that if they work, they could prove to be the ideal cancer therapy. The concept is for the most part not to *prevent* cancer (although there are some vaccines that are attempting that) but rather to get the body's own immune system to fight the cancer off.

By stimulating the immune system so that it recognizes the cancer cells are aberrant and don't belong in the body, the same cells that kill off invading bacteria and viruses would attack and destroy tumor cells.

Theoretically, this would happen with few side effects, such as destroying normal cells, because of the immune system's specificity. So far, there have been some promising prostate cancer vaccine results.

tient is infected with the modified virus. Ideally, his immune system responds to the virus and becomes sensitized to cancer cells containing PSA, destroying these cells.

BIOLOGICAL THERAPY

Biological therapy (also called biotherapy and immunotherapy) is a treatment designed to stimulate or restore the immune system's ability to fight infection and disease.

Biological therapy uses substances called biological response modifiers (BRMs). The body normally produces these substances in small amounts in response to infection and disease. Using advanced laboratory techniques, scientists can produce BRMs in large amounts for the treatment of cancer and other diseases. Biological therapy agents include monoclonal antibodies, interferon, interleukin-2 (IL-2), and CSF, GM-CSF, and G-CSF factors.

GENE THERAPY: THE FUTURE OF PROSTATE CANCER TREATMENT?

Despite the high prevalence of prostate cancer, little is known about the genetic predisposition of some men to the disease. However, that situation is changing even as you read these words. Six possible sites for prostate cancer genes have been identified on the human genome.

Not only has the Human Genome Project provided basic information about the human genome, it has refined the techniques available to scientists who study genetics. Many of these techniques are applicable to prostate cancer cell research.

DNA is the molecule that carries the instructions for nearly everything our cells do. Some people develop certain types of cancer because of inherited or acquired DNA mutations. Scientists have made great progress in recent years understanding how certain changes in DNA can cause normal prostate cells to grow abnormally and become cancerous.

Scientists have observed that genetic abnormalities increase as a man's cancer progresses. Genetic mutations in the primary tumor are carried on by the metastatic tumors that arise from it. Mutant cell genes contain "instructions" for allowing abnormal cell growth and division.

Genes that direct cell growth and division are called oncogenes. Genes that suppress cell growth or proliferation are called, logically enough, tumor suppressor genes. Cancers can be caused by DNA mutations that activate oncogenes or deactivate tumor suppressor genes. Scientists have identified the p53 tumor suppressor gene, which codes for proteins involved in the cell cycle.

Genetic profiling of prostate cancer patients will offer opportunities to tailor treatments most likely to be effective for men with particular genetic profiles.

Genes that appear to be responsible for a man's inherited tendency to develop prostate cancer include:

- **HPC1** (hereditary prostate cancer gene 1). There is a susceptibility "spot" for prostate cancer on chromosome 1, called HPC1. The next step will be to clone this hereditary prostate cancer gene. Once researchers map the sequence, they will be able to search databases to compare the HPC1 gene product to previously characterized proteins from humans and other animals. This should provide strong clues as to how HPC1 functions in the cell.
- **HPC2** (also known as ELAC2).
- **HPCX** This is connected to cancers of the prostate and brain.

- **EMSP1** This may play a role in the tendency of prostate cancer to spread to the bone.

Many scientists consider the prostate gland an ideal candidate for gene therapy. The number of clinical trials utilizing gene therapy methods for prostate cancer is increasing rapidly. Current prostate cancer gene treatment strategies include immunotherapy and corrective approaches (replacement of deleted or mutated genes).

Gene therapy as a treatment approach for prostate cancer needs to address three major issues:

- Deciding what genes to insert
- Deciding how to deliver those genes
- Ensuring that the therapeutic genes will actually be "expressed" at the site of cancer

CYTOREDUCTIVE GENE THERAPY AND CORRECTIVE GENE THERAPY

Cytoreductive gene therapy seeks to directly destroy malignant cells with toxic genes, or to bolster genes that stimulate immune response in order to indirectly destroy malignant cells. Corrective gene therapy replaces or inactivates defective genes with tumor suppressor genes. Vectors are the "UPS trucks" that deliver and insert cloned or engineered DNA or RNA sequences into the target cells. Vectors are categorized as viral and nonviral. Nonviral vectors offer advantages with respect to safety and ease of production. Viral vectors promote stable integration and a steady level of therapeutic expression.

PROSTATE CANCER AND GENETIC RISK

Studying identical and nonidentical twins is an interesting way to separate genetic factors from environmental factors when looking at disease development.

Identical twins have the exact same genes; nonidentical twins have about half the same genes. If a given disease were caused by purely genetic factors, it would seem only reasonable that identical twins would develop the same disease, in the same part of the body, at around the same time in their lives, assuming similar exposure to environmental triggers. For example, if prostate cancer were a purely genetic disease, identical twins would develop it at much the same time and to much the same degree.

QUEST FOR THE TEST: PROTEIN PCa-24—SUCCESSOR TO THE PSA?

Proteins provide the structure and functional framework for cellular life. Proteins are complex organic compounds required for the structure, function, and regulation of the body's cells, tissues, and organs. Each protein has unique functions. In effect, protein interaction provides a definition of an individual's state of wellness or disease.

Has a new protein marker for prostate cancer been identified? It's possible, according to a study published in the medical journal *Cancer*. A cellular protein, identified as PCa-24 and unique to prostate cancer cells, has been discovered by a Harvard research team using proteomics—the branch of genetics that studies all proteins produced by a cell. PCa-24 could lead to a screening test that clearly distinguishes between prostate cancer and benign prostatic hyperplasia without a biopsy.

The Harvard team stated that PCa-24 did not exist in any of the noncancerous tissue (normal prostate cells nor cells of BPH specimens), but it was present in sixteen of the seventeen cancerous tissues (94 percent of the epithelial cells from prostate cancer). While blood tests of live human patients have just begun and scientists know relatively little about PCa-24 except for its size, so far the protein seems to predict cancer with impressive accuracy. If this biomarker is as promising as it seems, a blood test could be commercially available within as little as four years.

Proteomics is the next phase in the complex process of understanding cellular biochemistry and the mechanisms of disease. The main tool for proteomics research is called a mass spectrometer. These machines have been around for years, but better software has dramatically improved their capabilities, allowing them to screen thousands of blood samples quickly and accurately.

At the Clinical Proteomics Program, a joint effort of the National Cancer Institute and the Food and Drug Administration, instead of looking for single proteins that could indicate the presence of cancer, researchers are examining hundreds and even thousands of proteins in the body, training a powerful computer to find subtle patterns that indicate cancer.

The Bioinformatics Unit of the Institute for Cancer Prevention, headed by N. K. Narayanan, Ph.D., is using cutting-edge research disciplines such as molecular biology and genomics with the hope that they may have a major impact on the way diseases are diagnosed, prevented, treated, and managed.

Seeking to unlock the genetic connection of various cancer types, researchers from the Karolinska Institute in Sweden studied more than 44,000 pairs of identical twins from Denmark, Finland, and Sweden. The findings of this large-scale study were published in *The New England Journal of Medicine*.

274 THE PROSTATE HEALTH PROGRAM

IL-2 GENE THERAPY

According to a report in the journal *Human Gene Therapy*, researchers at UCLA's Jonsson Cancer Center have shown that gene-derived immunotherapy may be a powerful weapon against locally advanced prostate cancer.

Using an ultrasound guidance system, a gene expressing interleukin 2 (IL-2) was injected directly into the prostate. IL-2 is a hormonelike substance that stimulates the immune system to form killer cells called lymphocytes.

More than half the patients showed reduced PSA levels as a result of the therapy. The study proved for the first time that IL-2 is active against prostate cancer. It was even hoped that this therapy might eventually eliminate the need for radical prostatectomy.

More than 10,000 cancers were discovered within the study group. Researchers found that if one identical twin developed cancer, the odds of the other twin developing the same cancer were less than 15 percent. Based on their findings, environmental factors were seen to have a greater influence overall on cancer incidence than genetic factors. However, among all the cancers, prostate cancer was seen to have the most substantial genetic connection.

According to the research, cancers that seem to be most influenced by genetics are:

Prostate cancer: 42 percent
Colorectal cancer: 35 percent
Stomach cancer: 28 percent
Breast cancer: 27 percent
Lung cancer: 26 percent

While the estimated genetic contribution for prostate cancer seems high, the study remains an interesting one. This is especially true when you consider that some day scientists will likely be able to determine the exact genetic contribution to prostate cancer, as well as to all other cancers.

GENETIC FINGERPRINTING

The critical question is, How do we tell which prostate cancer is the somnolent, slow-growing one and which is the one that will grow, spread and become life-threatening? That is an area of intense research, primarily by looking at the genetic "fingerprint" of the prostate tumor.

Researchers have extracted the DNA and proteins from prostate cancers and layered them onto "gene chips" about the size of a large postage stamp. Even at that small size, the chip contains hundreds of thousands of sites where the tumor materials can bind with fluorescent markers. A sensitive machine reads the intensity of light coming from the fluorescent markers, indicating the presence and quantity of each of the many compounds in the tumor.

A computer analyzes the result. It's not the level of any *one* compound that tells the story; it's the *pattern* of the *thousands* of tumor compounds that may be predictive of the cancer's aggressiveness.

While it's still too early to use genetic fingerprinting as a routine clinical tool, it does appear that soon we will have a way of characterizing prostate, as well as other cancers, to determine their aggressiveness, their likelihood of spreading, and even which treatments will be most effective.

SURGERY

RADICAL PROSTATECTOMY

The aim of radical prostatectomy—removal of the prostate gland (as well as the capsule surrounding it, and the seminal vesicles)—is to cure the cancer by removing all cancer-affected tissue from the body. Radical prostatectomy is usually recommended for men under seventy who have localized prostate cancer and no other major health problems.

There is a distinct risk of nerve damage in surgery—albeit a less prevalent risk in this era of "nerve-sparing" procedures—that might leave the patient incontinent (especially in the short term), impotent, or both.

The simple truth is that prostate surgery can cause a lot of problems. And the majority of prostate cancer patients live for a number of years whether they have surgery or not. In fact, some researchers believe surgery does not change long-term survival odds all that much.

Here's what usually happens: Under anesthetic, an incision is made in the lower abdomen. Lymph nodes close to the prostate are removed and are examined by a pathologist. If the lymph nodes are cancerous, the operation will be stopped, because it is clear that the cancer has already spread from the prostate, and just removing the prostate doesn't address or impact those "escaped" cells: a localized cure is no longer possible. If no cancer is detected in the lymph nodes, the operation will in all likelihood proceed.

Modern, innovative nerve-sparing operations have the advantage of minimizing damage to the nerves that assist with erection. Such

SIDE EFFECTS AND COMPLICATIONS OF RADICAL PROSTATECTOMY: IS IT WORTH IT?

As with any major surgery, radical prostatectomy has its share of complications and side effects—perhaps more than its share:

- **Impotence.** If the nerves surrounding the prostate are damaged—less likely these days—erectile dysfunction will result.
- **Dry orgasms.** These are orgasms unaccompanied by ejaculate. Two structures responsible for much of the fluid in ejaculate—the prostate and the seminal vesicles—are removed in radical prostatectomy. The vas deferens (the tube which transports sperm from the testicles) is also disrupted.
- **Incontinence.** Injury to nerves and surgical impact on the urethra can result in temporary and (more rarely) permanent incontinence.
- **Excessive hemorrhaging.** The prostate gland is surrounded by a dense complex of blood vessels. Significant blood loss is a possibility; blood transfusions may be necessary.
- **Partial bladder neck obstruction.** Scar tissue forms when the urethral stump is sutured to the bladder neck, sometimes causing difficulty in urinating.
- **Infection.** Infection is a consideration in any major operation.
- **Rectal tears.** Again, consider the close proximity of the rectum to the prostate gland. A colostomy may be necessary while the rectum heals.
- **Blood clots.** These may develop in the legs or in deep pelvic veins (deep venous thrombosis). The clot may break loose and travel to the lungs (pulmonary embolism), causing breathing difficulty or, if the clot is large, sudden death.

operations greatly reduce the risk of impotence and incontinence. Even in a worst-case scenario, nerve-sparing surgery significantly increases the likelihood that impotence and incontinence will only be temporary.

Once the prostate is removed, the urethra is joined to the bladder to ensure proper urine flow. A catheter (a narrow tube held in place by a small balloon in the bladder) drains urine so that the joined area can have time to heal. The patient is in the hospital for about four to seven days; the catheter is generally removed after one to three weeks. Most men return to work four to six weeks following surgery.

LAPAROSCOPIC RADICAL PROSTATECTOMY (LRP)

Laparoscopic radical prostatectomy is touted to have benefits over conventional radical prostatectomy. The most obvious difference between LRP and "open" radical prostatectomy is that only small abdominal incisions are involved, as opposed to one large one. A voice-controlled surgical robot is sometimes used to hold the laparoscope (a long fiber-optic tube with a magnifying lens, attached to a camera). The laparoscope is inserted through a small incision along with specially designed instruments that are also inserted into small incisions to cut out and remove the prostate.

LRP produces a reduced level of discomfort and pain. The elimination of major incisions and incisional pain also improves and speeds postoperative function, lessening the amount of time spent in the hospital and the time the catheter has to stay in. LRP also reduces blood loss, offers improved visualization of the patient's anatomy, and presents less trauma to the body. A claimed reduction in complications such as impotence and incontinence has yet to be proven.

RADICAL RETROPUBIC PROSTATECTOMY
(RETROPUBIC SURGERY)

This is the classic or standard operation. The surgeon removes the prostate and nearby lymph nodes through an incision in the abdomen that starts just below the umbilicus and continues down to the pubic bone. The patient's bowel is retracted up and to the side to expose the lymph nodes in the drainage area of the prostate. The lymph nodes are removed and studied by a pathologist if the cancer is aggressive with a high likelihood of nodal disease. If cancer is found in the nodes, the prostate will not be removed.

RADICAL PERINEAL PROSTATECTOMY

The patient lies on his back with his legs in stirrups (similar to the ones in a gynecologist's office) that place them over and behind the body. The prostate gland is gradually separated from the rectum, bladder, urethra, and vas deferens through an incision between the scrotum and the anus (the area known as the perineum). The seminal vesicles are removed along with the prostate.

The vas deferens is divided and tied off. The bladder is reconnected to the urethra. While the patient is still under anesthesia, a Foley catheter—a hollow, flexible tube used to drain urine—is inserted into the penis, through the urethra, and into the bladder. The catheter is left in place for two to three weeks, or until the bladder-urethra connection heals.

TRANSURETHRAL RESECTION OF THE PROSTATE (TURP)

TURP is a common procedure for men with *noncancerous* enlargement of the prostate gland. Prostate cancer is sometimes discovered during a TURP procedure for BPH.

In some cases, transurethral resection is also used as a palliative option for elderly prostate cancer sufferers who are also experiencing other serious diseases. It is less invasive and less traumatic than radical prostatectomy, recovery time is shorter, and the side effects are much less substantial.

However, there is an all-important proviso: TURP is intended to relieve the *symptoms* caused by a cancer tumor, primarily to remove cancerous tissue that blocks urine flow. Unlike radical prostatectomy, *its goal is not to cure or eliminate the cancer.*

With TURP, the doctor removes only part of the prostate. An instrument called a resectoscope is inserted into the penis through the urethra. Tissue is cut from the prostate by electricity passing through a small wire loop on the end of the resectoscope.

A TURP operation takes about an hour, with a typical hospital stay of a day or two. A catheter is inserted after surgery for an average of two or three days to facilitate urination.

PELVIC LYMPHADENECTOMY

An exploratory procedure to remove lymph nodes in the pelvis to see if they contain cancer. If the lymph nodes do contain cancer, the doctor will not remove the prostate, and will recommend other, non-localized treatment, possibly hormonal therapy.

CRYOTHERAPY

This is also known as cryosurgery and cryoablation. To a large degree, the jury is still out on the effectiveness of this alternative to conventional surgery and radiation therapy. Recent data indicates its effectiveness. It seems to be comparable to radiation therapy in its cancer cure ratio. The new generation cryosurgical machines have good side-effect profiles. Clinical trials comparing cryotherapy's success rate and side effects to those of other forms of therapy—surgical, hormonal, chemopreventive—conducted in a randomized, controlled manner will help answer vital questions about this therapy. And it's not just cryotherapy as an isolated treatment that's being studied. For example, a clinical trial is in progress to study the effect of cryotherapy combined with radiation on recurrent cancer.

The cryosurgeon tries to avoid damaging healthy tissue by placing probes, known as cryoprobes, in direct contact with the prostate cancer tumor in order to freeze it. These probes are inserted into the prostate under ultrasound control. Liquid nitrogen or, more recently, argon gas is then passed through the probe.

Proponents of cryotherapy claim there are fewer complications than with prostatectomy. Some researchers dispute this claim. Impotence following cryotherapy reportedly occurs more often than it does after radical prostatectomy. Extreme cold destroys the cancer cells, but it may freeze and damage nerves and healthy tissue near the prostate, causing impotence.

There are other complications. Freezing may damage the bladder and the intestines, leading to pain, a very uncomfortable burning sensation, and a persistent need to empty the bladder and bowels (most men reportedly do eventually recover normal bowel and bladder function). A fistula (abnormal opening) between the rectum and bladder develops in about 2 percent of men after cryosurgery, possibly requiring surgical repair. About 50 percent of men notice a temporary swelling of their penis and scrotum, usually lasting for a few weeks.

TREATING THE COMPLICATIONS OF PROSTATE CANCER

BOWEL DISORDERS

Bowel disorders are a moderately common result of radiation treatment for prostate cancer. Up to 20 percent of men who receive external beam radiation therapy for prostate cancer experience gastrointestinal problems that can include constipation, blood in the stool, diarrhea, cramps, or urgency to have a bowel movement. Diarrhea and constipation are also side effects of certain medications.

For diarrhea, follow the Prostate Health Pyramid dietary recommendations, being careful to eliminate as much fat from your diet as you can.

For constipation and gas, probiotics, buckthorn, Beano, epsom salts, and senna may help. Ask your physician about specific remedies he recommends for you.

A simple walking regimen can be a very effective ally against constipation (as well as fatigue).

FATIGUE AND WEAKNESS

Fatigue is a common side effect of prostate cancer treatment—whether radiation therapy, chemotherapy, or surgery. Most symptoms of fatigue will stop soon after treatment ends, although in some cases fatigue will persist for quite some time.

Physical activity and other strength-building techniques (see Chapter 8) can help combat fatigue, but don't forget to get enough rest. Even healthy individuals often fail to get sufficient rest. Learn to pace yourself and plan your activities to conserve energy.

Lower red blood cell count is a common side effect of chemotherapy. This will lead to fatigue. Ask your physician to recommend drugs that will boost your red blood cell count.

NAUSEA

Antiemetic drugs are effective against the nausea and vomiting caused by chemotherapy.

Stick to a bland diet if you experience considerable nausea for a prolonged period. Try eating more slowly; eat several smaller meals throughout the day.

Fresh ginger and caraway seed (brewed in a tea) are effective folk remedies for nausea. You might also want to try licorice tea, arrowroot, or kudzu.

Acupuncture can be used to offset nausea as well as pain.

RELIEVING AND TREATING PAIN

Prostate cancer may cause pain in its more advanced stages. Since quality of life is an important issue, the patient will want to seek out the best pain relief possible, with minimal side effects.

Pain can result from the cancer itself (for example, when a tumor causes pressure on organs, nerves, or bones), or it can derive from cancer treatment (such as discomfort after a radical prostatectomy). Given the medicines, treatments, and technologies available, even advanced prostate cancer pain is usually manageable.

BISPHOSPHONATES TO COMBAT BONE PAIN

Bisphosphonates (BPNs) are used to treat osteoporosis, or thinning of bone. They are also used to treat hypercalcemia (elevated calcium blood levels), a complication of breast and other cancers. Other trials are investigating whether bisphosphonates (specifically clodronate) can slow the development of metastatic cancer in bone.

When prostate cancer spreads to bone, it weakens the bone and causes substantial pain. Bone fractures become much more likely. Researchers are testing the efficacy of bisphosphonates to relieve pain caused by prostate cancer that has spread to bone. There is even some clinical indication that bisphosphonates may slow the growth of prostate cancer.

Bisphosphonates do, however, have certain side effects. Ibandronate has been found to cause nausea and diarrhea. Zoledronic acid (Zometa) can cause fatigue, muscle aches, swelling in the feet and legs, and anemia.

PAIN MEDICATIONS

Medicines that relieve pain are called analgesics. Analgesics act on the nervous system and elsewhere to provide temporary relief. Nonprescription (over-the-counter) pain relievers include aspirin, acetaminophen, and ibuprofen. Aspirin and ibuprofen are types of nonsteroidal anti-inflammatories (NSAIDs).

Opioids are the most widely used prescription pain relievers and may be prescribed in ways that relieve pain while minimizing side effects such as drowsiness and risk of addiction. These include codeine, hydromorphone, methadone, and morphine.

Stronger nonsteroidal anti-inflammatory drugs (NSAIDs) are another group of prescription pain relievers, including Naprosyn, Nalfon, and Trilisate. These are useful for moderate to severe pain and may be especially helpful in treating cancer that has spread to the bone.

Advanced prostate cancer patients are treated with any number of chemotherapeutic drugs, which do not cure the disease, but do ease the pain and other symptoms. The toxicity or side effects of chemotherapeutic agents, as balanced against the potential pain-relieving benefits, must always be considered.

BLOCKING NERVE PATHWAYS

When certain substances are injected into or around a nerve, that nerve is no longer able to transmit pain. Numbness in the area of the nerve distribution and loss of feeling is the result of a nerve block. Patients are more likely to sustain injury to the area because they no longer have the protective reflexes of pain, pressure and temperature.

A local anesthetic, which may be combined with cortisone, provides temporary pain relief. For longer-lasting pain relief, phenol or alcohol can be injected to actually destroy the nerves carrying pain signals.

Neurological interventions are nerve blocks where surgery is performed to implant devices that deliver drugs to block nerves.

ELECTRICAL NERVE STIMULATION

A transcutaneous electric nerve stimulation (TENS) unit applies a mild electrical current to selected areas of the skin via a small power pack connected to two electrodes. These subtle impulses appear to intercept or "confuse" pain messages. The pain relief reportedly lasts even after the current is shut off.

RADIOTHERAPY AND STRONTIUM THERAPY TO RELIEVE BONE PAIN

Radiotherapy may be effective in relieving bone pain associated with prostate cancer. Local or whole body radiation therapy may increase the effectiveness of pain medication and other noninvasive therapies by reducing tumor size. A single injection of a radioactive agent may relieve pain when cancer has spread extensively to bone.

Strontium is injected into the bloodstream to help control bone pain in patients with advanced metastatic prostate cancer that no longer responds to hormonal therapy. Strontium is incorporated into bone, where it delivers radiation. Injection of strontium can also be combined with external beam radiation therapy.

SURGERY FOR PAIN RELIEF

Surgery may be used in a palliative manner rather than in a curative way. This could include removal of all or part of a tumor when the cancer has already metastasized, in order to reduce pain, or to relieve the symptoms of obstruction or compression caused by the tumor.

Surgery may also be used to destroy a nerve or nerves that are part of the pain pathway. A neurosurgeon may cut a nerve close to the spinal cord (rhizotomy) or bundles of nerves in the spinal cord itself (cordotomy).

THE INTERVENTIONAL MRI: AN MRI THAT HELPS DELIVER ANESTHESIA

Scientists from Stanford University Medical School have developed a type of magnetic resonance imaging (MRI) that guides regional anesthesia more accurately. The physician can observe the precise trajectory and depth of the needle to monitor exact distribution of pain medication.

The interventional MRI (iMRI) design resembles an open magnet. The physician and the radiologist stand between the two "magnet prongs," on either side of the patient. The procedure takes from forty-five minutes to two-plus hours. Pain relief reportedly lasts anywhere from weeks to months. The iMRI unit permits physicians to target needles and catheters in regions that were hitherto inaccessible.

THE INSTITUTE FOR CANCER PREVENTION'S PROSTATE CANCER SYMPTOM AND TREATMENT CHARTS

These charts will give you the Institute for Cancer Prevention recommendations and options for treating prostate cancer. They will help you become a more informed and interactive partner with your physician in the treatment decision process. *Please note that there is no current consensus on prostate cancer treatment.* Some physicians and other medical institutions may have different recommendations.

Guidelines should not be confused with professional medical advice. This treatment chart is not meant to suggest a specific course of action to replace a personal consultation with your primary care physician. It will help you develop questions to ask your physician and familiarize you with possible treatment strategies. You should discuss the full range of treatment options with your physician, coming to an informed decision only as a result of this consultation. You might want to consider a consultation with another doctor as well. Whatever decision you come to, be sure to inform your doctor of any and all treatments and medications you are taking.

The Institute for Cancer Prevention has found the choices recommended in this treatment chart to be effective options for many patients. They take into consideration specific risk factors such as age, overall health, and grade and stage of the cancer. The stage of the cancer has an especially strong influence on recommended course of treatment.

SYMPTOMS OF PROSTATE CANCER AND OTHER PROSTATE CONDITIONS

Prostate cancer usually does not exhibit overt symptoms in its early stage. When symptoms finally do become apparent, the cancer is often at an intermediate to advanced stage.

In these stages, prostate cancer often exhibits symptoms similar to those of benign enlargement. These symptoms include difficulty urinating, weak or interrupted urine stream, and frequent urination. If you exhibit any of these symptoms, have a DRE and a PSA blood test.

Many prostate symptoms are the result of benign conditions such as benign prostatic hyperplasia (BPH, enlarged prostate), prostatitis or prostatodynia (see Chapters 10 through 12). Contact your primary care physician if you exhibit any of the symptoms listed below. Even if these symptoms are not indicative of prostate cancer, they do indicate that something may be wrong with your prostate or your lower urinary tract.

	Symptom Diagnosis	**More Information**
Do you feel the need to urinate frequently? NO YES ➤	Not an indicator of prostate cancer (although it may be a red flag). May not be related to a prostate problem at all, although is a common symptom of enlarged prostate, prostatitis, or prostatodynia. Frequent urination may also stem from a lower urinary tract condition or from other conditions, such as diabetes.	Chapter 2, pp. 22–23; Chapter 3, pp. 35–36; Chapter 10, pp. 185–187; Chapter 11, pp. 199–204; Chapter 12, pp. 223–224; Chapter 13, pp. 249–252
Do you ever wake up two or more times during the night to urinate? NO YES ➤	Common symptom of an enlarged prostate.	Chapter 3, pp. 35–36; Chapter 12, pp. 199–204

(continued on next page)

Symptom Diagnosis **More Information**

**Do you ever
get the feeling
that your bladder
is not completely
empty even
though you've
finished urinating?**

Chapter 2, pp. 22–23;
Chapter 3, pp. 35–36;

NO   YES ━━━▶ May indicate an enlarged prostate.   Chapter 11, pp. 199–204

**Do you have a
sensation that your
bladder is full, even
though you may not
urinate?**

May be a symptom of BPH,

NO   YES ━━━▶ prostatitis, or prostatodynia.   Chapters 10, 11, 12

**Do you often
experience dribbling
after urinating?**

Chapter 2, pp. 22–23;

NO   YES ━━━▶ Probably a symptom of BPH.   Chapter 11

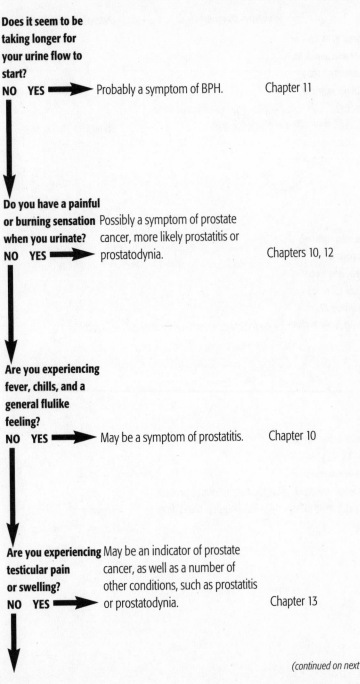

Does it seem to be taking longer for your urine flow to start?

NO   YES ➡️ Probably a symptom of BPH.   Chapter 11

Do you have a painful or burning sensation when you urinate?

NO   YES ➡️ Possibly a symptom of prostate cancer, more likely prostatitis or prostatodynia.   Chapters 10, 12

Are you experiencing fever, chills, and a general flulike feeling?

NO   YES ➡️ May be a symptom of prostatitis.   Chapter 10

Are you experiencing testicular pain or swelling?

NO   YES ➡️ May be an indicator of prostate cancer, as well as a number of other conditions, such as prostatitis or prostatodynia.   Chapter 13

(continued on next page)

	Symptom Diagnosis	**More Information**

**Do you ever feel a
sudden urgency to
urinate that may
come on without
warning?**
NO   YES ➡ May be a symptom of BPH or
prostatodynia.   Chapters 11, 12

**Have you noticed
that your urine
stream has become
weaker or more
intermittent?**
NO   YES ➡ Likely indicates an enlarged prostate.   Chapter 11

**Is there a discharge
at the tip of your
penis emanating
from your urethra?**   May be a symptom of prostatitis
NO   YES ➡ or a sexually transmitted disease.   Chapter 10

**Are you experiencing
painful ejaculation?**   May be a symptom of prostatitis,
NO   YES ━━▶   prostatodynia, or prostate cancer.   Chapters 10, 11, 13

**Are you experiencing   While this could be a symptom of
marked incontinence?**   prostate cancer, it may be due to
NO   YES ━━▶   any number of other factors.   Chapters 9, 13

**Are you experiencing   A common side effect of prostate
erectile dysfunction   cancer, and a symptom of the
(impotence)?**   advanced disease, as well as of   · Chapter 9, pp. 169–176;
NO   YES ━━▶   prostate conditions such as   Chapter 10,
prostatitis and prostatodynia.   Chapter 12

**Do you have blood   While this could be a symptom of
in your urine?**   prostate cancer, it could be a symptom
NO   YES ━━▶   of prostatitis, a urinary tract infection,
or any number of other things.   Chapters 10, 13

(continued on next page)

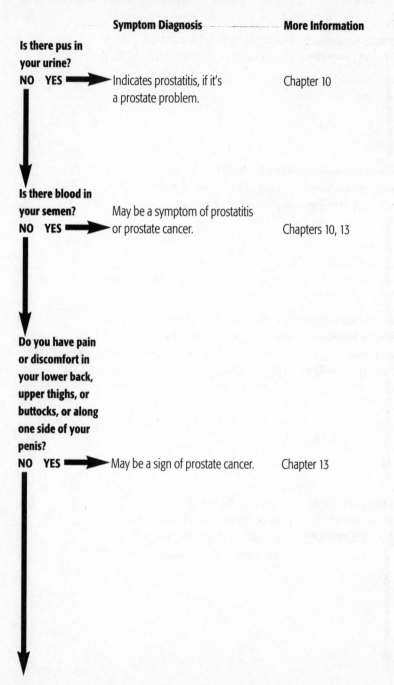

Symptom Diagnosis ——————— **More Information**

Is there pus in
your urine?
NO   YES ➡ Indicates prostatitis, if it's   Chapter 10
          a prostate problem.

Is there blood in
your semen?   May be a symptom of prostatitis
NO   YES ➡ or prostate cancer.   Chapters 10, 13

Do you have pain
or discomfort in
your lower back,
upper thighs, or
buttocks, or along
one side of your
penis?
NO   YES ➡ May be a sign of prostate cancer.   Chapter 13

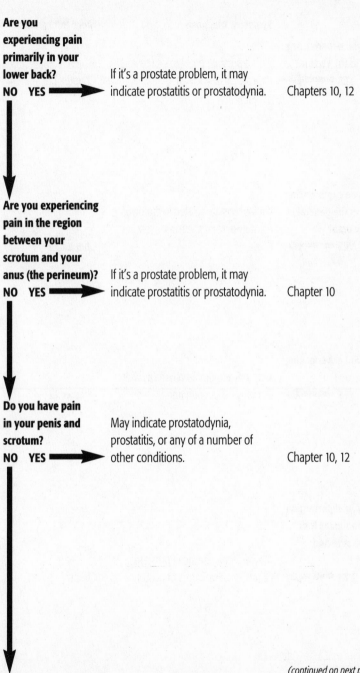

Are you experiencing pain primarily in your lower back?
NO   YES ➡️   If it's a prostate problem, it may indicate prostatitis or prostatodynia.   Chapters 10, 12

Are you experiencing pain in the region between your scrotum and your anus (the perineum)?
NO   YES ➡️   If it's a prostate problem, it may indicate prostatitis or prostatodynia.   Chapter 10

Do you have pain in your penis and scrotum?
NO   YES ➡️   May indicate prostatodynia, prostatitis, or any of a number of other conditions.   Chapter 10, 12

(continued on next page)

	Symptom Diagnosis	More Information

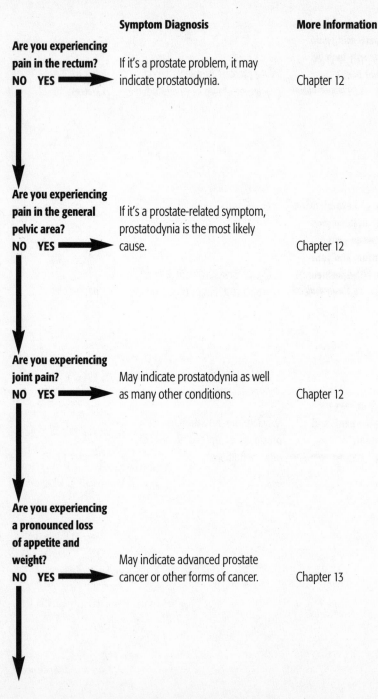

Are you experiencing pain in the rectum?
NO   YES ➤ If it's a prostate problem, it may indicate prostatodynia.   Chapter 12

Are you experiencing pain in the general pelvic area?
NO   YES ➤ If it's a prostate-related symptom, prostatodynia is the most likely cause.   Chapter 12

Are you experiencing joint pain?
NO   YES ➤ May indicate prostatodynia as well as many other conditions.   Chapter 12

Are you experiencing a pronounced loss of appetite and weight?
NO   YES ➤ May indicate advanced prostate cancer or other forms of cancer.   Chapter 13

Is your PSA level elevated?

NO   YES ➡ May stem from any number of factors, but it may be a sign that cancer is present in your prostate gland. Further PSA testing is indicated, and a biopsy may be necessary.

Chapter 1, pp. 10–13;
Chapter 3, pp. 37–40;
Chapter 13, pp. 241–243

⬇

It is not likely that you have prostate cancer, although a false-negative PSA reading is possible, and early-stage prostate cancer does not exhibit symptoms.

WHEN PROSTATE CANCER IS FOUND: TREATMENT OPTIONS BASED ON THE STAGE AND GRADE OF THE CANCER

When you are diagnosed with prostate cancer, your doctor needs to know the stage (extent) of the disease. Cancer stage is determined by a number of factors. These include: size and location of the tumor; whether the cancer is localized or has spread (metastasized); and how far it has spread beyond the prostate. In staging, the letter "T" stands for tumor; "N" stands for lymph nodes; and "M" stands for metastasis.

In Stage I, the tumor is located within the prostate only, exhibits no symptoms, and is too small to be detected by a digital rectal exam (DRE). In Stage II, the tumor is still located only within the prostate, but it is large enough to be felt by a DRE, and some symptoms may be present. Stage III tumors have spread from the prostate into the immediate surrounding area, including the seminal vesicles. In Stage IV, the cancer has spread from the pelvic area to distant parts of the body. Bone pain, weight loss, and fatigue are common symptoms of Stage IV cancers.

See chapter 13 for a further discussion of staging, as well as a detailed analysis of the Gleason grading system.

A combination of therapies is very common in the treatment of prostate cancer. Hormonal therapy, surgery, radiation therapy, and chemotherapy may be combined or employed at different stages of treatment, especially when the cancer is advanced.

In all stages of prostate cancer, the Prostate Health Pyramid, the Transition Diet, and the Healthy Prostate Fitness Regimen can be very helpful as adjunct therapies in managing the disease, meaning you can follow these programs in addition to therapies recommended by your doctor. Lifestyle changes or modifications (for example: stopping smoking, limiting your alcohol intake, or stopping drinking altogether) also fall into the category of adjunct therapies.

Alternative therapies may also be considered for all stages of prostate cancer, with this important proviso: Consult with your physician before employing any alternative therapy. Alternative therapies may even be counterproductive under certain circumstances.

	Treatment Course	More Information
Does your biopsy show atypical cells or PIN (prostatic intraepithelial neoplasia)? **NO YES** ➤	Repeat biopsies; adjunct therapies (diet, exercise, lifestyle).	Chapter 3, pp. 37–40; Chapters 4–8, 14, 16

Have you been diagnosed with Stage I prostate cancer? Tumors are categorized as T1, N0, M0, G1, Stage A.

NO   YES ➤ Watchful waiting; surgery; adjunct therapies (diet, exercise, lifestyle); radiation therapy (external beam radiation or brachytherapy) in some cases.

Chapter 1, pp. 6–13;
Chapter 3;
Chapters 4–8, 14, 16

Have you been diagnosed with Stage II prostate cancer, in which tumors are categorized as T1, N0, M0, G2, 3, or 4?

NO   YES ➤ Watchful waiting; surgery; adjunct therapies (diet, exercise, lifestyle); radiation therapy (external beam radiation or brachytherapy).

Chapter 1, pp. 6–13;
Chapter 3, pp. 37–40;
Chapters 4–8, 13, 14

(continued on next page)

	Treatment Course	**More Information**
Have you been diagnosed with Stage II prostate cancer in which tumors are categorized as T2, N0, M0, any Gleason grade, A2, B1, or B2? NO YES ➡️	Close watchful waiting; surgery; radiation therapy (external beam radiation or brachytherapy); adjunct therapies (diet, exercise, lifestyle).	Chapter 1, pp. 6–13; Chapter 2, pp. 22–23; Chapters 4–8, 13, 14, 16
Have you been diagnosed with Stage III prostate cancer? Tumors are categorized as T3, N0, M0, any G (Stage C). NO YES ➡️	External beam radiotherapy; hormonal treatment (orchiectomy or androgen-suppressing drugs) combined with radiation therapy; hormonal therapy alone; watchful waiting in a very select number of patients; radical prosta-tectomy combined with pelvic lymph-adenectomy; adjunct therapies (diet, exercise, lifestyle); clinical trials using experimental therapies; treatments to relieve urinary tract symptoms and other palliative treatments.	Chapter 1, pp. 6–13; Chapter 2, pp. 22–23; Chapters 13, 14, 16

Have you been diagnosed with Stage IV prostate cancer where the tumor is categorized as T4, N0, M0, any T, N1 through N3, M0, any G (Stage D1, D2)?
NO   YES ➡

Orchiectomy or antiandrogen therapy; LHRH agonists; leuprolide combined with an antiandrogen; radical prostatectomy and orchiectomy; chemotherapy; experimental clinical trials; treatments for urinary tract blockage and other symptoms; treatments for pain, including corticosteroids; radiation therapy for bone metastasis; chemotherapy for palliative effect; adjunct therapies (diet, exercise, lifestyle); alternative therapies in very select cases.

Chapter 1, pp. 6–13; Chapter 2, pp. 22–23; Chapter 14
Chapter 16

Have you been diagnosed with Stage IV prostate cancer, where the tumor is categorized as T, any N, M1, any G (stage D2)?
NO   YES ➡

Orchiectomy alone or with an antiandrogen; leuprolide (or other LHRH agonist); leuprolide and an antiandrogen; chemotherapy; pain relief; treatment for urinary tract symptoms (including transurethral resection); treatment for bone metastasis, including strontium radioisotopes; adjunct therapies (diet, exercise, lifestyle); alternative therapies in very select cases.

Chapter 13, pp. 243–248; Chapter 14

(continued on next page)

	Treatment Course	**More Information**
Have you been diagnosed with recurrent prostate cancer? **NO YES** ➤	Radiation and hormone therapy; adjunct therapies (diet, exercise); clinical trials; prostatectomy or hormonal therapy after radiation treatment has failed; alternative therapies in very select cases.	Chapter 13, pp. 243–248; Chapter 14

15. African Americans and Prostate Cancer

Stopping the Crisis

The four most prevalent cancers among men and women of all racial and ethnic groups are lung/bronchial cancer, prostate cancer, breast cancer, and colorectal cancer. One statistic stands out quite dramatically in the sobering morass of cancer statistics. It is a statistic that has received far too little attention both in the mainstream medical community and in the media—but it can no longer be ignored.

African-American men have the highest prostate cancer rate in the world and the lowest survival rate. According to American Cancer Society statistics, approximately 18,500 African-American men are diagnosed with prostate cancer every year, and about 6,100 a year die from it. African-American males are 1.5 times more likely to develop prostate cancer and 2 to 3 times more likely to die of it than white American males.

Early screening for prostate cancer is much publicized in the majority media these days. Until quite recently, little media attention was targeted specifically at African-American men. This situation is doubly unfortunate, since the difference in the stage of prostate cancer at the time of diagnosis is actually widening between African Americans and white Americans, with African Americans initially diagnosed at a more advanced stage of the disease. Only 66 percent of African-American men diagnosed with prostate cancer survive for five years after the initial diagnosis, compared to 81 percent of white men. The stage at which the cancer is detected is the primary reason for this disparity.

Although black men have substantially higher incidence and mortality rates for prostate cancer than white men, mortality rates for prostate cancer are at an all-time low for both white and black Americans. Among black men, mortality rates were the lowest since those rates were first compiled and recorded in 1969. The record low rate for black men was best reflected in the fifty-to-sixty-nine age group, a prime demographic for incidence of prostate cancer in African-American men.

In order to stop the prostate cancer crisis in the African-American community rather than merely allay it, **there is an urgent need for earlier screening among African-American males.** This is the number one priority in the Institute for Cancer Prevention's ten-step plan to prevent and combat prostate cancer in African-American men. It is the key to stemming the tide of this insidious health crisis.

RACE AND AGE

In every age group, blacks have a higher incidence of prostate cancer than whites. Among younger men—in whom prostate cancer incidence is usually quite low—blacks have a substantially higher occurrence of the disease than whites.

A MORE AGGRESSIVE INCIDENCE OF THE DISEASE

Equally alarming is research showing that men of African descent usually develop a more aggressive form of prostate cancer. This disparity cannot be explained away as the result of inferior treatment. Studies indicate that blacks get a more virulent form of the disease and have a lower survival rate than whites even when there is equal access to good health care. When income and education are on a similar level, African Americans still compare unfavorably to whites on virtually all statistical levels related to the disease.

BLACK MEN AND PROSTATE CANCER: A GRIM PICTURE

- Many African-American men continue to remain unaware even that they are at greater risk of developing prostate cancer than other groups are.
- African Americans are less likely to take advantage of early prostate cancer screening than other men.
- At initial diagnosis, African Americans have higher PSA levels and a higher grade of clinical-stage tumors than other groups.
- African-American men with prostate cancer have a significantly worse prognosis than white men. They are more likely than white men to have metastasized disease, bone pain, less successful recovery, higher PSA levels, and a higher Gleason score.

HOW MUCH DOES RACE HAVE TO DO WITH IT?

Is risk factor number one simply a matter of being of African descent?

It is undeniable that clinical prostate cancer and mortality rates differ sharply by race. The lowest incidence of prostate cancer is for Chinese living in China, followed in ascending order by other Asians, South Americans, Southern Europeans, and Northern Europeans. Overall, men of African origin have the highest rate in the world. Within the United States, African Americans have the highest mortality rate; Asians, Pacific Islanders, and American Indians the lowest. It is important to note that autopsy studies show a similar rate of prostate cancer in all ethnic groups; it is the rate of progression to clinical disease that differs by group.

However, the racial risk factor may not loom quite as large as has been previously suspected—if black men adopt a preventive prostate health program.

SIMILARITIES IN RECURRENT CANCERS
AMONG BLACKS AND WHITES

A study in *The Journal of Urology* examined whether African-American men had a worse prognosis for prostate cancer after recurrence than white men. Researchers reviewed the medical records of 955 men who underwent surgery for localized prostate cancer. In all,

127 Caucasian men and 37 African Americans experienced cancer recurrence.

Researchers tested prostate-specific antigen velocity for this subgroup. PSA velocity measures the rate of protein level increase. The higher the velocity, the more rapid the increase in prostate cancer. When analyzed in terms of race, researchers found no difference in PSA velocity between blacks and whites with recurrent prostate cancer. The results of the study suggest that the reason for the higher incidence in and mortality of prostate cancer among African Americans may be due not to a discrepancy in the tumor growth rate between blacks and whites but to other factors, some of which may be modifiable.

The primary question remains unanswered: Is prostate cancer in African Americans simply more aggressive by nature?

A recent study provides a clue or two. Studying medical records from military health facilities, researchers were able to track trends in prostate cancer care in 797 patients from 1988 to 1999. In the group studied, 587 patients were white; 195 were African-American.

Pronounced improvements in findings for African-American men were evident over the passage of time. PSA levels at the time of initial diagnosis decreased dramatically over the ten-year course of the study, indicating that cancers were being discovered earlier. In the last year of the study, PSA levels at diagnosis for African Americans and Caucasians were virtually identical, in stark contrast to the divergent levels found at the onset of the study.

A GREATER INCIDENCE OF HIGH-GRADE PIN IN AFRICAN AMERICANS

Biopsies of PIN (prostatic intraepithelial neoplasia) lesions in blacks and whites suggest that race might play a role in the incidence and rate of growth of prostate tumors.

PINs are premalignant lesions considered markers for the development of prostate cancer. High-grade PIN (HGPIN) lesions are thought of as precursors of cancer.

Scientists have found more HGPIN among African Americans than among whites, even as early as age thirty, and through to age seventy-plus. When African Americans exhibited HGPINs, they also developed more aggressive tumors than their white counterparts.

PROSTATE CANCER MORTALITY RATES
AMONG BLACK ETHNICITIES

While it is well known that blacks have higher prostate cancer mortality rates than whites, recent data indicates that there may be mortality differences within the black race itself.

A study looked at the influence of birthplace on cancer mortality rates among black New Yorkers. It found that Caribbean-born men living in New York had the highest prostate mortality rate. The incidence of the disease in Jamaican-born New Yorkers was also more clinically significant and more lethal than in American-born black New Yorkers.

POSSIBLE CAUSATIVES AND RISK FACTORS
OTHER THAN RACE

HORMONES

Hormonal levels and other hormonal factors may vary between racial and ethnic groups. Researchers at the University of Southern California compared testosterone levels of African-American men in Los Angeles with a like group of white men in Los Angeles. Daily variations in testosterone level as well as lifestyle factors that affect testosterone were taken into account. Even so, researchers still found testosterone levels in African Americans to be, on average, about 15 percent higher than in their white counterparts. The assumption would be that African Americans are at higher risk with higher testosterone levels. However, when a similar study examined Japanese men, their testosterone levels were comparable to those of whites, but their incidence of prostate cancer was markedly lower.

The study then turned its attention to DHT (dihydrotestosterone), the most powerful male hormone. Since DHT can't be measured directly in the prostate, researchers looked at a surrogate marker that *can* be measured with a blood test and that would indicate how much DHT was being produced. The Japanese had low levels of this agent, meaning that on average they were not producing as much DHT as either black or white men. Other studies have measured serum androgens (male hormones) in older men of different races. They have found that the amount of DHT relative to the amount of testosterone was highest in African Americans, intermediate in whites, and lowest in Asians.

There are demonstrable racial differences in levels of an androgen enzyme which converts testosterone to DHT. Called 5alpha-reductase, it is found in the prostate, with African Americans having the highest amount of activity when it comes to converting testosterone to DHT (dihydrotestosterone). Development of prostate cancer may be dependent on production of DHT.

Other studies are looking at additional androgens that may be important in prostate cancer progression, such as estradiol.

FAMILY HISTORY AND GENETIC FACTORS

A family history of prostate cancer—common among African Americans—is associated with a two-to-three-times increase in risk of getting the disease.

Recent research has found some evidence of possible genetic predisposition among blacks for prostate cancer. The highly aggressive nature of prostate cancer in African Americans may be linked to the bcl-2 gene, which inhibits what is normally the programmed death of cancer cells, called apoptosis. The protein produced by this gene creates a survival advantage for malignant over normal cells. It also bolsters resistance to radiation and chemotherapy.

Researchers found a connection between bcl-2 and the more aggressive prostate cancer tumors experienced by blacks. Tumor growth is more rapid when fewer cells are "instructed" to die.

We must also consider overall effects of specific alterations in DNA. Free-radical damage to mitochondrial DNA is a major factor in cellular aging and cancer incidence. Specific mutations can serve as inheritable factors that might predispose African Americans to prostate cancer.

Genes produce an enzyme called PADRPR, needed to repair naturally occurring breaks in DNA and to control cell growth. If PADRPR production is somehow altered, the result may be cancer. Research suggests that African-American men may be more susceptible to alteration of this enzyme.

Scientists at the National Genome Research Institute mapped the location of a gene associated with increased risk of prostate cancer, estimating that alterations in this gene (HPC1) are responsible for one third or more of the cancer that runs in families. Approximately one in every 500 men is believed to possess an altered version of the HPC1 gene. Initial studies suggest that HPC1 may play a role in early onset of prostate cancer among blacks.

Researchers also found that mutations in the gene MSR1 (macrophage scavenger receptor 1) were more common in white men with a risk factor for hereditary prostate cancer compared to white men who had no such family history. In African-American men, a different mutation of the same gene was six times as common in those with a hereditary risk factor. What is especially significant is that this mutation is associated with a more dangerous form of prostate cancer that spreads quickly, typical of African-American men.

ENVIRONMENTAL FACTORS

Environmental exposures related to farming, particularly work involving herbicides and poultry, may be related to prostate cancer risk, especially among southern and midwestern blacks.

BLACK OR WHITE, IT'S STILL A GUY THING

Many men—black as well as white—fear that prostate cancer treatment such as surgery and radiation will lead to impotence and infertility (as indeed may be the case). Most men—black and white—are notorious for ignoring their health and avoiding medical checkups.

BLACK SKIN, VITAMIN D, AND ULTRAVIOLET LIGHT

The farther north in the United States you live, the higher your risk of prostate cancer. Epidemiologists have analyzed the relationship between the incidence of prostate cancer and the amount of ultraviolet light residents of various regions of the country are exposed to. Prostate cancer mortality rates are highest where the average amount of ultraviolet light is lowest.

Ultraviolet light provides the first step in the body's production of vitamin D. Some research indicates that lower vitamin D levels may help set the stage for prostate cancer. This constitutes even more of a potential risk factor for prostate cancer in black men, since they absorb less ultraviolet light due to melanin pigment in their skin. Black men who live in northern climates would have an even higher risk for prostate cancer than their southern counterparts.

IS CAVEOLIN-1 A KEY TO THE MYSTERY?

A protein linked to the spread of prostate cancer may explain why African-American men frequently have a more aggressive form of prostate cancer. Researchers at Baylor College of Medicine in Houston found a twofold difference in the amount of the protein caveolin-1 in African Americans with prostate cancer. Caveolin-1 is a protein specifically associated with virulent disease. The study, reported in *Clinical Cancer Research*, was a follow-up of an earlier study in which a link had been found between caveolin-1 and the spread of prostate cancer to other parts of the body.

Prostate cancer samples from equal numbers of African-American and Caucasian men were studied for a variety of biomarkers associated with presence of prostate cancer. Only caveolin-1 levels showed a pronounced difference between the two groups.

This research could lead to development of a blood test to determine caveolin-1 levels, which could become a useful screening tool for African-American men, helping to predict the aggressiveness of their cancer and thus tailor their treatment accordingly.

THE INSTITUTE FOR CANCER PREVENTION'S TEN-STEP PLAN TO PREVENT AND COMBAT PROSTATE CANCER IN AFRICAN AMERICANS

Deaths from prostate cancer have decreased among both white and black men since the mid-1990s.

Building on this encouraging news, the Institute for Cancer Prevention's ten-step plan to combat black prostate cancer is a unique, proactive way to bridge the prostate cancer racial gap, helping to ensure that American black men get their fair share of preventive attention and equal medical treatment when prostate cancer does occur.

1. *Screen early for prostate cancer.*

The Institute for Cancer Prevention strongly recommends that African-American men have a PSA test every year after age forty, ten years earlier than other racial groups. African-American men with a family history of prostate cancer—two or more men in the family experiencing the disease or who are in remission; families with two or more generations who have had prostate cancer; families with any members diagnosed with prostate cancer before the age of seventy— are doubly at risk for the disease. These men need to begin screening

AFRICAN AMERICANS AND THE PERCENT FREE PROSTATE-SPECIFIC ANTIGEN TEST

A study of predominantly Caucasian men indicated that the percent free prostate-specific antigen test (%fPSA for short) can be a more effective variant of the traditional prostate-specific antigen test (PSA).

A second test focused exclusively on African Americans. Results were encouraging, indicating that the %fPSA test works equally well for blacks as it does for whites. This simple blood test (see Chapter 3) can detect elevated PSA levels before any other symptoms appear. The %fPSA test analyzes the percent of PSA that floats freely in the blood and is not bound to other proteins. Higher amounts of free PSA are linked to a lower risk of prostate cancer.

The %fPSA test is generally given as a follow-up to men who have exhibited elevated levels in a standard PSA test. It helps determine whether even slightly elevated PSA levels are early warning signs of prostate cancer or simply signs of an enlarged prostate. The test can reduce the need for stressful and inconvenient biopsies.

for the disease at an even earlier age, preferably thirty-five. **Because prostate cancer in African Americans is generally not as slow-growing as it is in their white counterparts, the combination of earlier diagnosis and effective treatment is especially beneficial.**

2. *Recognize that medical care inequities continue to exist for African Americans.*

An increased risk of prostate cancer is a given for any man with a family history of the disease. Most studies of hereditary incidence of prostate disease focus on white Americans. Few clinical studies have attempted to obtain a definitive picture of the hereditary nature of black prostate cancer.

Many American black men are at a disadvantage in that, due to slavery—the African Diaspora—they are limited in how far they can trace their family history. Postslavery black generations were subjected to inadequate medical record keeping, inferior medical treatment, and other indignities.

A number of African Americans continue to harbor a deep mistrust of the medical profession due to historic bias and past racist maltreatment. Some blacks as young as age fifty are old enough to remember the Jim Crow era, with its segregated hospitals and its separate but very unequal medical facilities.

3. *The dietary recommendations of the Prostate Health Pyramid and the principles of the Transition Diet should be followed.*

A high-fiber, low-fat diet is the key to prostate health. The high-fat diet followed not just by blacks but by many Americans has been shown to be a likely risk factor for prostate cancer.

In a National Cancer Institute–sponsored study, an increased risk of prostate cancer was found to be associated with a high intake of saturated fat in blacks, whites, and Asian Americans. The study also found that adolescents' diet may account for differences in prostate cancer incidence among racial and ethnic groups.

4. *Lose the extra weight!*

Obesity is a major problem in the African-American community. Obesity is a well-known prostate cancer risk. It's not enough to just eat right—you have to work on getting rid of those extra pounds as well.

5. *Support and lobby for a dramatic increase in clinical research focusing on the incidence and nature of prostate cancer in African-American men.*

Lack of research funding is a major barrier to understanding how prostate cancer develops, specifically in African Americans. Research should center on potential causes, race-specific and general risk factors, preventive measures, and the most effective treatment modalities for African-American men. African Americans should be involved in all phases of research design and execution of these projects.

6. *Educate yourself—and be educated—about the unusually high incidence of prostate cancer in the black community and the acute need for preventive measures to lower the rate and severity of the disease.*

Afrocentric radio stations, the BET cable channel, and magazines geared toward the black community are three primary conduits for getting the prostate health message out. The Internet and local community and church organizations can also play a major educational role. Black celebrities such as Harry Belafonte have already done their part to get the word out, but many more celebrities can be enlisted—and not just black men who have had prostate cancer. Promotional TV and radio spots featuring some of today's beautiful music divas would be very persuasive indeed.

7. *Get the word out on prostate health to other African Americans.*

Every African American, male as well as female, can spread the word in their community: "I [he] just got screened for prostate cancer. Have you been tested?" Sometimes the most effective way to get the message out is on a one-man-at-a-time basis.

8. *Consider participating in clinical research trials.*

It's the best way to be in the forefront of innovative and potentially effective new treatment modalities.

9. *Exercise a minimum of thirty minutes a day, 3–5 times a week.*

See the Healthy Prostate Fitness Regimen in Chapter 8 for a detailed rundown of the best way to go about it.

10. *Stop smoking and reduce your consumption of alcoholic beverages as general health enhancement measures.*

THE AFRICAN-AMERICAN HEALTH SCORECARD: PROSTATE CANCER IS ONLY PART OF THE PICTURE

To get a sense of the overall reality, the African-American prostate cancer epidemic must be seen within the context of other dismal health statistics relating to both African-American men and African-American women. According to an article in *The New England Journal of Medicine,* the health status of African Americans has actually worsened in the past fifteen years, compared to that of white Americans.

- African Americans between the ages of forty-five and fifty-five have four to five times the stroke death rate of whites.
- African Americans have the highest incidence and mortality

AFRICAN AMERICANS AND THE AFTEREFFECTS OF PROSTATE CANCER SURGERY AND RADIATION TREATMENT

Duke University Medical Center initiated an ongoing study looking at some of the typical symptoms and problems African Americans face after treatment for prostate cancer. Problems surveyed included incontinence, impotence, pain following surgical intervention or radiation therapy, and psychological readjustment after therapy.

The study found that African-American men are significantly more likely than Caucasians to develop side effects during treatment. They are also notably less satisfied with their level of medical care and postoperative treatment and with the quality of their primary care physician.

rates from the four leading cancers, except for breast cancer, where the incidence in black women is lower than in whites but black mortality is higher.

• One in four black women over the age of fifty-five, and one in four black men between the ages of fifty-five and seventy-four, has diabetes.

• Cerebrovascular disease (most commonly, stroke) is twice as high among African-American men as it is among white men, and twice as high among African-American women as it is among white women.

• The rate of new AIDS cases for African Americans is more than eight times as high as it is for whites.

HISPANIC MEN AND PROSTATE CANCER: NO EASY ANSWERS

Latinos recently became the largest minority group in the United States, surpassing African Americans. In the year 2000, there were approximately 32.5 million Hispanic Americans, making up 11.8 percent of the population. It is estimated that by the year 2050 Latinos will make up 25 percent or more of the population. Any discussion of the Hispanic or Latino population must emphasize that it encompasses all racial groups and comprises distinct national cultures, and cultures within cultures. We must be careful not to generalize or stereotype. Monolithic pronouncements surely do not apply when it comes to Hispanics and prostate cancer—or to Hispanics and any other aspect of life.

Prostate cancer is the second leading type of cancer among Hispanic American men. Latinos in general have higher prostate cancer rates than, for example, Asians or Native Americans. On the whole, Hispanics born in the United States have higher cancer risks than foreign-born Hispanics who live in the same region. There is an urgent need for a large-scale clinical study to shed some light on why this may be so.

The prostate cancer incidence rate for Puerto Ricans and Cuban Americans is very close to that of non-Hispanic white Americans. Age-adjusted mortality rates for prostate cancer are lower among Cubans born in the United States than they are among Cubans in Cuba, where there is a relatively high mortality rate.

Among Hispanics in the United States, the incidence of prostate cancer is significantly lower only among Mexican Americans. It is a little-known fact that prostate cancer is far more common in the United States than in Mexico. When comparisons of prostate cancer rates are made between the United States and other countries, it is Asian countries such as Japan and China that are most often cited.

In one respect, Hispanic-American men are just like non-Hispanic white and African-American men: They have been reluctant to participate in prostate cancer screening programs. As we said earlier in this chapter, sometimes it's just a guy thing.

V.

ALTERNATIVES

16. Alternative Treatments

Outside the Realm

Given the many treatment options for various diseases of the prostate, it might seem strange that patients seek out forms of therapy that are totally outside of conventional medicine. Yet alternative treatments are used by an increasing number of men in the United States who find them an economical choice for treating their condition. A recent survey in the United States found that between one quarter and one third of men with prostate cancer made use of these therapies. They were typically younger patients with higher levels of income or education, or patients with a more advanced state of cancer. Alternative therapies offer a new world of options for men who are suffering with various kinds of prostate disease.

What Is Conventional (Allopathic) Medicine?

When we speak of "medicine" in the United States, we refer to a medical system that has been developed in Western Europe and America over the last two or three hundred years. This system uses the scientific method of observation and controlled experimentation to diagnose and treat illness. This type of medicine came to be called allopathy, meaning "other disease"; that is, illness that was caused by something outside the body.

There are critics who claim that conventional medicine has its limitations. Critics argue that mainstream medicine often treats only symptoms and not the underlying causes of disease. High-tech surgical procedures can be overly intrusive, do not always work, and are capable of causing major complications or even death.

Some patients feel that modern Western medicine does not focus enough on non-disease-specific aspects of health such as diet and psychological and environmental factors and emphasizes complex treatments of disease symptoms over simple prevention.

Orthodox Western medicine has regarded alternative medicine with a mixture of skepticism, suspicion, or outright hostility. Because most alternative therapies have not been scientifically evaluated, many doctors are hesitant to recommend them.

Over the last few decades, however, the use of alternative therapies has increased dramatically for a variety of reasons. During the 1960s and 1970s, America was exposed to Eastern religious and philosophical systems such as yoga and Zen Buddhism, which in turn led to an interest in traditional medical systems from China and India that predate Western medicine by thousands of years. Experimentation with alternate lifestyles included an interest in "new age" alternative medical treatments, including massage and bodywork, acupressure, aromatherapy, and macrobiotic diets, among others.

In October 1991, Congress mandated the creation of the Office of Alternative Medicine at the National Institutes of Health. This became the National Center for Complementary and Alternative Medicine (NCCAM) in 1998. The office evaluates and disseminates information about the effectiveness of all forms of alternative therapy. The Richard and Hinda Rosenthal Center for Complementary and Alternative Medicine was recently established at the prestigious Columbia University College of Physicians and Surgeons, and other medical schools around the country have followed suit. An increasing number of HMOs and medical insurance companies are starting to provide coverage for some alternative therapies.

WHAT IS ALTERNATIVE MEDICINE?

"Alternative medicine" is a blanket term that covers a wide variety of treatments that are outside the orbit of mainstream medicine. Some of these therapies are thousands of years old; some are products of the space age. Despite their variety, most types of alternative medicine have a number of points in common:

- Prevention of disease is emphasized over the treatment of symptoms. Diet, exercise, and overall mental outlook are important.
- Alternative medicine practitioners view the mind and the body as integral parts of a single entity and treat both. They approach each patient as an integrated whole. This is sometimes called the holistic approach.
- Alternative medicine practitioners believe that the body is capable of healing itself.
- Alternative medicine practitioners also believe that good health is a harmonious state, not merely the absence of disease, and that the patient must play an active role in maintaining it.
- Many therapies involve the cleansing of toxic environmental substances from the body.
- The therapies do not use any form of surgery.

TYPES OF ALTERNATIVE THERAPIES

Some forms of alternative medicine are not too far from mainstream science, such as dietary therapies and techniques designed to relieve stress, anxiety, and dysfunctional mental states. Others are completely alien to the Western scientific worldview and rely instead on exotic theories of health and disease, mysterious diagnostic techniques, and obscure forms of treatment.

Not all alternative therapies claim to provide remedies for problems relating to prostate health. The following is a list of some therapies that some people believe have a positive impact on certain prostate conditions:

Homeopathy. This is a European system of medicine that involves taking controlled doses of highly diluted toxic substances as an alternative to using conventional prescription drugs.

Traditional Chinese medicine. Based on centuries-old traditions, Chinese medicine employs practices such as acupuncture, meditation, and herbs to promote good health.

Chiropractic medicine/osteopathic medicine. Although these therapies do not directly impact on prostate health, they emphasize balance, stability, and a normally functioning structural framework that can positively affect the prostate.

Ayurvedic medicine. This is a system of alternative medicine based on practices derived from the ancient traditions of India.

Herbalism. Medicinal herbs derived from traditional folk medicines from various parts of the world are used as a substitute or in addition to conventional prescription drugs to promote health.

Nutrition therapies. These therapies treat illness by making significant, sometimes radical, adjustments to the patient's diet.

Bodywork. Massage and other physical manipulation techniques are used to provide drug-free relief from a variety of neuromuscular problems.

Naturopathy. This type of therapy emphasizes the ability of the body to heal itself naturally and uses an integrative approach that employs techniques from many different types of alternative medicine.

Patients who have serious illnesses that have not responded well to conventional medical therapy, or adventurous souls whose symptoms are not severe, may be inclined to consider one (or more) of these alternative treatments, but they should be approached with caution and in consultation with your doctor.

THE PLACEBO EFFECT

At the heart of the controversy over alternative medicines is the so-called placebo effect. Over the years, medical researchers have noticed that a certain percentage of patients will report relief from their symptoms even when given false or bogus treatments or placebos. Almost any kind of treatment can produce a positive response if the patient believes it will help. Ordinary sugar pills will provide relief from symptoms in roughly a third of patients during most clinical drug trials. Hooking patients up to an impressive-looking machine that does absolutely nothing relieves pain in more than half of experimental subjects.

This tendency to react positively to bogus treatment is called the placebo effect, and these types of patients are referred to as placebo responders. Results like these lead mainstream doctors to suspect that at least some of the claims and testimonials made by the proponents of alternative medicine are due to the placebo effect, because these treatments have not been held up to scientific scrutiny.

In order to overcome this effect, modern medicine attempts to hold itself to a higher standard. The aim of scientific medical research is to find treatments that work better than a placebo. Clinical trials for new treatments typically involve recruiting a large number of subjects, half of whom are given a placebo while the other half receives the actual medicine. This is done under controlled conditions so that neither the experimenters nor the patients know who is getting the real medicine and who is taking the placebo. This is called a double-blind procedure, or more specifically a randomized (because of how patients are assigned to each group), double-blind, placebo-controlled clinical trial. The treatment will be judged effective only if it can score significantly above the number of the patients who respond to the placebo. The placebo effect is built into the structure of the experiment. Although placebos can produce actual physical changes in the body (such as lowering blood pressure), they can't cure serious illnesses such as massive infections or cancer. "Mind over matter" has its limitations.

The majority of alternative treatments have never been evaluated in a scientific manner, but proponents of alternative medicine point out that (to quote a statement issued by the NIH in 1992), "not all alternative medical practices are amenable to traditional scientific evaluation, and some may require development of new methods to evaluate their efficacy and safety."

There is no guarantee that any medical practice, conventional or alternative, will actually be effective in treating your condition. Medical quackery is rampant, especially in the age of the Internet. Do lots of research, consult with your doctor, and exercise a healthy skepticism before embarking on any alternative treatment program.

A WORD OF CAUTION
While alternative therapies may hold a great deal of promise for treating your condition, there are some matters that are best left to conventional medicine. One area where orthodox medicine has a definite edge is in diagnosis. Alternative practitioners do not generally have the diagnostic skills of an M.D., nor do they have access to

sophisticated, high-tech diagnostic testing techniques such as MRI, CAT scan, or EEG. If you are concerned about any serious medical condition, you should consult a mainstream doctor immediately to ensure a proper diagnosis before turning to alternative medicine.

You should also take care that the specific type of alternative therapy you have selected is appropriate for treating your condition. Alternative therapies may work well on certain types of problems but may not be able to do anything for your prostate. Some of these therapies may even be harmful for patients with certain medical conditions.

Herbal remedies should be used with caution. Because of the popular notion that herbs are natural, many people believe that they are safer than conventional drugs, but in reality some of them can be dangerous or even deadly. Herbs such as the popular but now banned diet aid ephedra and the sedative kava have caused fatalities when abused or used incorrectly. Using combinations of herbs can increase the risk because different substances are introduced into the body at once.

Unlike over-the-counter or prescription medications, herbal preparations are not standardized and contain varying amounts, if any, of active ingredients, which makes their potency uncertain. While manufactured drugs usually contain only one active ingredient derived from a plant source, the whole plant may contain a num-

ARE HERBAL MEDICATIONS REALLY SAFER? THE CASE OF PC-SPES

In February 2002, the FDA took a popular herbal remedy for prostate cancer called PC-SPES off the market. According to the manufacturer, PC-SPES contained a mixture of saw palmetto, licorice, chrysanthemum, and a number of Chinese herbs. The formula, which had been sold since 1996, seemed to provide some relief for men with advanced prostate cancer, although clinical trials of the medication had never been conducted.

Unfortunately, it was discovered that this elixir contained more than just herbs. Capsules of PC-SPES were analyzed by the FDA and found to contain several prescription drugs, including the anticlotting agent warfarin, the hormone diethylstilbestrol (DES), and the anti-inflammatory indomethacin. These drugs can cause serious side effects in some patients and can interfere with the action of other prescription medications. Because of these contamination problems, PC-SPES was withdrawn from the market and the U.S. manufacturer, Botanic Labs, went out of business a short time later.

ber of other active ingredients, some of which may not be helpful, or may even be harmful, for your condition. Herbal remedies can also interfere with the effects of prescription medications for heart problems and bleeding disorders and can affect liver and kidney functions. Always talk to your doctor about any herbal medicines you plan to take, whether or not you are already taking one or more prescription drugs on a regular basis.

HOMEOPATHY: SOMETHING FOR NOTHING?

A SHORT HISTORY OF HOMEOPATHY

In the 1790s, a respected German physician named Dr. Samuel Hahnemann devised a therapeutic system called homeopathy or homeopathic medicine. In particular, he wanted to discover medicines that were safer and less toxic than the crude medications that were then being used.

Hahnemann experimented with a botanical medicine derived from the bark of a Peruvian tree called cinchona. Cinchona bark

---

SERIOUS CONDITIONS THAT REQUIRE A CONVENTIONAL DOCTOR'S CARE

Alternative medicines cannot cure every illness and are not appropriate for treating many severe disorders. You should see an M.D. immediately if you suspect that you have any potentially damaging or life-threatening condition, including:

- Asthma
- Cancer
- Coronary artery disease
- Diabetes
- Eye disorders
- Fractures or dislocations
- High blood pressure
- High fever
- Infections
- Irregular heartbeat
- Poisoning
- Stroke

contains the alkaloid quinine, a drug commonly used to treat malaria. Hahnemann found that after giving himself controlled doses of cinchona he developed the symptoms of malaria.

Over the next fourteen years, he tested hundreds of animal, vegetable, and mineral substances on himself and others. On the basis of these experiments he developed his Law of Similars, which held that substances that produce symptoms in healthy people can effectively treat the same symptoms in sick people. Hahnemann created a system of medicine based on the principle of "like cures like." Because many of the substances he tested were poisonous, he devised a method of tempering their toxicity by diluting them many times. According to his Law of Potentization, a medicine's effectiveness was directly proportional to how many times it had been diluted. These watered-down medications were thought to work on the "vital force" of the patient in order to effect a cure. Like allopathic medicine, homeopathic practices were aimed at treating the symptoms of disease, rather than the causes of disease.

Homeopathic medicine was introduced into the United States in the 1830s. From the start, homeopathy was surrounded by controversy. It flew in the face of the germ theory of disease advocated by French chemist Louis Pasteur, which stated that invisible microorganisms, rather than imbalances in the patient's vital force, caused infectious illnesses. As Pasteur's techniques for treating disease were proven to be effective, the appeal of homeopathic medicine waned.

Another controversy concerned Hahnemann's Law of Potentization, directly contradicted by a fundamental principle of pharmacology called the dose-response relationship, which states that the larger the dose of a drug, the greater its effect. As a rule, homeopathic medicines are so dilute that only a single molecule or less of the original disease-causing substance is present.

Homeopathic practitioners respond to this criticism by claiming that, although their medicines may not be pharmacologically active, they are biologically active—that although their presence cannot be detected in the medicine, they can still cause effects within the body.

Today there are about five thousand doctors in the United States who use homeopathic medicine as part of their practice. A 1993 report in *The New England Journal of Medicine* suggested that as many as 2.5 million Americans have used homeopathic medications.

ABOUT HOMEOPATHIC MEDICATIONS

Instructions for the use of homeopathic medicines are set forth in the bible of homeopathy, *The Homeopathic Pharmacopoeia*. This book, first published in 1897 and updated regularly, is a catalog of homeopathic treatments for various symptoms and illnesses. The medicines are prepared from hundreds of different plant, animal, and mineral substances. Some of these are derived from familiar herbs, such as garlic or chamomile, but others are far more exotic. Some of these ingredients, such as mercury or belladonna, are highly toxic and would be poisonous if taken in high dosages. Homeopathic medicines are considered safe because in some cases the active ingredient has been diluted to the point that it is no longer physically present.

HOMEOPATHIC METHODS OF DIAGNOSIS

Homeopathic diagnostic procedures center around a detailed analysis of symptoms. Symptoms are seen by homeopaths as the body's way of externalizing disease. Unlike mainstream doctors, they believe that symptoms are patient-specific, not disease-specific. Patients are asked in great detail about aspects of their lifestyle, their occupation, their diet, family history, and emotional problems. They are asked about every nuance of their disease symptoms in order to analyze their symptom complex. Two patients with identical symptoms may be diagnosed and treated differently by the same homeopath.

Once the diagnosis is complete, the practitioner will prescribe one or more homeopathic medications to treat the patient's condition. In the United States, all homeopathic medicines are sold over the counter and therefore no prescription is required to obtain them (although they might have to be ordered by mail from a health food outlet). In general, they tend to be less expensive than conventional medications. All remedies are assigned Latin names. Homeopathic medicines may have to be taken for a longer period of time than conventional medications.

Prostate Cancer

Prostate cancer is such a serious condition that homeopathic medicine may be used as an addition to—but not as a substitute

OUTRIGHT QUACKERY AND FRAUD

The fact that some practitioners of alternative healing say that the Western scientific method may be inappropriate for the subtleties of alternative methods may well have a kernel of truth to it.

But it also creates a perfect environment for outright quackery and fraud. Beware the practitioner who says, "I know this hasn't proven to be safe or effective by doctors, but they just don't understand how this works" or some variation on that theme. The fact is, if something really works, it should be testable in some scientific way.

And remember, while homeopathic medicines are so dilute that they are unlikely to cause any harm, the harm can come if you use these medicines instead of conventional treatments for serious conditions such as cancer.

for—orthodox medical treatment. Nonetheless, there are a number of homeopathic remedies that are used in treating the symptoms of prostate cancer. *Such homeopathic preparations and remedies, however, remain scientifically unproven and are not recommended by the authors.*

- Stony hard prostate; inability to have erections but high sex drive; intermittent urination in old people; urine flows and stops; weight like a stone in perineum: *Conium maculatum*
- Cancer with hematuria: *Crotalus horridus*
- Incontinence of urine; complete dissipation of strength and general emaciation: *Iodatum*
- Discharge of prostatic fluid before urinating; several organs flabby, torpid; aversion to coitus: *Psorinium*
- Intense sexual activity leading to debility; symptoms worse in hot weather, after sleep and after relaxation; involuntary urinary dribbling: *Selenium*
- Offensive sweat around genitals: *Sulfur*
- Pain, burning sensation of urination or ejaculation; intense sexual problems; frequent and urgent desire to urinate: *Thuja occidentalis*

In addition to these standard medications, there has been some experimental medical research into the possibility of treating prostate cancer with a homeopathic preparation of human growth hormone (HGH).

TRADITIONAL CHINESE MEDICINE

Traditional Chinese medicine has come to America and has finally been welcomed in the Western world as an effective system of alternative therapy. An estimated 12 million patient visits a year are made to practitioners of Chinese medicine in the United States, and the number is growing. Traditional medicine is still widely practiced in many regions of China today and is frequently the only type of medicine available to millions of Chinese citizens.

THE TAO OF CHINESE MEDICINE

The origins of traditional Chinese medicine are said to go back 4,500 years.

Understanding Chinese medicine involves understanding certain Chinese philosophical concepts. The Chinese believe in *tao*, a wholeness that pervades the universe and connects all things. The *tao*, in turn, is divided into two complementary yet opposite phenomena called *yin* and *yang* that should exist in a constant flux of balance and harmony. *Yin* embodies the passive or "feminine" qualities of softness, darkness, coldness and wetness, while *yang* comprises the "masculine" qualities of hardness, brightness, heat and dryness. Nothing is all *yin* or all *yang*, but everything contains a mixture of these two opposing qualities.

Within the human body, *yin* and *yang* manifest themselves as part of *qi* (pronounced "chee"), which is thought to be the life force or vital force that permeates all living human beings. Qi is an intangible force that flows through our bodies and makes us alive. *Yin* and *yang* also manifest themselves inside the body as blood and moisture. These fluid substances distribute the force of *qi* throughout the body. *Qi*, blood, and moisture are all subject to *yin/yang* influences from our environment. These include the five basic elements (wood, fire, earth, metal, and water); the five seasons (spring, summer, late summer, autumn, and winter); and the five climates (wind, heat, dampness, dryness, and cold). These three sets of forces exert an influence on the twelve major internal organs of the body, the *zangfu.*

Disease is thought to occur when there is an imbalance between the forces of *yin* and *yang* in the body that causes a dysfunction of the patient's *qi.*

DIAGNOSIS

Like other forms of holistic treatment, Chinese medicine is dedicated to treating the whole person. The doctor takes a detailed case history, asking patients about their symptoms and about other aspects of their lifestyle, including their sleep patterns, food preferences, and work and social environments in order to determine their general physical, mental, and emotional state of health.

After the interview, the Chinese physician utilizes a complex technique designed to evaluate the workings of a patient's organs by feeling the pulse, called pulse diagnosis. An experienced Chinese physicians can distinguish up to thirty-two different pulse patterns. Using pulse diagnosis, the physician can monitor the balance and flow of *qi* through the patient's meridians and corresponding organs.

Another technique that may be employed is tongue diagnosis. The appearance of the patient's tongue is said to indicate much about the nature, intensity, and location of diseases within the body.

TREATMENT OPTIONS

While Western medicine treats patients with the same diagnosis similarly, Chinese medicine treats patients individually. Chinese medicine utilizes two principal types of treatment. The most ancient of these consists of Chinese herbal remedies designed to restore harmony and vigor to the patient's *qi.* The other is acupuncture, the practice of inserting needles at specific points on the patient's meridians in order to restore the proper flow of *qi* through the internal organs. In addition to acupuncture and herbal preparations, other treatment options may include meditation, special diets, and therapeutic exercise regimes such as tai chi or *quigong.*

ACUPUNCTURE

Acupuncture is a technique that involves inserting special needles into the patient's body at special points along the twelve meridians that pass close to the skin. The insertion of needles at these points strengthens *qi* or disperses *qi* that has become stagnant or blocked. In theory, there are between 360 and 2,000 acupuncture points on the body, but in practice, about 150 are typically used.

Acupuncture needles are solid, not hollow; extremely thin; and typically between half an inch and four inches in length. They are usually made of stainless steel or copper but can also be made of gold, silver, or wood. The needles should be carefully sterilized before use, and some practitioners use disposable needles to prevent the transmission of disease. During treatment, the patient lies on a couch while the needles are placed at the proper points. Great care is taken to avoid blood vessels and major organs. The insertion of the needles should be virtually painless, and the patient should feel nothing more than a pinprick as the skin is broken, followed by some sensation as the needle goes deeper. The needles are inserted to a depth of a quarter inch to three inches and are usually left inside the patient's body for about twenty minutes and then removed. It usually takes about six to twelve sessions for an acupuncturist to get results.

Sometimes a low-voltage electrical current is passed through the needles to treat pain. Another variation is called moxibustion, in which small quantities of an herb called moxa (Chinese mugwort) are placed on a receptacle on top of the needles and burned. A variation of acupuncture technique that uses massage in place of needles is known as acupressure.

ABOUT CHINESE HERBS

Unlike Western herbal medicines, Chinese herbs are categorized not by their pharmacological effects but according to the Chinese theory of herbs as "energy medicines." Specific herbs are selected in order to correct imbalances in the patient's *qi*. Herbs are classified based on five qualities: color; nature (warming, cooling, neutral); taste (sour, bitter, sweet, bland, spicy, salty); configuration (shape, texture, moisture); and property (dispersing, consolidating, purging, tonifying). They can be taken as a tea brewed from the dried plants or in liquid extract or pill form. Chinese herbal preparations, unlike their Western counterparts, are not standardized, and some products have been found to contain contaminants, including lead.

CHINESE MEDICINES FOR THE PROSTATE

Because of the severity of the disease, acupuncture and Chinese herbal remedies are not generally considered appropriate treatments for prostate cancer. Some recent studies have suggested that acupuncture can help to relieve the physical and mental stress associated with cancer treatments and improve the patient's overall quality of life. It has proven to be especially useful in pain management.

Chinese medicine does provide treatment options for benign enlargement of the prostate (BPH) and prostatitis. Both of these conditions are further broken down into two or more syndromes according to the specific cause of the disease. Each syndrome has its own therapeutic principle and treatment regimen. The following are sample treatments for men with prostate disorders. Bear in mind that according to the principles of Chinese medicine, every person receives a unique diagnosis and treatment. Notify your physician if you are considering any of these treatments.

Benign Prostatic Hyperplasia (BPH)

SYNDROME A: DAMP-HEAT TYPE

Herbal therapeutic principle: Clearing away pathenogenic heat and dampness; removing blood stasis

Chinese herbs used: Pyrrosia leaf; windweed rhizome; Chinese pink herbs; philodendron bark

Acupuncture therapeutic principle: Regulating circulation of *qi* and blood

Acupuncture treatment: Acupuncture at *ren* and *du* meridian points twenty to thirty minutes; moxibustion at each point ten to fifteen minutes

SYNDROME B: KIDNEY DEFICIENCY TYPE

Herbal therapeutic principle: Warming and reinforcing *yin/yang* in the kidney; promoting urination

Chinese herbs used: Dogwood fruit (*Cornus officinalis seib.*); Chinese yam (*Dioscorea*); Oriental water plantain root (*Alisma orientalis*); Achyranthes root (*Atractylodes lancea*)

Acupuncture treatment: At *ren*, spleen, and bladder meridians

Prostatitis

SYNDROME A: STASIS-STAGNANCY TYPE

Herbal therapeutic principle: Promoting blood circulation; removing blood stasis and promoting the flow of *qi* to remove stagnancy

Chinese herbs used: Red sage root (*Radix salvia miltiorrhizae*); lycopus herb; red peony root (*Radix paeoniae rubra*); dahurian angelica root (*Radix angelicae dahuricae*); dandelion

SYNDROME B: DAMP-HEAT TYPE

Herbal therapeutic principle: Clearing away pathenogenic heat and dampness

Chinese herbs used: Philodendron bark; patrinia (*Patrinia heterophylla*); atractylodes root (*Atractylodes lancea*); Oriental water plantain root (*Alisma orientalis*)

SYNDROME C: KIDNEY-DEFICIENCY TYPE

Herbal therapeutic principle: Warming the kidney, supplementing *qi*, removing pathenogenic dampness and heat

Chinese herbs used: Curculingo root; epimedium (*Epimedium brevicor*); Chinese yam (*Dioscoria*); philodendron bark; dandelion

Other Chinese herbs used to treat the prostate include:

- **Reishi:** This herb is derived from a mushroom, *Gandomera lucidum*, and is used to treat a variety of ailments
- **Huang quin:** Known in the West as Baikal skullcap (*Scutellaria baicalensis*)
- **Dong ling cao fang** (*Rabdosia rubescens*)
- **Da qing ye:** Dyer's woad (*Isatis tinctoria*)
- **Mu dan pi:** tree peony bark (*Moutan cortex radicis*)
- **Paris rhizome** (*Rhizoma paridis polyphylla*)
- **Bai hua she cao:** Oldenlandia (*Herba hedyotis diffusa*)
- **Panax ginseng:** A popular herb widely used as a tonic and to increase male sexual potency

Again, be cautious with the use of Chinese herbs. Remember that Chinese herbal medicines are prescribed using an entirely different set of treatment criteria than their Western counterparts. Packaged herbal preparations are not usually manufactured in the United States according to standardized practices, which means that potencies may vary and medicines may be contaminated with foreign substances.

CHIROPRACTIC MEDICINE AND OSTEOPATHIC MEDICINE

In chiropractic medicine, the body is viewed as a functional unit. In theory, maximal balance and stability in the spinal column and skeletal framework result in the body's functioning at its healthiest level. This balance and stability affect tissues and internal organs. Abnormal posture, position, or structure of the skeletal framework can lead to tissue breakdown, disease and pain. Chiropractic medicine is not a cure for any condition; it is purported to be a restorative therapy.

Osteopathic medicine (there is a D.O. instead of an M.D. after the doctor's name, even though both have four-year medical school training) emphasizes that the musculoskeletal system plays a key role in disease prevention, overall wellness, and recovery from disease. While it does not focus on prostate-specific remedies, osteopathic medicine believes that alignment of mind, spirit, and body is key to prostate health. Osteopathic physicians stress the importance of preventive health care and the body's ability to heal itself. They integrate accepted allopathic treatments into body manipulation techniques known as osteopathic manipulative treatment (OMT).

AYURVEDA: THE OLDEST MEDICINE?

Another ancient Oriental system of alternative medicine that has recently been transplanted to the West is Ayurvedic medicine from India. Ayurvedic medicine was first popularized in America by the Maharishi Mahesh Yogi—guru to the Beatles and various other celebrities—in the early 1970s. More recently, media savants such as Dr. Andrew Weil and Dr. Deepak Chopra have brought the principles of Ayurvedic medicine to an audience of millions in America and Europe through their writings and lectures.

HEALING ARTS FROM ANCIENT INDIA

Like traditional Chinese medicine, Ayurvedic medicine traces its ancestry back thousands of years. Proponents of Ayurveda claim that it is the oldest system of natural healing on Earth, and that it is the common root of many of today's other medical traditions. About four thousand years ago, a group of holy men in ancient India composed the ancient Hindu philosophical and spiritual texts called the Vedas. These Vedic texts set forth the principles of the four main branches of sacred knowledge: philosophy, yoga, astrology, and medicine.

The term "Ayurveda" is a combination of two words in Sanskrit, the ancient holy language of India, *ayus*, meaning "life," and *vid*, or "knowledge." Ayurvedic medicine is still practiced in India today by about 80 percent of the population who do not have access to Western medicine. It employs a combination of various treatments, including diet, meditation, massage, and herbal remedies.

PRANA AND THE FIVE ELEMENTS

Like other systems of alternative medicine, Ayurveda is built upon the concept of healing the individual's "life force." The Ayurvedic term for this is *prana*, which is described as the vital force that enlivens the human body and exists inside all living things. The concept of prana is roughly equivalent to that of *qi* in traditional Chinese medicine. *Prana* can also be thought of as a kind of nutrient that can be taken into the body through the breath in order to restore life energy to the patient. Ayurveda uses a variety of breathing exercises called *pranayama* to bring *prana* inside the body to promote healing.

According to Ayurvedic teachings, *prana* is manifested in the five basic elements—earth, water, air, fire, and ether (space)—that make up all things in the universe and also permeate the human body. Each of these elements is connected to a specific part and function of the body. Earth influences the solid components of the body, such as bones, skin, nails, and hair. Water controls blood, digestive enzymes, and other fluids. Fire fuels digestion, thinking, and other bodily processes. Air regulates breathing and the nervous system. Space, or ether, governs the hollow cavities within the body such as the mouth, nose, and respiratory tract.

These five elements are constantly interacting with one another within the body in a series of complex life processes. When the five elements are in harmony, the body is healthy, but if they are out of balance, disease can occur. Ayurvedic physicians believe that most disease results from the buildup of a substance called *ama*, a kind of liquid sludge created by the combination of poorly digested food and an imbalance of the body's digestive enzymes.

HOW'S YOUR *DOSHA*?

In Ayurvedic medicine, each individual has a unique constitution, called the *pakriti*. The *pakriti* is a pattern that is formed at the moment of conception and is composed of varying amounts of three forces or *doshas*. The three *doshas* represent manifestations of the five elements and their influences in the body. The balance of the three forces determines a person's overall body type, or *tridosha*.

Sometimes one of the *doshas* will predominate over the others, but some people can have a more complex situation in which there are equal influences of multiple *doshas*.

DIAGNOSIS AND TREATMENT

An Ayurvedic medical examination will begin by having you fill out a simple questionnaire. You will be asked about your sleep patterns, eating habits, emotional and psychological health, and other aspects of your lifestyle.

After completing the questionnaire, the patient is given a physical examination. Ayurvedic physicians pay particular attention to the condition of the patient's skin and nails. Like Chinese medicine, Ayurveda employs the techniques of pulse and tongue diagnosis. Ayurvedic medicine also employs the technique of urine analysis, in which the color and consistency of the patient's urine are analyzed to determine the balance of the *tridosha*.

AYURVEDIC DIET THERAPY

Diet therapy is considered an important component of Ayurvedic treatment. Once the patient's *tridosha* has been mapped, the physician will recommend a diet of foods designed to counteract a specific condition of the *doshas* that is perceived to be out of balance. Each patient is assigned a special diet that corresponds to his individual therapeutic needs.

MASSAGE AND MEDITATION

Ayurvedic massage, called *abhyanga,* works by stimulating a system of 107 points (called *marma* points) on the surface of the body in order to rebalance the *doshas.* Massage is also used to break up toxic substances and move them out of the body. Medicinal oils may be used to restore the flow of *prana* energy throughout the body. Frequent self-massage with sesame oil may also be encouraged.

Meditation is used for stress reduction and to increase the body's awareness of itself. *Pranayama* breathing exercises are used to relax the nervous system and breathe in healing *prana* energy. One technique involves alternating breaths between the right and left nostrils. Hatha yoga exercises may also be recommended.

DETOXIFY WITH *PANCHAKARMA*

Panchakarma is an intensive treatment program that is designed to purge various supposedly toxic substances from the body. The procedure takes place over a period of several days in a special, spa-like facility and may be performed once or twice a year.

AYURVEDIC HERBAL MEDICINES

Unlike Western allopathic medicine, in which single active ingredients are isolated from herbs and refined into pure pharmaceuticals, Ayurvedic medicine uses herbs in their natural state and usually in combination with several other whole herbs in herbal formulas called *rasayanas.* These formulas can contain ten or twenty different herbs, and each herb contain hundreds of active substances.

Rasayanas should be prescribed by an Ayurvedic physician, but these preparations are starting to become available to the general public on the Internet and through health-food outlets for self-medication. As with any "medicine," extreme caution is the rule when considering self-medication. The majority of them are made in India and are not manufactured under standardized conditions.

AYURVEDIC TREATMENTS FOR PROSTATE HEALTH

According to Ayurvedic thinking, prostate problems arise because of natural changes in the *doshas* that occur as a man's body ages. During this transitional period the *vatta dosha* begins to dominate the *tridosha*. The dry quality of the *vatta dosha* causes testosterone production to fluctuate, leading to enlargement of the prostate (BPH). Because prostate enlargement is caused by an imbalance of the *vatta dosha*, the patient must avoid eating *vatta*-aggravating foods. These include dry, light, and cold foods with astringent, bitter, or pungent tastes. Conversely, a *vatta*-fortifying diet consisting of warm, oily foods with sweet, sour, and salty tastes will help restore the balance of the *doshas*.

Certain vegetables are recommended for prostate health, including asparagus and daikon radish, as well as grains such as amaranth and quinoa, which are high in protein and zinc.

SUMMING IT ALL UP

Ayurvedic medicine is not recognized as a medical discipline in the United States, and there is currently no system for licensing Ayurvedic practitioners. This means, among other things, that treatments are not covered by medical insurance.

Ayurvedic herbal preparations are not standardized and often consist of ten or twenty different herbs containing a large number of active ingredients. With a few exceptions, none of these substances has undergone clinical trials that could validate either their effectiveness or their potential dangers. Consult with your doctor about any Ayurvedic medicines you may be taking, especially if you are already taking conventional medication for prostate or other medical conditions.

BACK TO MOTHER NATURE: HERBS AND THE PROSTATE

Herbs provide a wealth of medicinal substances. More than 120 commonly prescribed pharmaceuticals are extracted from ninety species of plants. About 25 percent of all over-the-counter and prescription drugs used in the United States are derived from plant sources. Plants have provided many safe and effective allopathic medicines over the last two hundred years, including:

- Aspirin (from willow bark)
- Penicillin (from mold)

MAK-4, MAK-5, AND OTHER HERBAL REMEDIES FOR THE PROSTATE

In 1993, Dr. Hari Sharma, a pathologist at the Ohio State University College of Medicine, conducted basic research on two Ayurvedic herbal formulas manufactured by the Maharishi Mahesh Yogi's manufacturing company. These herbal *rasayana*s, called Maharishi Amrit Kalash–4 and –5 (abbreviated as MAK-4 and MAK-5) are versions of a traditional Ayurvedic metabolic tonic used to combat cancer and other diseases. The study showed that the MAK-4 and MAK-5 preparations shrank tumors in mice, increased immune cell production, and inhibited the formation of cancer cells in human lung tissue.

Upon analysis, MAK-4 was found to contain raw sugar, ghee (clarified butter), Indian gallnut, Indian gooseberry, dried catkins, Indian pennywort, honey, nutgrass, white sandalwood, butterfly pea, shoeflower, aloewood, licorice, cardamom, cinnamon, and turmeric. MAK-5 contains black musale, heart-leaved moonseed, butterfly pea, licorice, elephant creeper, Indian wild pepper, *Gymnema aurentiacum, Sphaerantus indicus,* and *Vanda spatulatum.* Several of the herbs from these MAK formulas are used in Ayurvedic medicine to treat prostate problems, including white sandalwood, heart-leaved moonseed, turmeric, and licorice.

There are a number of Ayurvedic preparations designed specifically to treat enlarged prostate and prostatitis. Many of these formulas contain the Indian herbs *gugqulu* (*Commiphora mukul*), *gokshur* (*Tribulus terrestris*), and *kachnar* (*Bauhinia variegata*). Other Ayurvedic prostate remedies used to treat BPH contain Indian sarsaparilla, *Mimosa pudica, Argyreia speciosa, Orchis mascula, Ocimum sanctum,* black pepper (*Piper nigrum*), and *Asphalatum punjabinum.* Consult your doctor if you are considering taking any of these substances.

- Morphine and codeine (from the opium poppy)
- Digitalis (from foxglove)
- Ephedrine (from the ephedra plant)
- Quinine (from the cinchona plant)
- Taxol (anticancer drug; from the yew tree)

The use of herbal supplements in the United States is growing by an estimated 10 to 15 percent a year. Americans spend more than $4 billion a year on various "natural" health products (excluding homeopathic medicines and teas).

In the United States, medical herbalism is not licensed as a professional practice. Herbs are used as self-medication outside the context of medical treatment. Herbal preparations are sold as over-the-counter medications in drugstores and health food stores and through Internet mail-order companies.

HERBS FOR THE PROSTATE

Saw Palmetto (*Serenoa repens*)

The berries of the saw palmetto plant have been used to treat impotence for centuries by the Seminole Indians of southern Florida. Preparations of saw palmetto are now sold in pill form as a medicine for enlarged prostate (BPH). The active ingredients in saw palmetto are the phytosterols beta-sitosterol, campesterol, stigmasterol, and cycloarterol. The herb is thought to inhibit 5alpha-reductase, the enzyme that converts testosterone to dihydrotestosterone, thought to be the hormone responsible for causing the prostate to enlarge.

NATURAL DOES NOT ALWAYS MEAN SAFE

I have often heard people speak of using a "natural" supplement in terms that tell me they are clearly not taking the herb, vitamin, or mineral seriously enough. They often say, "Well, it's natural, so it can't do me any harm, and it might do some good. At least it's not one of those toxic 'drugs.'"

They're half right; it might do some good. But as far as the rest of it goes, they may well be wrong.

Do not make the mistake of thinking that because something is "natural" that it cannot do you any harm. Anything that is strong enough to do you any good can by definition be strong enough to do harm under certain circumstances.

And think of what "natural" means: made by nature. There are many things that are natural that can do plenty of harm. Poison ivy, many mushrooms, snake venom, arsenic, and bacteria and viruses are as natural as medicinal herbs, yet I wouldn't voluntarily take any of them (although arsenic is being tested as a treatment for prostate cancer). Kava, ephedra, and the amino acid tryptophan have all been linked to deaths, yet I have heard some people refer to all of them as "safe and natural."

Again, "natural" does not necessarily equal "safe," especially when natural remedies are taken in combination with other supplements or with conventional drugs. Remember to discuss *everything* you're taking with your doctor!

Although the data from clinical trials on the effectiveness of saw palmetto is mixed, it is thought to be similar in its effects to the prescription drug finasteride (Proscar). Unlike Proscar, however, saw palmetto does not cause impotence. Like Proscar, it may artificially lower PSA levels, which could interfere with diagnosing prostate cancer. It is also much less expensive than Proscar and does not require a doctor's prescription. Saw palmetto is considered safe for general use and has no serious side effects. Users do, however, sometimes experience stomachache, diarrhea, and constipation.

There are currently many different herbal preparations that contain saw palmetto. If you plan to use it, you should purchase products that are advertised as containing "fatty acid" or "lipophilic extract," as these are the only parts of the saw palmetto berries that are effective.

African Plum (*Pygeum africanum*)

For centuries, the native peoples of central and southern Africa have used the powdered bark of an evergreen tree to make a tea used to treat urinary disorders. More recently, pygeum has been used as a popular herbal medicine in France and Italy to treat BPH. Pygeum contains beta-sitosterol, the same phytosterol substance found in saw palmetto. It also contains ferulic esters, compounds that combat prostate enlargement by reducing the levels of prolactin, a substance that produces testosterone and pentacyclic terpenes, which also help reduce swelling.

African Star Grass (*Hypoxis rooperi*)

Traditional South African herbalists have long recommended the root of African star grass as a remedy for enlarged prostate. It has been used in European herbal prostate formulas for years. This herb also contains beta-sitosterol and other phytosterols.

Stinging Nettle (*Urtica dioica*)

The root of this plant has been used by European folk healers for centuries to treat the urinary symptoms of BPH. Unlike saw palmetto and other herbs that work to shrink the prostate physically, stinging nettle produces a diuretic effect that relieves urinary symptoms such as frequent urination and weak urinary flow. It's best when taken in combination with saw palmetto or pygeum. Note that only the nettle root is effective and that preparations made from other parts of the plant have no effect on the prostate.

Radix Urticae

This plant has long been used as a prostate remedy by the folk healers of Eastern Europe. Little is known about the action of this herb on the prostate, but some European clinical studies have shown that *Radix urticae* has beneficial effects on BPH, possibly by influencing the activity of the sex-hormone-binding globulin in its relationship to testosterone.

Pumpkin Seed (*Cucurbita pepo*)

Pumpkin seeds have been used as a folk medicine to treat BPH in Turkey, Bulgaria, and Ukraine, where the traditional treatment is a handful of seeds a day. The seeds have been found to contain antioxidants and anti-inflammatory substances. Like stinging nettle, pumpkin seeds appear to work on urinary symptoms but do not actually shrink the prostate. For this reason, it is best to supplement their use with saw palmetto or pygeum. An extract of pumpkin seed oil can be used in place of eating the whole seeds.

Cernilton

In 1959, a Swedish urologist found that a preparation of rye flower pollen extract was effective in treating BPH. He developed an herbal remedy containing rye pollen called Cernilton, which became a popular prostate remedy in Scandinavia and England. Researchers are not sure how Cernilton affects the prostate, but it may have antioxidant qualities. Besides BPH, Cernilton has been used to treat noninfectious prostatitis and prostatodynia. Note: People with pollen allergies should not use Cernilton.

Other Herbs

The popular herbal cold remedy echinacea, derived from the roots of the plant *Echinacea purpurea*, may provide an effective treatment for BPH. Chimaphila is used as a homeopathic herb to treat the prostate. A plant called unicorn root (*Aletrius farinosa*), used primarily by herbalists as an aphrodisiac, may also have beneficial effects on prostate health. Some other common herbs that may be useful to your prostate health are chamomile, comfrey, cranberry, garlic, goldenseal, juniper, marshmallow, and valerian.

Be cautious with herbal medications and discuss their use with your doctor.

AN ALTERNATIVE DIET THERAPY FOR THE PROSTATE

The Institute for Cancer Prevention believes that a diet following the Prostate Health Pyramid substantially lowers the risk of prostate cancer and can help in managing the disease after it has been diagnosed. Other diets are still controversial and have not been scientifically proven to be effective. These diets are often aimed at curing or preventing various types of cancer. There is anecdotal evidence that a few may be effective in individual cases. You should keep in mind, however, that some forms of dietary therapy may even be hazardous to your overall health.

THE INTEGRATIVE APPROACH

I did a story on pediatric cancer therapy and interviewed oncologists at Columbia-Presbyterian's Babies and Children's Hospital who had taken a survey of the parents of their patients. They found that some parents were giving their kids alternative treatments in addition to the medications the oncologists had prescribed.

This is entirely understandable, as parents want to make sure they're doing absolutely everything possible for their sick child. But the doctors also found that a fair number of the supplements the parents were giving their child could either interact negatively, causing side effects, or actually interfere with the conventional medications the child was taking.

The oncologists I spoke with said they didn't object to the parents giving supplements; they just wanted to know so that they could manage the child's cancer appropriately.

Finally, you may choose to forgo conventional treatment altogether in favor of alternative therapy. If you do choose alternatives, I urge you to consider a combination—what we now call an integrative approach. Treatments for prostate cancer, while not perfect, are effective and can even be curative. It would be tragic to pass up something that might have cured you in favor of an unproven therapy. The alternative is to use both approaches. Just be sure to tell your doctor about the combination of treatments you're considering.

MACROBIOTIC DIET

This is the most widely followed alternative nutritional program in the United States. The term macrobiotic is derived from the Greek words *makros,* meaning "long," and *bios,* meaning "life." Originally called the Zen macrobiotic diet, this dietary regimen is based on ideas of *yin* and *yang* derived from traditional Chinese medicine. It could be called a radical vegetarian diet because in addition to avoiding meat, fish, and animal products, macrobiotic diets also prohibit certain vegetables, such as potatoes, tomatoes, eggplant, peppers, asparagus, spinach, beets, zucchini, and avocado.

The Macrobiotic Diet Food Pyramid

Although there are variations on the basic formula, most macrobiotic diets consist almost entirely of plant food sources in the following proportions:

- 50 to 60 percent whole grains
- 25 to 30 percent fresh vegetables
- 5 to 10 percent beans, soy-based products and sea vegetables
- 5 to 10 percent soups (miso soup; vegetable, grain, seaweed, or bean soup)
- Occasional treats: one to three times a week, a serving of seeds, nuts, fruits, or fish

Few mainstream nutritionists endorse the macrobiotic diet. The limited selection of foods can easily lead to serious nutritional deficiencies. For instance, it's easy to develop a vitamin B12 deficiency because this B vitamin is found mostly in animal sources. Taking a vitamin supplement will help correct this.

PHYSICAL THERAPY (BODYWORK)

The use of massage as a medical therapy goes back to the Greek physician Hippocrates, who prescribed it as part of the healing process and even wrote a book about it. While no longer part of standard urologic practice, massage and more intensive forms of bodywork can provide prostate health benefits for men suffering from noninfectious prostatitis and prostatodynia.

RELEASING THE TRIGGER

To treat chronic nonbacterial prostatitis and prostatodynia as a tension disorder, doctors have borrowed techniques from physical therapy called soft-tissue mobilization or myofascial release. This procedure involves having a physical therapist massage the trigger points in the pelvic area, stretching the tender, contracted muscle tissue. The aim of the procedure is to deactivate the tender and painful trigger points and to restore the chronically contracted tissues in the pelvic floor muscles back to a normal state.

A study at Stanford University Medical Center evaluated this approach to treating CNP and prostatodynia and sought to establish standard protocols for using myofascial release techniques to treat these disorders. In addition to myofascial release treatments, subjects in the study will also be trained in techniques designed to relax the pelvic muscles.

Besides specialized myofascial release techniques, standard body massage is thought to stimulate blood flow throughout the body and relax the muscles surrounding the pelvic area.

ROLFING

This is a technique of deep-tissue massage that seeks to relax and loosen the fascia, or membranes that surround the muscles, rather than the muscles themselves. It was first devised by Ida Rolf, a biochemist and physiologist, in the 1970s. Rolfing is sometimes referred to as structural integration therapy.

In order to break up knots in the fascia and "reset" the muscles, Rolfers apply slow, sliding pressure with their knuckles, thumbs, fingers, elbows, and knees while the subject is lying on a mat or massage table. Unlike standard massage, Rolfing procedures are not mild or relaxing but cause a degree of discomfort or pain. Some men suffering from prostatitis or prostatodynia have reported relief from their symptoms after undergoing Rolfing treatments.

BIOFEEDBACK AND HYPNOSIS

Biofeedback is a technique that teaches you to relax your pelvic muscles by using a machine that monitors muscle tension and gives you feedback when the muscles are properly relaxed.

Hypnosis is a mental technique that uses the power of suggestion to put you in a trancelike state. Hypnotherapy has been found to be effective in treating a variety of problems that hinge on emotions, habits and the body's involuntary responses. This type of therapy may be effective in treating type A personality problems that lead to muscle tensions thought to contribute to prostatitis and prostatodynia.

HYDROTHERAPY

Sitz baths have already been mentioned in connection with treating BPH and prostatitis. The therapy simply involves sitting in a tub containing warm or hot water for fifteen to thirty minutes one or more times a day. This is intended to increase circulation in the prostate area. Some people find hot tubs useful for this purpose. Instead of a tub, special sitz bath equipment can be used that immerses only the hips or buttocks in water or in a gentle saline solution. Hot jets of water playing on the lower back and perineum (the area between the anus and the scrotum) can also be employed. Another technique involves taking alternate hot and ice-cold sitz baths or taking a cold shower after having a hot sitz bath.

HEAT THERAPY

Orthodox medicine already uses heat energy to heal the prostate. TUMT, or transurethral microwave therapy, uses surgical techniques to direct microwave heat to treat BPH by shrinking enlarged prostate tissue. Naturopathic heat treatments are considerably less intrusive and possibly less effective. Hot compresses can be applied

---

NATUROPATHIC MEDICINE

Naturopathy is the most inclusive system of alternative medicine. Naturopathy embraces all facets of alternative medicine and treatment. Naturopathic practitioners are cross-trained in homeopathy, Ayurveda, Chinese medicine, bodywork, and a number of other alternative therapies.

The central organizing principle of naturopathic medicine is a belief in the natural power of the human body to heal itself. It rejects the use of synthetic drugs and invasive procedures and stresses the restorative powers of nature. It seeks to find the underlying causes of disease and attempts to treat the whole person, stressing the use of mental discipline to eliminate bad habits that can lead to disease. Homeopathy also embraces stress reduction techniques and detoxification regimes as part of its overall treatment strategy.

to the prostate area. Home therapy units are currently being marketed that are designed to gently raise the internal body temperature via a probe device that is inserted into the rectum.

A FINAL WORD ON ALTERNATIVE THERAPIES

Although some complementary or integrative therapies may, in fact, be effective, the vast majority of health insurers do not cover alternative therapies. This not only complicates obtaining treatment but inhibits research as well. However, this situation is changing due to the advent of managed care, which emphasizes the use of any therapy that can be effective.

Another factor that may limit your access to alternative medicine is geography. If you don't live near a big city or major population center, you may not have access to specialized therapies. The Internet can help hook you up with alternative practitioners and allow access to medicines and medical equipment that may not be available in your area.

The use of alternative medicine is growing rapidly as the barriers between conventional and unconventional medicine dissolve. An integrative approach may ultimately provide the best possible medicine for your prostate.

ABOUT THE INSTITUTE FOR CANCER PREVENTION

390 Fifth Ave., 3rd Floor
New York, NY 10018
Tel.: 212-551-2500
Fax: 212-687-2339
www.ifcp.us

"Prevention is the best cure."

The Institute for Cancer Prevention (IFCP) is the world's leading institute for cancer prevention research. IFCP is an official National Cancer Institute designated Cancer Center, the *only* NCI-designated Cancer Center in America devoted specifically to the prevention of cancer. Originally known as the American Health Foundation, IFCP was incorporated in 1969 as a nonprofit organization to engage in research and education in the field of preventive medicine, and ultimately to foster research breakthroughs to change the way preventive medicine is practiced. The Foundation was in the forefront in the research that exposed the dangers of smoking and in alerting the public to those dangers.

The Institute publishes *Preventive Medicine* (Elsevier), the leading journal in its field—an original scientific journal devoted to the prevention of diseases, and is now producing a major scientific reference work on all aspects of preventive medicine. The Institute conducts cutting-edge research in cancer prevention and in a number of critical areas in health at its research facility in Valhalla, New York, and oversees other important research at laboratories and clinics across the country.

IFCP launched the first annual National Cancer Prevention Month in 2003, as a dramatic means of educating the public about the primary role of prevention in the fight against cancer. In October 2003, the U.S. Senate passed a resolution declaring February 2004 National Cancer Prevention Month. The resolution was introduced by Senator Ernest F. Hollings (Democrat, South Carolina). Prostate cancer prevention and control is a major focus of this month.

RESEARCH RECORD

IFCP scientists are engaged in an impressive range of studies aimed at understanding the basis for cancer, and discovering why some people are more susceptible to specific cancers—with the overall goal of preventing these cancers. Outstanding current IFCP research and research highlights of the past thirty-five years include:

- Ongoing studies to increase comprehension of how the body's own healing mechanism works at the molecular level, one of the most exciting areas of research into the causes, prevention and treatment of cancers.
- The isolation and synthesizing of compounds designed for improved cancer prevention, leading to the possibility of new chemopreventive chemicals for cancer prevention by natural and synthetic products.
- Prominent studies on the beneficial effects of soy, garlic, zinc, tea, and low-fat diets, and their impact on prostate and other cancers.
- A landmark study concluding that dietary fat levels significantly influence the development of colon and breast cancer.
- Publication of the first major-scale laboratory study on the identification of carcinogens in tobacco smoke, pointing to the dangers of secondary smoke.
- Statistical evidence that smokers face an increased risk of bladder cancer.
- The IFCP's participation in the Dolphins and Human Health Study, in which dolphins are studied for the earliest signs of environmental degradation that compromises the dolphin immune system, which is very much like our own. This study has far-reaching implications for cancer prevention, as well as for health on this planet. The findings of this study will be helpful in predicting and preventing major health threats to humans, including potential carcinogens.
- A laboratory study demonstrating that high dietary fat intake affects hormonal levels in women, increasing their risk for breast cancer.
- IFCP scientists were the first to show in the laboratory that diets rich in omega-3 fatty acids (the ones plentiful in some fish and fish oil) do not increase the risk of colon cancer, and in fact may lower that risk.
- IFCP's ongoing effort to determine whether a low-fat diet can prevent breast cancer recurrence led to the formation of the landmark Women's Intervention Nutrition Study (WINS), the largest such investigatory initiative ever undertaken in the area of women's health and breast cancer recurrence prevention
- IFCP was the first to show that some nonsteroidal anti-inflammatory drugs (NSAIDs) are a strong chemopreventive against colon cancer.
- IFCP biochemists reported that components found in cruciferous vegetables have the chemopreventive potency to inhibit cancer develop-

ment. IFCP continues to identify potential anticancer agents in fruits and vegetables, as well as in related synthetic compounds.

THE NEXT FRONTIER

The next frontier in cancer prevention is called proteomics, the study of proteins. The Institute is undertaking ambitious studies that explore the essence of this most intricate element of life, probing deep inside the cell where malignancies begin. The aim is to manipulate the cell's own proteins to repair the cells before they develop malignancies. While proteomics may be one of the most powerful expressions of the potentialities of preventive medicine to date, the IFCP will continue to find new and increasingly powerful ways to illustrate that prevention is—without doubt—the best cure, and the medical wave of the future.

For more information about the Institute for Cancer Prevention, see the Institute's website, www.ifcp.us. To learn about opportunities for getting involved as a benefactor or as a volunteer, contact Robert Thompson, vice president, Development, at 212-551-2557, or rthompso@ifcp.us.

INDEX

ABOUT THE AUTHORS

Daniel W. Nixon, M.D., is the president of the Institute for Cancer Prevention and the editor-in-chief of the journal *Preventive Medicine*. Formerly the associate director for Cancer Control and Prevention at the Medical University of South Carolina/Hollings Cancer Center, Dr. Nixon has written dozens of scholarly papers and is the author of *The Cancer Recovery Eating Plan: The Right Foods to Help Fuel Your Recovery*. He lives in New York City.

Max Gomez, Ph.D., has been the Health and Science editor of WNBC, NBC's flagship station in New York, since 1991. His health reports are carried on NBC stations both nationally and internationally. Dr. Gomez has been honored with four New York Emmy Awards, two Philadelphia Emmys, a UPI Best Documentary Award, and an Excellence in Time of Crisis award from New York City. He was named the American Health Foundation's Man of the Year in 1986 for his contributions to public awareness of vital health issues. He lives in Westchester County, New York.